W9-BVY-000

DATE DUE

SEP 1 8 2004		
GAYLORD		PRINTED IN U.S.A.

Fourth Edition

HOSPITAL
ORGANIZATION
ᴬᴺᴰ MANAGEMENT
Text and Readings

Kurt Darr, JD, ScD, FACHE

Professor of Health Services Administration
Department of Health Services Administration
The George Washington University
Washington, DC

Jonathon S. Rakich, PhD

Professor of Management
   and Health Services Administration
College of Business Administration
The University of Akron
Akron, Ohio

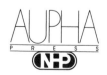

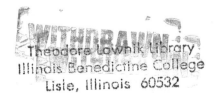

Published by
National Health Publishing
99 Painters Mill Road
Owings Mills, Maryland 21117
(301) 363–6400

A division of Williams & Wilkins

AUPHA Press is a joint venture between National Health Publishing
and the Association of University Programs in Health Administration.

© National Health Publishing 1989

Printed in the United States of America
First Printing

Acquisitions Editor: Sara Mansure Sides
Developmental Editor: Cindy Konits
Production Coordinator: Karen Babcock
Copyeditor: Michael Treadway
Designer: Sandy Renovetz
Compositor: Absolutely Your Type
Printer: Edwards Brothers

ISBN: 0-910591-08-3
LC: 88–062517

Leon I. Gintzig

1916 - 1984

Educator, innovator, friend

Contents

Foreword to the Fourth Edition

The decade of the 1980s for many practicing hospital executives has been one of future shock—that malady described by Alvin Tofler as the shattering stress and disorientation induced in individuals by subjecting them to too much change in too short a time. The 1980s have been a turbulent time for hospital executives as the result of increased pressures of budgetary constraints in the public and private financing sectors and an overriding concern about use of the nation's resources for health care. Responses to these pressures include trends toward competition; new forms of regulation; development of new kinds of accountability; and growing concern over the quality of patient care.

Hospital executives have been receiving conflicting signals from a variety of publics. The public expects hospitals to act more like businesses, but at the same time, expects them to continue to serve patient and community needs compassionately. Out of all this ambiguity is one clear trend: the emergence of both a new business language and behavior. No previous generation of hospital executives has experienced this different entrepreneurial behavior. As a result, innovations are tried and mistakes are made.

Many health care professionals wonder about the changes in hospital organization and management due to increased emphasis on hospital governance and the need to develop standards for medical and business ethics. Corporate values and business ethics are being discussed more frequently. Also, here has been growing concern throughout this decade over access to hospital and medical care for the thirty-seven million Americans who lack any form of health insurance. The public policy debate over this matter heightens as the 1980s close. For hospitals, the stakes are high.

This book helps the reader to understand these changing times. It is a solid reference and source of insight for practicing executives as well as individuals considering a career in hospital organization and management. It contains some of the timeless classics and at the same time is made current by some of the most important writings of the 1980s. It is a valuable reference to keep on the desk top—the kind of book one can pick up at any time and learn something new. The volume is another important contribution by Professors Darr and Rakich to the literature of hospital administration. They are to be commended for their professional leadership.

Richard J. Davidson
President and Chief Executive Officer
The Maryland Hospital Association
Baltimore, Maryland

Foreword to the Third Edition

For the health services industry, the 1980s may be characterized as the decade of the administrator. As we move into this era, the major problems and issues to be faced are clearly administrative in nature: the need for cost containment in the face of continuing economic uncertainty; heightened demand for quality assurance from an increasingly sophisticated public; and the imperative of careful service planning in the face of limited resources, to mention only three.

This new edition by Jonathon Rakich and Kurt Darr of a well-planned and organized collection of readings is particularly timely. The selections offer a good balance of information on hospital structure, internal management methods, and current policy issues confronting the contemporary hospital. A majority of the articles in this third edition are new, reflecting both rapid change in the field of health administration practice and an ever richer literature by students of the field. Articles from the two earlier editions which deal with general management principles and techniques still applicable today are retained. The book is enhanced by carefully developed introductory material and supplementary bibliographic references offering additional depth of study to the interested reader.

This volume will be equally useful as a general reference for the practicing administrator and as an instructional resource for university courses in hospital organization and management. The editors' continued contributions to our field are most welcome.

Charles J. Austin, Ph.D.
Vice-President for Academic Affairs
    and Professor of Management
Georgia Southern College
Statesboro, Georgia

Foreword to the Second Edition

As one astute observer has already pointed out, many of the modern disciplines possess a long history, but a short past. Health care management is very much a member of that family.

Twenty years ago the total body of literature on hospital administration was fully within a single individual's capacity to review, and even perhaps to own. Today, that body reflects an explosive and relentless expansion similar in magnitude to that which began among the professional medical specialties much earlier. If one thing becomes necessary in the face of this avalanche of material—both good and bad—it is the exercise of selectivity.

In this volume two young authors offer—above all—an expertly selected range of material. As with the initial edition in 1972, selectivity marks each element of all of its parts.

Those of us engaged in management of modern health care institutions owe our compliments to Jonathon Rakich and Kurt Darr, as well as to the contributors of the selected, original articles. Taken as a whole, this volume instructs, enlightens, and provokes. It will prove inspiring to some, and useful to all.

L. R. Jordan, FACHA
President
Miami Valley Hospital
Dayton, Ohio

Preface

A different strategy was used in preparing the fourth edition of this book. Although a few classic articles were retained, virtually all the rest are new. The editors were fortunate in being able to draw from the increasing richness of journals in the hospital and health services administration field. A special effort was made to choose concise, hard-hitting articles that provide essential information about how hospitals are organized and managed. The content of the articles chosen ranges from the pragmatic to the philosophical and from the classic to the avant-garde.

The book has three parts: "Hospital Organization," "Management Functions," and "Environmental Factors and Ethics." The revised interstitial material links the parts and relates them to the general systems conceptual framework. The interstitial material also provides essential background, context, and data that reflect the field's dynamism and competitiveness. To benefit readers wishing to examine a subject in greater depth, bibliographies are included at the end of each part introduction. To enhance selection and ease of use, each section within the three parts is preceded by a brief statement about the articles in it. The subject index is unique to books of this type and will be a valuable time-saver.

This book is usable as both a reference and a primer. Busy hospital managers often do not have time to read the current literature. In one volume, this book provides 45 articles, offering easy access to a wide range of subjects about hospital organization and management. Faculty and students in graduate and undergraduate hospital and health services administration programs will find this a valuable source. Those pursuing baccalaureate education in the allied health professions, especially nursing, will have coursework and assignments concerning the problems and issues included here. The book can also serve as a reference for faculty lectures and class discussion.

We are proud of the reputation and reception this book has enjoyed in the field since the first edition was published in 1972. We hope this fourth edition will continue to contribute to improving the management of acute care hospitals.

Kurt Darr

Jonathon S. Rakich

Acknowledgements

In preparing this fourth edition we have continued to receive and count on the support and encouragement of our wives, Anne Darr and Tana Rakich. We are in their debt.

We thank the editors and staff of *American Journal of Infection Control, Federation of American Hospitals Review, HIMSS Journal, Health Care, Health Care Financing Review, Health Care Management Review, Health Care Strategic Management, Health Management Forum, Health Management Quarterly, Health Matrix, Health Progress, Healthcare Executive, Hospital Forum, Hospital & Health Services Administration, Hospitals, Inquiry,* the Macmillan Publishing Company, *Modern Healthcare Magazine, Nursing Management, QRB, Risk Management, The Hospital Medical Staff, The New England Journal of Medicine,* and *Trustee,* for permission to reprint the articles and excerpts contained in this book.

A special thanks is owed the authors whose works appear in this compilation.

Our employers provided organizational support and an environment in which our work could be undertaken and successfully completed. At the George Washington University we acknowledge and thank Richard F. Southby, Ph.D., Chairman of the Department of Health Services Administration and Norma Maine Loeser, D.B.A., Dean of the School of Government and Business Administration; at the University of Akron we acknowledge and thank Alan G. Krigline, Ph.D., Head of the Department of Management and James W. Dunlap, Ph.D., Dean of the College of Business Administration.

We are grateful to those who provided research and clerical assistance: Norma Pearson—research librarian at the University of Akron, Laura Rosenthal, Barbara Lucas, and Julie Sweet.

Last, but certainly not least, we want to thank the responsive and effective staff at National Health Publishing and especially Jackie Karkos, Sara Sides, Cindy Konits, and Karen Babcock.

Introduction

Background

Health care — the total system to provide, finance, and promote societal health — has changed markedly during the twentieth century. It is moving in two directions simultaneously. There is great emphasis on wellness and prevention, but advances in diagnosis and treatment in both acute and restorative care have dramatically improved efficacy. Public policy has become much more interventionist in the last two decades. Health services, that component of the health care system composed of the practitioners and organizations providing care, has also undergone change — smoothly at times, turbulently at others.

Contemporary acute care hospitals bear little resemblance to those of 70 years ago. They face different environments, new rules, and greater accountability to multiple constituents. Microeconomics and financing are dominant considerations. Management structure and practices have changed dramatically. As a result, the hospital is appreciably different, yet its mission and societal responsibilities remain basically the same: to provide quality patient care. An observation made in 1924 applies today:

> The hospital occupies a strategic mid-position and has open to it a great opportunity and a corresponding obligation, not as an institution for the salvage of human wreckage, but as a coordinator of activities — professional, economic, and social — in their application upon the problems of health.[1]

The acute care hospital is a unique and highly complex organizational entity. To the community it is an important social and economic asset; to patients it is a place to receive care; to physicians it is a place to treat patients; to employees it is a place to work; and to its managers, it is a multifaceted organization embracing clinical, financial, ancillary, and support activities. It is a place where sophisticated equipment, technology, and personnel are organized to provide health services.

Advances in technology and medical science have caused the acute care hospital to become the central and primary provider organization in health services delivery. In a variety of ways the acute care hospital interacts with and influences other provider organizations: skilled nursing facilities, ambulatory services centers, medical group practices, home health and visiting nursing agencies, and a host of supporting entities, including prenatal care, senior citizen nutritional centers, substance abuse centers, and mental health outpatient and inpatient facilities. This role has been further emphasized as hospitals restructure and vertically and horizontally integrate their services. By most measures hospitals are the predominant provider entity and a linchpin in other delivery arrangements such as health maintenance organizations (HMOs) and preferred provider organizations (PPOs).

This book is about managing acute care hospitals. The subject is divided into three parts:

Part I, "Hospital Organization," presents the acute care hospital triad: the governing body, the chief executive officer (CEO) and senior management, the medical staff organization (MSO), and the relationships among them, as well as contemporary management issues and alternate forms of organization.

Part II, "Management Functions," includes macrolevel information about acute care hospital strategic planning and marketing, as well as microlevel intraorganizational material concerned with resource allocation, utilization, and control, including quality assurance and risk management and organizational change.

Part III, "Environmental Factors and Ethics," includes information on competition and entrepreneurship, policy issues and ethics, and the effects of, and a look, at the future of the acute care hospital in the health services system.

This book defines health care to mean *all* of society's private and public efforts to seek or retain health. Health services are defined as those public or private activities that primarily assist individuals in regaining health and, to a lesser extent, in preventing disease and disability. Health services are delivered in a variety of settings; the focus here is on how acute care hospitals organize and provide them.

Hospital Data

Before 1900, acute care hospitals were few in number, had few beds and high mortality rates, and were stigmatized as institutions that cared for the poor. A primary role was to separate the sick from the well. It is estimated there were approximately 800 hospitals of all types in the United States in the 1880s.[2] During the next 30 years, the number grew rapidly to reach 4,359 in 1909 and an all-time peak of 7,370 in 1924. A hospital of the 1920s was very different from its predecessors. It was usually owned by physician investors and had an average of 110 beds. By comparison, a typical hospital of 1986 had 189 beds and was likely to be owned by a not-for-profit corporation.[3]

World War II began the era in which acute care hospitals gained preeminence in health services delivery. The financial exigencies of the Great Depression were over. The 1946 Hospital Survey and Construction Act (the Hill-Burton Act) fostered the upgrading and expansion of not-for-profit hospitals. Advances in medical technology, more prevalent third-party hospitalization insurance, and increasing physician specialization were concurrent trends.

Table i-1 presents data on American Hospital Association (AHA)-registered hospitals, beds, admissions, occupancy rates, outpatient visits, full-time equivalent employees (FTEs), and population per 100 beds for selected years. The data show that the number of hospitals of all types increased from 6,788 in 1950 to 7,156 in 1975, and decreased to 6,841 in 1986.[4] The number of beds similarly increased, peaked, and declined, with far fewer beds (1.29 million) in 1986 than in 1950 (1.46 million),[5] for an 11 percent decrease in the bed inventory. During the same period, the U.S. population increased by 59 percent, from 152 million to 242 million,[6] and the number of annual inpatient admissions increased by 90 percent, from 18.5 million to 35.2 million.[7] This was possible because of a decrease in the average length of stay. Change in the location of service is evident and is reflected in Fig. i-1: Outpatient visits increased 134 percent, from 125.[8] million in 1965 to 294.6 million in 1986.[8] Stated another way, the average American made an outpatient visit at a hospital 1.2 times in 1986, versus 0.6 times in 1965. Note, too, that the downward trend of inpatient admissions that began in 1980 has continued.

Finally, advances in medical technology (e.g., intensive and coronary care, nuclear medicine, electronic fetal monitoring, coronary bypass surgery) improved the quality of care and required higher staffing levels and better trained personnel. To support this new technology, the average hospital had 283 FTEs per 100 beds in 1986 versus 115 in 1965.[9] Taken alone, acute care hospitals have an even higher ratio: 309 FTEs per 100 beds.[10]

Classification of Hospitals

Hospitals are categorized in several ways: for example, by length of stay (short-term or long-term), type of service, and type of control. Length of stay is categorized according to whether patients stay fewer than 30 days (short-term or acute) or 30 days or more (long-term). Approximately 85 percent of U.S. hospitals are short-term. Type of service denotes whether the hospital is "general," providing a broad range of medical and surgical services, or "special," providing rehabilitative, maternity, psychiatric, or pediatric services only. The third classification breaks hospitals down by type of control or ownership: not-for-profit, for-profit (investor-owned), or governmental (federal, state, local, or hospital authority). In 1986 approximately 49 percent of the nation's short-term general and other special hospitals were non-governmental not-for-profit hospitals, 12 percent were investor-owned, and 23 percent were controlled by state and local governments.[11] The remaining 16 percent either were federally owned or were psychiatric hospitals, tuberculosis and other respiratory disease hospitals, or long-term general and other special hospitals, whether nongovernmental not-for-profit, investor-owned, or owned by state or local government.

Table i-2 shows hospitals by type of control, number of beds, and admissions for selected years. By far the largest group is the nonfederal, short-term general and other special hospital. This category is also known as the community hospital and contains 83 percent of all hospitals, 76 percent of all

Table i-1. AHA-Registered Hospitals, Beds, Admissions, Occupancy Rates, Outpatient Visits, Personnel, and Population per 100 Beds, Selected Years.

Year	Number of AHA-Registered Hospitals	Number of Beds (in thousands)	Number of Admissions (in thousands)	Occupancy Rate (%)	Outpatient Visits (in thousands)	FTE Personnel (in thousands)	FTE Personnel per 100 Beds	Population per 100 Beds
1950	6,788	1,456	18,483	86.0	NA	1,058	72.6	10,440
1955	6,956	1,604	21,073	85.0	NA	1,301	81.0	10,350
1960	6,876	1,658	25,024	84.6	NA	1,598	96.4	10,900
1965	7,123	1,704	28,812	82.3	125,793	1,952	114.5	11,380
1970	7,123	1,616	31,759	80.3	181,370	2,537	156.9	12,620
1975	7,156	1,466	36,157	76.7	254,844	3,023	206.2	14,530
1980	6,965	1,365	38,892	77.7	262,951	3,492	255.8	16,285
1985	6,872	1,318	36,304	69.0	282,140	3,625	275.0	18,149
1986	6,841	1,290	35,219	68.4	294,634	3,647	282.7	18,759

Sources: American Hospital Association, *Hospital Statistics, 1987 Edition* (Chicago: American Hospital Association, 1987), Table 1, p. 2; U.S. Bureau of the Census, *Statistical Abstract of the United States: 1987.* 107th ed. (Washington, DC: U.S. Bureau of the Census, 1986), p. 8.

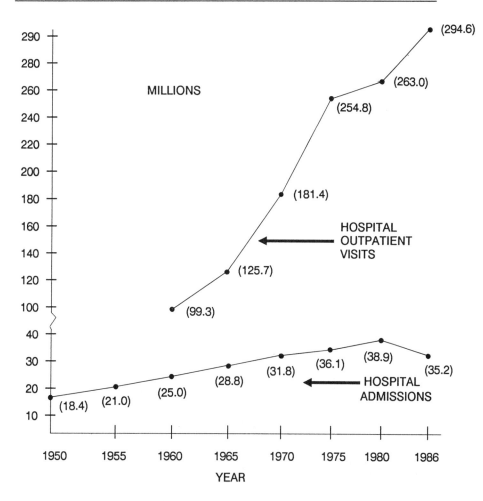

Figure i-1. Hospital Admissions and Outpatient Visits, Selected Years. Data from American Hospital Association, *Hospital Statistics, 1987 Edition,* (Chicago: American Hospital Association, 1987), Table 2, p. 1.

beds, and 92 percent of all inpatient admissions.[12] In 1986, this category included not-for-profit, investor-owned, and state and local government hospitals. Of all nonfederal, short-term general and other special hospitals, not-for-profit hospitals (nongovernmental not-for-profit hospitals, and state and local government-owned hospitals) account for 89 percent of beds and 90 percent of admissions, whereas investor-owned hospitals account for 11 percent of

Table i-2. AHA-Registered U.S. Hospitals by Control Categories, Beds, and Admissions.

	Year				
	1965	**1970**	**1975**	**1980**	**1986**
I. TOTAL U.S.	[SUM OF II, III, AND IV]				
Number of hospitals	7,123	7,123	7,156	6,965	6,841
Number of beds (in thousands)	1,704	1,616	1,466	1,365	1,290
Number of admissions					
(in thousands)	28,812	31,759	36,157	38,892	35,219
II. FEDERAL					
Number of hospitals	443	408	382	359	342
Number of beds (in thousands)	174	161	132	117	111
Number of admissions					
(in thousands)	1,640	1,741	1,913	2,044	2,117
III. NONFEDERAL, LONG-TERM					
Number of hospitals	944	856	795	702	71
Number of beds (in thousands)	788	607	387	256	197
Number of admissions					
(in thousands)	709	766	724	652	692
IV. NONFEDERAL, SHORT-TERM GENERAL	[SUM OF A, B, and C]				
(A. Not-for-profit, B. Investor-owned, and C. State and local government-owned).					
Number of hospitals	5,736	5,859	5,979	5,904	5,728
[% of total U.S.]	[80.5]	[82.2]	[83.5]	[84.8]	[83.7]
Number of beds (in thousands)	741	849	947	992	982
[% of total U.S.] [43.5]	[52.5]	[64.6]	[72.6]	[76.1]	
Number of admissions					
(in thousands) 26,462	29,252	33,519	36,198	32,410	
[% of total U.S.]	[91.8]	[92.1]	[92.7]	[93.0]	[92.0]
A. Not-For-Profit					
Number of hospitals	3,426	3,386	3,364	3,339	3,338
[% of nonfederal, short-term]	[59.7]	[57.8]	[56.3]	[56.5]	[58.3]
Number of beds (in thousands)	515	592	659	693	690
[% of nonfederal, short-term]	[69.5]	[69.8]	[69.6]	[69.8]	[70.3]
Number of admissions					
(in thousands)	19,001	20,948	23,735	25,576	23,492
[% of nonfederal, short-term]	[71.8]	[71.6]	[70.8]	[70.7]	[72.5]

Table i-2, continued.

	Year				
	1965	**1970**	**1975**	**1980**	**1986**
B. Investor-Owned					
Number of hospitals	857	769	775	730	834
[% of nonfederal, short-term]	[14.9]	[13.1]	[13.0]	[12.4]	[14.6]
Number of beds (in thousands)	47	53	73	87	107
[% of nonfederal, short-term]	[6.3]	[6.3]	[7.7]	[8.8]	[10.9]
Number of admissions					
(in thousands)	1,844	2,031	2,646	3,165	3,231
[% of nonfederal, short-term]	[7.0]	[7.0]	[7.9]	[8.7]	[9.9]
C. State and Local Government-Owned					
Number of hospitals	1,453	1,704	1,840	1,835	1,556
[% of nonfederal, short-term]	[25.3]	[29.1]	[30.8]	[31.1]	[27.2]
Number of beds (in thousands)	179	204	215	212	185
[% of nonfederal, short-term]	[24.2]	[24.1]	[22.7]	[21.4]	[18.8]
Number of admissions					
(in thousands) 5,617	6,273	7,138	7,458	5,687	
[% of nonfederal, short-term]	[21.2]	[21.4]	[21.3]	[20.6]	[17.6]

Source: American Hospital Association, *Hospital Statistics, 1987 Edition* (Chicago: American Hospital Association, 1987), pp. 3-6.

beds and 10 percent of admissions.[13] Table i-2 shows that the not-for-profit, short-term, general acute hospital continues as the nation's predominant type.

Health Care and Hospital Services Expenditures

Society's commitment to health is readily shown by how total expenditures for health care as a percentage of gross national product (GNP) have risen steadily from 4.0 percent in 1940 ($4 billion) to 10.9 percent in 1986 ($458 billion). Forecasts for 1990, 1995, and 2000 suggest further dramatic increases. Table i-3 shows the rapid increases in U.S. health care expenditures from 1940 to 1985. Fig. i-2 presents data on total health care expenditures and the hospital services component.

Public Initiatives and Health Care Costs

Nations cannot allocate ever-increasing resources to health care and simultaneously maintain infrastructures such as education, social services, and income maintenance. Consequently, public officials in the United States

Table i-3. Total United States Health Care Expenditures and as a Percent of GNP, Expenditures Per Capita, Percent of Expenditures Paid by Public or Private Sources; and Hospital Expenditures, Total and as a Percent of All United States Health Care Expenditures.

Calendar Year	U.S. Health Care Expenditures ($ billions)	Expenditures as a Percent of GNP	Expenditures Per Capita	Percent of Expenditures: Private	Percent of Expenditures: Public	Hospital Service Expenditures ($ billions)	Hospital Service Expenditures As a Percent of All Health Care Expenditures
1940	$ 4.0	4.0%	$ 29	79.7%	20.3%	$ 1.0	25.4%
1950	12.7	4.5	82	72.8	27.2	3.9	30.4
1955	17.7	4.4	105	74.3	25.7	5.9	33.2
1960	26.9	5.3	146	75.3	24.7	9.9	33.8
1965	43.0	6.2	217	75.1	24.9	13.9	32.4
1970	74.7	7.6	358	62.8	37.2	27.8	37.2
1975	132.7	8.6	603	57.7	42.3	52.1	39.2
1980	247.2	9.4	1,067	57.8	42.2	99.0	40.3
1985	422.6	10.6	1,710	58.4	41.6	167.2	39.6
1986	458.2	10.9	1,837	58.6	41.4	179.6	39.2
1987	496.6	11.2	1,973	59.4	40.6	192.6	38.8
1990*	647.3	12.0	2,511	58.4	41.6	250.4	38.7
1995*	999.1	13.4	3,739	57.6	42.4	393.6	39.4
2000*	1,529.3	15.0	5,551	57.5	42.5	621.0	40.6

*Estimates

Source: "National Health Expenditures, 1987," *Health Care Financing Review*, Summer 1987, pp. 24-25.

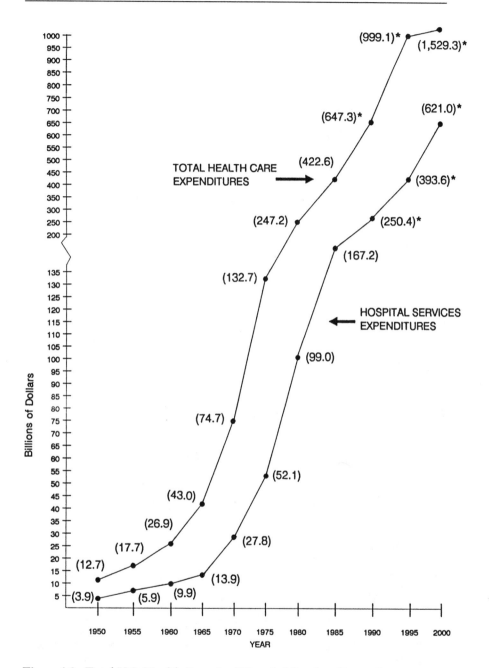

Figure i-2. Total U.S. Health Care And Hospital Services Expenditures, Selected Calendar Years. Asterisks denote estimates. Data from "National Health Expenditures, 1987," *Health Care Financing Review* (Summer): 25, 1987.

and Western Europe are being forced to make policy decisions about resource allocation. One outcome has been the initiative to decrease the proportion of health services expenditures, or at least keep them from increasing as rapidly.

State and federal public policy during the past three decades focused on expediency in health services delivery: doing that which had to be done to solve immediate problems and adding to prior solutions incrementally as needed. Throughout, however, the solutions sought to maintain the status quo. Federal initiatives prior to 1965 improved the supply of health services by enhancing institutional and manpower availability. During the Great Society years of President Johnson's administration, and specifically after 1965, federal initiatives caused a fundamental shift in demand for health services, and enactment of Medicare and Medicaid in 1965 substantially decreased the financial barriers to health care. The result has been greater amounts spent for health care, with an increasing percentage for acute care services. Further, more and more care is financed by public rather than private funds. Table i-3 shows that the percentage of health care expenditures from public sources decreased slightly from 1950 to 1965. In the succeeding 20 years it increased from 24.9 to 41.6 percent.[14]

The rapidly increasing federal fiscal burden for health services caused a major shift in federal public policy in the 1970s as initiatives to contain costs were enacted. The acute care hospital, as the most visible and costly provider, was the primary target for efforts aimed at controlling the supply of services. Included were certificate-of-need requirements, promotion of HMOs, utilization and rate review, and health planning. Recent major changes have affected several initiatives of the 1970s: professional review organizations (PROs) have superseded professional standards review organizations (PSROs), federally-sponsored health planning has ended, and certificate-of-need has suffered significant setbacks in the states.

Federal initiatives of the 1980s have stressed cost control and, where possible, cost reduction. The mainstay is a prospective pricing system (PPS) based on diagnosis-related groups (DRGs). Under DRGs, a fixed sum is paid for the care of Medicare patients based on their diagnosis. In effect, the DRG system establishes a budget in which hospitals must meet their expenses — it is a form of financial risk sharing.

Competition among hospitals is a phenomenon of the 1980s. Advocates see it as the way to bring marketplace pricing discipline into health services delivery. They argue that it is a way to reduce both the demand and the supply side of the equation. The result sought is reduced cost of services, as well as reduced demand because of greater attention to utilization. Deregulation has been traumatic for hospitals because it has forced them to reevaluate (1) their traditional role in health services, (2) the types and intensity of services provided, (3) their willingness to ally with others (e.g., in multi-institutional arrangements), and (4) downsizing as a survival strategy. The rapid growth of competing medical plans such as PPOs and independent practice arrangements (IPAs) suggests the effects of competition.

The contemporary hospital functions in a turbulent environment. Contradictory public policy initiatives such as increased supply before 1965, increased demand after 1965, decreased supply and funding after 1970, and cost control pressure in the 1980s have destabilized the system and traditional resource allocation activities. These changes have made management increasingly burdensome, internal organization more complex, and coping with the external environment a very difficult chore.

Hospital Organization and Management

This book uses a general systems theory model. Input-conversion-output occurs in the context of generic management activities; health services managers apply the functions of planning, organizing, staffing, directing, and controlling, as modified for their specific institutional setting. Those elements serving a linkage role are decision-making, communicating, integrating, mediating, and change. The relationships among managerial functions are shown in Fig. i-3.

The degree to which managers perform these functions depends on their position in the organizational hierarchy and their responsibility for resources. Yet, as managers perform their duties and engage in managerial functions, they do so in an organizational setting (the hospital) that utilizes resources (inputs) such as people and technology which are acquired, grouped, and converted to accomplish organization objectives (outputs), the most important of which is patient care. Fig. i-4 illustrates the input-conversion-output process, the hospital's conversion role, and its relationship to the external environment.

An integrated hospital organization and management model is shown in Fig. i-5 and serves as the basic conceptual framework of this book. The components in the model are identified by roman numerals and correspond to the book's three parts.

Part I, "Hospital Organization," is where inputs — resources from the external environment — are converted into outputs. Inputs include human and other resources such as technology, capital, equipment, and information. Outputs include patient care, community health status, education, and research. Part I of the book examines organizational arrangements, trends, and issues, as well as specific components: the governing body, the CEO and senior management, and the MSO.

The primary and linking managerial functions are presented in Part II, "Management Functions." Included are the subjects of strategic planning, objective and strategy formulation, and their interconnection with health care marketing; resource utilization and control, including quality assurance and risk management; and human resource dynamics and organizational change.

Part III, "Environmental Factors and Ethics," considers issues of competition, ethics, entrepreneurship, health policy, and the hospital's future. Nowhere have changes been more dramatic. The rites of passage have been formidable during the past two decades, and there are numerous predictions

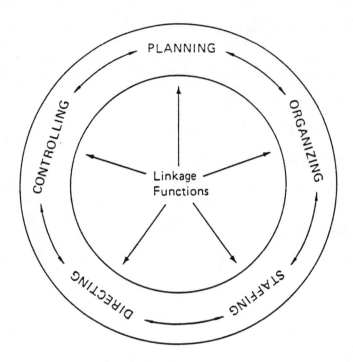

Figure i-3. Management Functions.

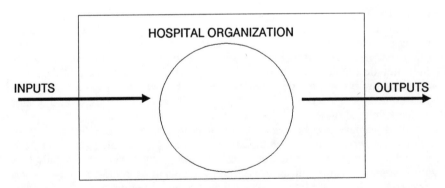

Figure i-4. The Input-Conversion-Output Model.

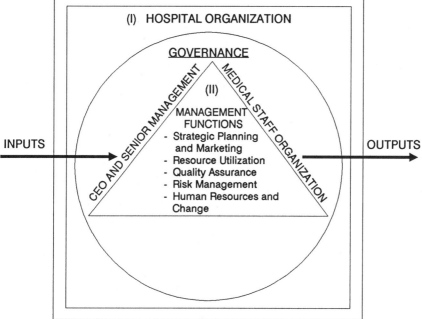
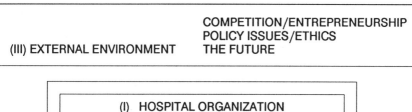

Figure i-5. Hospital Organization and Management Model.

for similar developments in the future. Changes in the external environment will challenge hospital managers as never before, and their skills will be put to the test. But never have managers been better prepared.

The Challenge of Hospital Management

Hospital managers face many challenges. They emerged from the 1970s bruised, but eager for the fray. Those who are successful will be more proactive in the 1990s and beyond. They are learning to influence, shape, and control the external environment. In the last decade, external influences were paramount. In the 1990s, both the external and the internal environment will challenge hospital managers. A major problem will be to do more with less.

Notes

1. Frank E. Chapman, *Hospital Organization and Operation* (New York: Macmillan, 1924).
2. Commission on Hospital Care, *Hospital Care in the United States* (New York: The Commonwealth Fund, 1947), p. 58.
3. American Hospital Association, *Hospital Statistics, 1987 Edition* (Chicago: American Hospital Association, 1987), p. 2.
4. *Ibid.*
5. *Ibid.*
6. U.S. Bureau of the Census, *Statistical Abstract of the United States: 1987.* 107th ed. (Washington, DC: U.S. Bureau of the Census, 1986), p. 8.
7. American Hospital Association, *Hospital Statistics, 1987 Edition*, p. 2.
8. *Ibid.*
9. *Ibid.*
10. *Ibid.*, p. 4.
11. *Ibid.*, p. 12.
12. *Ibid.*
13. *Ibid.*
14. "National Health Expenditures, 1986-2000." *Health Care Financing Review* Vol. 8, No. 4, p. 24.

Part I

Hospital Organization

Introduction

As they seek to perform their duties, hospital managers are no longer alone. Often this is to their benefit, but sometimes it is to their rue. They have been joined by operations researchers, engineers, accountants, attorneys, political scientists, economists, sociologists, and ethicists. Hospitals are the major recipient of increased attention because they are highly visible organizations, focal points for health services delivery, and, most importantly, because they consume 40 percent of the national health care budget.

Hospitals and their personnel at all levels are experiencing future shock. The old assumptions about hospitals have been challenged, and hospital managers face an environment with new rules. There are questions about the cost and efficacy of medical care, the desirability of receiving it, the fallibility of the physician, and the ability of the health care system to save people from imprudent life-styles, unhealthy environments, and genetic makeup. The problem is perhaps best stated as a crisis of confidence, and for many Americans it is an unpleasantly abrupt realization of the limits of modern medicine. Leaders in and out of the health services system contend that it has major problems, and public confidence has eroded. But the system will not collapse as some predict. It will continue to do as well as it can within its resource constraints as Americans enjoy the best medical care in the world.

Complexity of Hospitals

The general acute care hospital is one of the most complex organizations ever established. It has developed arrangements termed prototypical. For example, task teams composed of a variety of skilled professionals are commonplace. Some researchers studying hospitals have come away surprised that they function as well as they do.

Hospitals are complex for several reasons:

1. There is a wide diversity of objectives and goals among individuals, professional groups, and various subsystems. Hospital components are responsible for, or participate in, patient care, education, research, prevention, hotel-like accommodations, and intricate medical and surgical procedures. These activities sometimes conflict. Effective coordination is critical to minimize conflict and to obtain maximum support and coordination in achieving the hospital's mission.

2. Hospital personnel range from highly skilled and educated managers and physicians to unskilled and uneducated employees, some of whom may be illiterate. Enabling them to work together efficiently is a major responsibility of hospital managers. Unionization among more restive personnel complicates human resource management in hospitals.

3. Hospitals are operated continuously. This means high standby costs and causes personnel and scheduling problems.

4. Many components of hospital operation have dual lines of authority. Managers solve a wide variety of problems; physicians are responsible for patient care, education, and research. Most physicians practicing in hospitals are independent contractors over whom the hospital has no line authority in the management sense. This necessitates unique skills and special working relationships.

5. Hospitals deal with problems of life and death. This puts significant psychological and physical stresses on all personnel. The setting and outcome may cause consumers and their families to be hypercritical.

6. The major product is difficult to determine, and the quality of patient care rendered in hospitals has eluded precise measurement. There has been progress in determining what quality is, but many questions are unanswered, and there is disagreement among experts as to how and what should be measured.

These problems are inherent in managing the organization that a hospital must be. Advances in technology, economic and political pressures, and consumer demands add complexity and problems to hospital management at a rate equal to, or greater than, the rate at which managers solve them. The challenge has never been greater, nor is it likely to become any less.

Historical Development of Hospitals

Hospitals in Ancient Times

The earliest evidence of institutionalized care for the ill dates from about 1200 B.C., when patients were cared for in Greek temples. Hippocrates (460?-370? B.C.), the most prominent Greek physician, was instrumental in separating medicine from religion and philosophy. He is credited with using a rational approach to medicine, and the philosophical foundations of modern medicine are built on his work. Medical training gained importance in this era, as did recognition of environmental influences on health and disease. Religion, however, continued in a key role.

Greek medicine reached its zenith during the Golden Age of Greece, about 400 B.C., when the temples of Aesculapius emerged.[1] Considered among the earliest hospitals in Greek and Roman civilizations, the temples were used as both houses of worship and shelters for the ill. Patients were often ambulatory. Care in the Aesculapian temples emphasized exposure to the open air and sunshine and a regimen of rest, relaxation, baths, exercise, and proper diet. The temples were similar to modern-day spas—both mind and body were included in the recuperative process. Limited medication was prescribed.

The first hospitals evidencing modern features were found in ancient Egypt and India.[2] In Egypt, at approximately 600 B.C., medical care was often rendered in temples. Egyptian priest-physicians were among the first to prescribe practical drugs, and they performed limited surgery and set fractures. Between 273 and 232 B.C., hospitals called *cikista* were built in India. Hindu physicians were adept at surgery, and medications were administered. *Cikista* were noted for their cleanliness. Patients remained overnight and care was provided by attendants.

Hospitals and Christianity

The Christian era stressed humanitarianism. Ecclesiastic hotels were built adjacent to churches so priests could conveniently care for and offer solace to patients. By A.D. 500 almost every city in the old Roman Empire had church-related hospitals. Religious beliefs superseded scientific, Hippocratic knowledge in the treatment of patients, however. Emphasized above all else was the importance of compassion and caring, often at the expense of the little scientific knowledge that was available.

After the fall of Rome, and especially during the Middle Ages (A.D. 500-1450), hospitals were marked by increasingly strong religious influences. This was a bleak period for hospitals. Medical knowledge went unused, primarily because of social and religious pressures. Renewed emphasis on supernatural influences in health and disease occurred as Christianity gained a prominent role in guiding medical treatment.

The Middle East did not experience the decline in medicine that occurred in Western Europe during the Middle Ages. Mohammedan physicians used inhalation anesthesia, and they originated the use of many new drugs. Moslem countries had asylums for the mentally ill a thousand years before such institutions appeared in Europe.[3] Built in Cairo in the thirteenth century, Al-Mansur Hospital had separate wards for serious diseases, outpatient clinics, and homes for convalescence.[4]

The Renaissance

Scientific medicine was rediscovered during the Renaissance, beginning in the fourteenth century, and medicine was increasingly separated from religion. Ironically, although Christianity was a major inhibiting force in the earlier use of this knowledge, much of ancient medicine was recorded in books prepared and preserved in monasteries. As the works of the early Greeks were revived, sixteenth-century scholars applied it to develop new theories. The rebirth of interest in scientific medicine encouraged physicians to attempt procedures that exceeded the limits of science and their ability to prevent or understand the consequences. The hospital's reputation was not enhanced by these increasingly daring surgeons. During the late eighteenth and into the nineteenth century wound infection was ubiquitous; pus drainage was considered a sign of healing. Commonly used medical treatments were brutal by modern standards and included bleeding, purging, violent emetics, and cathartics. A good surgeon was one who operated quickly—the lack of anesthesia made the patient's pain unbearable and he was very difficult to control.

During this period, hospitals (the English word is derived from the Latin *hospes*, meaning host or guest) evolved from a religious to a medical orientation. The oldest hospital in Western Europe is the Hôtel Dieu in Paris. It was founded in A.D. 550 and rebuilt in the thirteenth century. Malcolm T. MacEachern, hospital historian, writer, and theorist,[5] describes it as similar to a modern facility. Its construction separated individuals with different diseases and in various stages of recovery. There was a unit for convalescing maternity patients. Departments with specialized functions were directed by a department head, and specific tasks concerned food, drugs, laundry, and dressings for wounds. A kind of governing body, the board of provisors, conducted semiannual inspections.

Period of Growth: 1860-1920

The first hospital in the United States, the Pennsylvania Hospital, was founded in 1751. In 1798 Congress established the Marine Hospital Service to care for merchant seamen. Medicine's limited effectiveness caused hospitals to have a poor image, however, and their number increased slowly. A rapid increase occurred from 1860 to 1920, however, and the number peaked at

7,370 in 1924. The growth occurred primarily because scientific advances made hospitalization safer and more effective.[6]

Efficacious surgery was significant in the emergence of modern hospitals, and in turn it relied on scientific advances made during the mid- and late-nineteenth century. Lister showed that antisepsis drastically reduced infection rates, and his work was followed by the widespread use of aseptic techniques. Koch's study of anthrax and tuberculosis and Pasteur's work with rabies and cholera in the 1880s provided a scientific theory to explain why antisepsis and asepsis prevented infection.[7] Other developments included the use of surgical anesthesia from the 1840s; Roentgen's discovery of X-rays in 1895;[8] blood typing in 1900, which permitted safer transfusions; successful electrocardiography in 1902; and the Curies' experimentation with radium. Such advances as these allowed surgeons to intervene in disease processes with decreasing mortality and increasing success. A site in which to focus this technology was needed. Hospitals, already established, offered the physical facility, equipment, personnel, and perhaps most importantly, an organizational framework in which to work.

During the nineteenth century, allopathic medicine was only one of many theories of disease causation and cure. It competed with homeopathy, osteopathy, chiropractic, and others. However, scientific developments, especially in microbiology and surgery, supported the radical interventionist approach of allopathy, whose theories hold that if the body deviates from normal functioning, vigorous remedies must be applied. As a result, allopathic medicine became dominant.

Before 1900 most medical schools were proprietary. Entrance and graduation requirements were minimal. Most had no laboratory facilities or clinical training. In 1893 the Johns Hopkins University Medical School was founded. Emphasizing biomedical sciences and modeled after German universities, it soon became the premier American medical school. It was the first to require an undergraduate degree for admission and four years of study, as compared with two years in most of the other 131 schools then in existence.[9] In 1910, Abraham Flexner, whose work was sponsored by the Carnegie Foundation, reported his evaluation of medical schools in the United States and Canada. Major deficiencies were low or nonexistent admission standards, poor facilities, inadequate staff, and lack of basic science in clinical instruction.[10] The Flexner report was heavily influenced by developments at Johns Hopkins, and it had a major effect on American medical education. It had a significant effect on hospitals because they were identified as essential to physician education.

Concurrent developments that shaped the hospital's role were the emergence of nursing as a profession, and changes in society's attitude toward hospitals. Before the Crimean War (1854-1856), when Florence Nightingale did her work, nursing was usually performed by religious orders. Nonsectarian nursing had low status and standards and attracted persons who sometimes abused and robbed their patients. However, in the mid- to late-1800s, advances in nursing included an expansion of its role in health care delivery and the establishment of nursing schools. Pioneers in English and American nursing, Florence Nightingale and Dorothea Dix, respectively, were instrumental in these changes. The first three schools of nursing in the United States were established in 1873; by 1890 there were 38; in 1910, 1,129.[11] These new professionals were considered the physician's handmaidens until the 1960s. In the past two decades, nursing has become increasingly assertive and has striven to achieve more participation and independence in hospitals.

Improvement in society's attitude toward acute care hospitals occurred slowly. Crowded and unsanitary conditions, high mortality rates, and meager medical resources deterred people from entering hospitals voluntarily. Industrialization and the resulting urbanization contributed in an unfortunate way to hospital growth, even before the advent of efficacious medicine. The new urban poor with medical problems had little choice but to enter hospitals, which became an important source of charity care. At the end of the 1800s and into the early 1900s, surgeons and physicians seeking to practice state-of-the-art medicine found it increasingly necessary to hospitalize private patients. The presence of middle-class, paying patients enhanced the respectability of hospitals at a time when the quality of medicine delivered enhanced their reputation.

Consolidation: 1920-1950

By 1920 the foundation had been laid for the contemporary hospital system, and the following 30 years brought refinement and consolidation. The increasing average size of hospitals probably improved the comprehensiveness and quality of care. Two developments with a major effect on hospitals during this period were accreditation and private health insurance.

The American College of Surgeons (ACS) was formed in 1913. Requirements for fellowship included the submission of 50 case histories of patients on whom surgery had been performed. When it was found that many surgeons could not submit cases because hospitals had inadequate patient records, ACS developed requirements for a "Hospital Standardization Program" in 1918, and hospitals that met the criteria were placed on the approved list.[12] The criteria included medical staff standards, quality and content of patient records, and a certain level of diagnostic and therapeutic equipment. The ACS continued this program singlehandedly until 1951, when its activities were transferred to the Joint Commission on Accreditation of Hospitals (JCAH), an organization that now includes the American Hospital Association, the American Medical Association, the American College of Surgeons, the American College of Physicians, and the American Dental Association. Malcolm MacEachern directed the ACS standardization program for almost three decades prior to 1950. There is no doubt the program improved quality of care. In 1987, the JCAH changed its name to the Joint Commission on Accreditation of Healthcare Organizations (JCAHO), although it uses the title "Joint Commission" in day-to-day operations. This name change reflects a broader mission to nonhospital service delivery organizations. The Joint Commission continues as a major force in developing and applying structure, process, and, more recently, outcome measures to the quality of health services, and in providing education and consultation.

A second major event affecting hospitals between 1920 and 1950 was the development of private hospitalization insurance. One of the earliest insurance agreements, that between Baylor University Hospital (Texas) and 1,500 teachers, was signed in 1929. For a fixed fee the hospital agreed to provide 21 days of hospitalization to subscribers.[13] By the mid-1940s, 87 plans covered 20 million people.[14] The effect was substantial: (1) Many hospitals avoided bankruptcy during the Depression; (2) insured individuals avoided financial disaster from major illness by spreading risk; (3) the concept of private-pay patients in hospitals became established; and (4) insurance ensured that general acute care hospitals would be the premier institution in health services delivery.

The general acute care hospitals established from 1900 through the end of World War II resulted primarily from private, voluntary action. Government participation at the federal level was limited to special groups—the armed forces, veterans, American Indians, and merchant mariners—and to psychiatric (long-term) hospitals at the state level. Local governments built some general acute care hospitals, but their numbers were dwarfed by the voluntary system.

Since World War II, general acute care hospitals have increased in number, and their reputation has improved significantly. Much of the wherewithal for these changes resulted from congressional willingness to fund several programs for new construction and remodeling of hospitals, education of physicians and other medical personnel, and funding for medical research and biomedical sciences.

From 1946 until the mid-1970s, the Hill-Burton program provided billions of dollars to general acute care hospitals, especially in rural areas, for expansion, bed replacement, and remodeling. Beginning in the early 1960s, Congress funded medical education programs, primarily for physicians and nurses. Currently, it is feared there will be too many physicians. Conversely, nurses are generally in short supply. From a modest beginning in cancer research in the 1930s, the National Institutes of Health (NIH) became preeminent in biomedical research. Technological advances tended to cause further centralization of acute care services in hospitals and improvements in quality, but at higher costs.

The 20 years from the end of World War II in 1945 until the passage of Medicare and Medicaid in 1965 brought managers the glory days of acute care hospitals. Third-party payors paid without too many questions, Hill-Burton provided new physical facilities, there were few regulators, and the supply of medical and paramedical personnel was usually adequate. Initially, the Medicare program seemed to provide a favorable environment for hospitals. With it, the federal government provided cost-based reimbursement for the elderly, a group typically underserved and underfunded. The reality was short-lived, however.

The external environment evolved from supportive to hostile and seemed to threaten the very existence of hospitals. During the 1970s, hospitals were included under federal labor legislation; safety and health act requirements; various wage and hour, civil rights, and equal employment opportunity laws; health planning legislation; professional standards review organizations; and certificate-of-need laws.

Ultimately, however, controls on reimbursement would become the bane of hospitals' existence. Initially, third-party payors, including the federal government, acted tentatively. By the early 1980s, however, drastic actions had been taken, and hospitals were put at economic risk for patient care decisions. For Medicare patients this was called prospective payment and was linked to diagnosis-related groups (DRGs). In theory, each diagnosis costs, on average, a fixed amount to treat. This is the payment hospitals receive. More costly care puts the hospital at financial risk; if care is less costly, the "profit" is the hospital's.

Changes in reimbursement are a major reason why hospitals are engaging in corporate restructuring, diversification, joint ventures with medical staff, backward and forward integration, and for-profit activities. A destabilized health services system means that hospitals must be competitive. This has generated hospital advertising, efforts to fully integrate the organization, and the offering of services in ways only recently unacceptable.

This radically changed environment holds a major challenge for hospital managers, and the future is linked primarily to economics. It is predicted that the next decade will find physician payments included in the basic DRG payment as well as a pronounced trend toward capitation payments—one fee paid for all health services provided to an individual. Such limits on hospital income mean that survival will require efficient and effective management.

Hospital Organization: The Triad

During their evolution, not-for-profit hospitals developed unique features. The most important is an arrangement called the triad, the foremost example of which is found in the voluntary not-for-profit community hospital,* which is typically owned by a private association. Teaching hospitals are similar, but their organizations are more complex. The triad includes the governing body, the chief executive officer (CEO), and the medical staff organization (MSO). In theory, the triad permits power sharing among the three. It is best characterized as an accommodation, however, and results from the independent contractor status of the physicians, who treat patients in the hospital, and the governing body's need to delegate responsibility for day-to-day operation to the CEO and senior managers. Despite shortcomings and challenges to its efficiency and desirability, the triad shown in Fig. I-1 is typical of privately and publicly owned not-for-profit acute care hospitals.

---

* The AHA defines community hospitals to include all nonfederal short-term general and other special hospitals, excluding hospital units of institutions, whose facilities and services are available to the public.

Often, adopting a "corporate structure" only superficially modifies the form, especially position titles, but little of substance changes.

New Models

The voluntary not-for-profit hospital continues to be the dominant type of acute care hospital, but others have increased rapidly in number. From a moribund condition in the 1960s, investor-owned hospitals have rebounded since the passage of Medicare. In 1987, the most recent year for which data are available, investor-owned corporations owned 1,375 hospitals with 164,079 beds.* In addition, they managed 352 not-for-profit hospitals with 45,437 beds. Owned and managed hospitals include community and noncommunity hospitals, but the former predominate.[15] In 1986, the AHA classified 3,338 hospitals with 689,685 beds as nongovernmental, not-for-profit community hospitals; 1,556 community hospitals with 185,139 beds were owned by state and local governments.[16]

Both not-for-profit and investor-owned hospitals that are part of a system tend to have similar relationships with corporate headquarters. Some management functions, such as purchasing, finance, and planning, are likely to be centralized. In some systems each hospital has a governing body to develop local policy within the corporate framework. Necessarily, a system reduces local autonomy. This is a price many freestanding hospitals are reluctant to pay. Except for the few acute care hospitals financially strong enough to remain independent, however, the era of stand-alone facilities appears to be ending.

Fiscal and regulatory pressures have forced governing bodies to rely increasingly on their chief executives, and this requires greater accountability from them. About 70 percent of CEOs are governing body members, often with a vote. Those who are on the governing body participate in policy development and decision-making at the highest level. Especially in larger hospitals, many CEOs concentrate on external relationships and problems; they delegate day-to-day operational responsibility to an associate called the chief operating officer (COO). The assignment of managerial tasks along internal and external lines has gained wide acceptance in larger hospitals, but more recently also in smaller facilities. Hospitals increasingly employ full-time, paid chiefs of medical staff, who often have the title of medical director. This physician may also be a voting member of the governing body. This provides important input at the hospital's policy level, but may raise other problems.

Features found in the corporate model form of acute care hospital organization are a greater role of the CEO and, occasionally, line accountability for MSO activities. The American College of Healthcare Executives (ACHE), formerly the American College of Hospital Administrators

---

* The discrepancy in totals between the AHA data in Table i-I and the Federation of American Health Systems data results from differences in the numbers of investor-owned hospitals reporting to each.

(ACHA), is on record as preferring the corporate structure through its endorsement of a 1974 ACHA task force report. The report recommended to the JCAHO (then the JCAH) that there be direct line accountability between the MSO and the CEO through a medical director. In the interim, the JCAHO has stressed MSO accountability to a greater extent, but has yet to recommend interposing the CEO between the MSO and the governing body. It is unlikely that JCAHO will include such a requirement soon. MSOs are very powerful and independent, and the JCAHO has a strong physician bias. It must be stressed, however, that even when physicians are independent contractors, their clinical practice is subject to peer review. Recommendations from this process are made to governing bodies increasingly aware of the peril of failing to act on identified problems. In hospitals where physicians are employed — Veterans Administration, military, university hospitals — there is greater line authority over them, at least as to the administrative aspects of hospital medical practice. Even here, however, physicians have significant freedom of action.

This causes a dilemma. Medical education stresses independence, a necessary and desirable trait in professional activity. Since MSOs in hospitals retain a high degree of independence, changes in behavior rely mainly on persuasion. Increasingly, however, this may be insufficient, and hospitals will have to be more aggressive in solving medical staff problems. Courts have found that even absent an employment relationship, the hospital, through its governing body, has corporate liability for medical practice. Inevitably this will result in increased control of physicians' activities and greater willingness by hospitals to use sanctions such as limitation on, or suspension of, clinical privileges. Attenuating or removing privileges is the most direct and drastic control hospitals have over physicians.

The Governing Body

Traditionally, hospitals relied on the business and professional expertise of governing body members, supplemented by managerial staff. This pattern predominates but is increasingly inadequate. Hospitals and business enterprise have numerous similarities, but the differences are great and warrant special expertise, which must be reflected in the governing body. Diverse pressures, including community interest, government regulation, third-party payors and prospective pricing, and malpractice claims, have caused the governing body to be scrutinized more closely. To better solve these problems, various proposals have been made to increase the competence of governing body members. Specialized seminars and continuing education are common. It has been suggested that the hospital managerial staff as well as consultants can provide the expertise to assist governing body members. Such proposals are misfocused. Community hospitals will be served best by adopting the business enterprise model, in which directors are paid for their time and knowledge. Paying directors will permit hospitals to obtain the expertise they need and ensure that members of governing bodies commit the time needed to be effective. High-quality policymaking is only a matter of chance if the governing body is marginally or inadequately informed. Ill-informed members only react to problems and can make no independent, positive contribution to policymaking and oversight responsibilities. Governing body members cannot match the technical expertise of management staff and consultants, but they must have a level of expertise about hospitals and their environment similar to that of the CEO. Furthermore, it is necessary that technical expertise be available as needed. A casual approach to hospital governance is long past.

Recent AHA data show that 22 percent of hospitals pay members of the governing body a per meeting or annual fee. This is a substantial increase from the level found by a similar study in 1979. Surprisingly, for-profit hospitals were found to compensate only half as often as other types. Other compensation has also increased significantly.[17] Paying governing body members is important because it will be more effective in getting maximum commitment and performance than requests for contributed time and expertise. This is true even if the service is disproportionate to the payment. Contributing time permits one to believe that the recipient (hospital) is being done a favor. The recipient, too, may feel that it should be grateful for whatever is received rather than critical, regardless of quality. Payment, however, enhances the governing body's psychological ability to hold members accountable for performance.

The future will witness a change from the historical source of governing body members, at least for those in the voluntary sector. Hospital-related expertise will be a vital consideration. Enhanced governing body accountability will result in a natural selection process. Individuals without the time and expertise to be effective will no longer participate, and nonchalant involvement will not be tolerated. Hospitals might also benefit by adopting a practice found in business enterprise: professional directors. These are persons skilled in guiding policy development and decision-making, but who have no permanent employment other than their several paid directorships.[18]

Often, the title "trustee" is used despite the absence of a trust for which the governing body is responsible. In such situations, "director" is the appropriate term. Both directors and true trustees are fiduciaries. Fiduciaries must safeguard the organization's assets, protect patients from harm, and not get any secret personal gain from their relationship. True trustees, however, are held to a more stringent legal standard. Conflicts of interest affecting hospital governing bodies have been the subject of journalistic and judicial inquiries. Court decisions establish nonfeasance as important as malfeasance.

Until the 1970s, the potential for conflict of interest raised objections to service on the governing body by members of a hospital's MSO. Similar concerns precluded service by CEOs. Although potential problems noted by such authors and practitioners as LeTourneau, MacEachern, and McGibony are still present, MSO members are now commonly on the governing body. It is believed that the benefits of coordination and cooperation, as well as involvement by physicians in policy development and implementation, outweigh potential disadvantages. Most governing bodies now include several members of the MSO; most also include the CEO.

The Chief Executive Officer

MacEachern identified Florence Nightingale as the first hospital administrator.[19] Since Nightingale did her work during the mid-nineteenth century, this makes the emergence of the hospital chief executive a relatively recent event. Hospital administration was identified as a distinct body of knowledge in 1934, when the University of Chicago established the first graduate program in the United States. The number of programs increased slowly during the next three decades, but rapid growth occurred in the mid-1960s. In 1987 there were 50 graduate education programs (45 in the United States and Puerto Rico, 5 in Canada) accredited by the Accrediting Commission on Education for the Health Services Administration. Nine more programs are affiliated with the programs' trade association, the Association of University Programs in Health Administration (AUPHA), and are eligible for accreditation. The number of undergraduate programs has grown from about a half-dozen in the late 1960s to the 32 currently affiliated with AUPHA.[20] Programs are found in a variety of academic settings: schools or departments of business, public health, public administration, economics, and medicine. Program content varies, but accreditation requires the inclusion of certain subject matter: social-behavioral and management sciences; individual, social, and environmental determinants of health and disease; elements of medical care; and application of administrative concepts and skills in specific health services organizations and programs. An unsolved problem is integrating and articulating undergraduate and graduate health services education.

Concerns have been voiced that the number of graduates will exceed the market's need for them. It is true that first jobs today are very unlikely to be at the assistant or associate level. Various studies and reports show, however, that demand for graduates of health services administration programs will outstrip supply during the next decade. For employers it is desirable that adequate numbers of candidates be available. As a matter of policy, the public will benefit from a ready supply of competent managers.

In the century since Florence Nightingale did her work, hospital administration has become a profession. This evolution has been significantly buttressed and reinforced by graduate education. There is no doubt that hospital managers have been professionalized by establishing associations, hierarchical prominence, and income, titles, and other accouterments. Governing bodies, staff, and physicians generally recognize the role and importance of hospital managers. However, hospital managers have been slow to achieve public recognition and status consistent with their roles, and there is evidence that some physicians do not consider managers their professional peers and colleagues as both groups strive to provide high-quality health services. The fault for this may lie as much with managers as with physicians. Energetically demonstrating competence is also a management skill. Furthermore, effectively involving physicians in hospital management enhances the outcome of problem solving and demonstrates the job's complexity and the specialized skills needed. However, it is regrettable that for many managers this interaction has been no more desirable than involvement of managers in MSO affairs has been desirable for physicians.

The ACHE is the most important professional association for hospital managers and the largest in the health services field. Currently, it has over 20,000 affiliates, including student associates. Its organization and levels of affiliation are similar to those of medical specialty societies, and unlike many health services associations it has stringent advancement requirements. Affiliations include nominee, member, and fellow, and these are separated by length of tenure and written and oral requirements. ACHE plays an important role because hospital managers are not licensed. Consequently, affiliation, especially as a fellow, is increasingly recognized as a necessary credential. The ACHE has a code of ethics that is applied by a standing committee composed of fellows. In addition to revising the code, it confidentially investigates complaints against affiliates and recommends disposition of these cases.

The Medical Staff Organization

A medical staff organization (MSO) is indispensible to the acute care hospital. Society has identified a special place and role for physicians, and through licensing it verifies their preparation. By virtue of their license, physicians exercise powers not given others. An example is prescribing controlled substances. A focus of this role is in hospitals, where patient care depends on physicians personally providing treatment, or directing and supervising others who do. This role, in addition to professional independence, economic power, and social status, necessitates relationships in the hospital that give physicians substantial power. The result is that managing acute care hospitals is immensely complex. The status of physicians as independent contractors has diminished somewhat as increasing numbers have become salaried, but in smaller community hospitals especially, they remain fiercely independent.

More frequently in the recent past, and for a variety of reasons, hospitals have sought to regulate their physicians. This control is no less significant than initial licensing, and it is used to limit the otherwise unlimited state license granted physicians. Through credentialing, hospitals determine the medical or surgical activities in which physicians on their staff may engage. These are known as clinical privileges. Quality assurance enables the hospital to judge the continued appropriateness of privileges that have been granted to individual physicians. Nowhere else does this occur. There is no ongoing, organized scrutiny of physicians in office practice and no effort to determine the quality of care provided there. In this regard it is fortunate, and in the patient's best interests, that technology necessitates centralizing acute medical practice in hospitals. Nonetheless, credentialing and monitoring are problem laden. The hospital must be willing to suspend or terminate the physicians unwilling or unable to comply with hospital standards.

All hospitals should have at least a part-time medical director. Chiefs of clinical services should be added as need demands and resources permit. The appointment of clinical managers such as a medical director and chiefs of service enhances MSO accountability, which ultimately improves quality of care. This model is suggested by the Joint Commission and by researchers. Physician managers may be paid or voluntary; however, from the standpoint of commitment and responsiveness, it is desirable that there be an economic arrangement. The same arguments apply here as to paid governing bodies.

The CEO and the governing body interact with clinical managers in the same fashion as with other technical experts. Nonphysician managers and governing body members are not competent to judge the quality of clinical decision-making and practice. Instead, managers and governing bodies receive information from clinical managers in order to make decisions that affect the hospital's clinical activities. The clearest example is that in which management and the governing body rely on clinical managers to recommend that a physician be granted privileges both for initial appointment and reappointment. This recommendation does not relieve the governing body of a need to inquire, to understand basic data, and to take action as indicated. In theory, this relationship is universally applied. Historically, however, management and governing bodies have been only tangentially involved and, more often than not, have been rubber stamps for the credentialing process.

Three factors have caused significant change in relations with hospital-based physicians, such as pathologists and radiologists: greater scrutiny by governance and management, especially as to the economic effect of contracts; increased pressure from outside agencies such as cost review commissions, the Health Care Financing Administration (HCFA, a part of the Department of Health and Human Services), and the Federal Trade Commission; and professional society policy and membership guidelines. Radiologists are likely to bill separately for services. Pathologists are more likely to be salaried now than they were in the past when compensation based on percentages of gross or net revenues were common. In addition, more of these specialists are available. This fact has several consequences: management is in a stronger bargaining position in any negotiations; more of these specialists will be salaried in the future; and costs of services might decrease, or at least increase less rapidly.

The Office of Management and Budget has recommended that all physician services be included in the DRG prospective pricing system (PPS). The Reagan administration's budget proposal for fiscal 1988 included radiologists, anesthesiologists, and pathologists, but vigorous opposition by hospitals and medical groups defeated the initiative.[21] Doubtless, the future will include this and similar efforts to reduce Medicare payments.

The physician surplus predicted for the 1990s seems less likely. Two reasons have been identified: medical schools have fewer applicants, and some specialty boards have begun reducing the number of approved residencies, thus reducing the number of entrants into the specialty. Whatever surplus occurs, however, offers hospital managers the opportunity to improve the organization and management of hospital-based physicians and MSOs generally. Governing bodies will be in a stronger position to structure MSO relationships to meet new hospital objectives. Energetic and competent managers will be prepared to take advantage of the opportunities this situation presents. For example, a physician surplus will allow hospitals to put clinical managers such as medical directors on salary. Ironically, similar pressure may come from physicians more generally as they seek income security. It is suggested that primary care physicians should be gatekeepers for access to specialists and hospitalization. An economic gatekeeping function will become mandatory for all physicians as the concept of managed care gains acceptance. Generally, such developments lend weight to efforts to tie specialists more closely to hospital practice.

An MSO enables the hospital to meet its social mission. However, the era in which physicians treated indigent patients in exchange for the opportunity to admit private patients to acute care hospitals is long past. Except for bad debts and a small amount of charity care, physicians are paid for all patients' services. What replaces the previous exchange of admitting privileges for charity care? How does the physician contribute to the hospital relationship? Surely, it must be more than availability of medical service. The annual income generated for an acute care hospital by various specialties ranges from $943,000 per year per physician in cardiovascular to $124,000 in ophthalmology.[22] But this economic symbiosis does not address the concerns of the third element in the equation: society, as represented by consumers of health services in hospitals.

This element is absent and perhaps the world is irretrievably changed. If so, and only economic relationships remain, it is time to consider whether physicians should pay to practice medicine in hospitals. The charges to these independent contractor physicians need be only modest, and physicians would certainly pass along these costs to patients. The modest income thus produced for the hospital would be insignificant. What is important is that the psychological commitment of being on staff is reinforced by the economic exchange. Although qualitatively different from the earlier relationship, it has the potential for more committed and involved physicians. In turn, it should have a salutary effect on physicians' performance, plus an incentive for hospitals to improve quality generally. The arrangement has the attributes of a contract with enforceable provisions. The economic relationship remains subordinated, however, to credentialing and quality assurance processes.

Whatever opportunities hospitals have in the decade ahead and however effectively they are used, the long-term trend in hospital-physician relationships will necessarily result in greater control exercised by hospitals. Increased demands for accountability from government, consumers, and third-party payors, as well as precepts of good management, demand it.

Conclusion

The acute care hospital is today and will remain among the most complex, fascinating, and challenging organizations ever developed. Hospitals have been thrust into a milieu in which those who lead them will have numerous opportunities to demonstrate their skills. It will take the dedicated and enlightened work of all involved to meet the challenge. As long as there are acute care hospitals, means to effectively and efficiently manage them can and will be found. For those who take up the gauntlet, the challenge is momentous.

Notes

1. Mary Risley, *House of Healing* (Garden City, NY: Doubleday, 1961), pp. 53-66.
2. *Ibid.*, pp. 29-52.
3. Malcolm T. MacEachern, *Hospital Organization and Management*, 3rd ed. (Berwyn, IL: Physicians Record Company, 1962), pp. 8-10.
4. *Ibid.*, p. 10.
5. *Ibid.*, pp. 8-10.
6. U.S. Department of Commerce, *Historical Statistics of the United States: Colonial Times to 1957* (Washington, DC, U.S. Government Printing Office, 1960), p. 35.
7. H.S. Hartzog, Jr., *Triumphs in Medicine* (New York: Doubleday, Page, 1927), pp. 161-163, 144-148.
8. Fielding H. Garrison, *History of Medicine*, 4th ed. (Philadelphia: W.B. Saunders, 1929), p. 721.
9. For data on the number of U.S. medical schools by sect (allopathic, homeopathic, and eclectic) for the years 1850-1920 see "Medical Education in the United States," *Journal of the American Medical Association* 79, no. 8 (August 19): 629-659, 1922.
10. A review of the Flexner report is strongly recommended. See Abraham Flexner, *Medical Education in the United States and Canada* (New York: The Carnegie Foundation, 1910).
11. U.S. Department of Commerce, *Historical Statistics*, p. 34.
12. Laura G. Jackson, *Hospital and Community* (New York: Macmillan, 1964), p. 357.
13. C. Rufus Rorem, *Non-Profit Hospital Service Plans* (Chicago: American Hospital Association, 1940), p. 9.
14. Nathan Sinai, Odin W. Anderson, and Melvin L. Dollar, *Health Insurance in the United States*, (New York: The Commonwealth Fund, 1946), p. 44.
15. Federation of American Health Systems, "Federation of American Health Systems 1988 Directory of Investor-owned Hospitals, Hospital Management Companies and Health Systems," *FAHS Review*, p. 7, 1987.
16. American Hospital Association, *Hospital Statistics, 1987 Edition* (Chicago, American Hospital Association, 1987), p. 12.
17. Joan L. Rehm and Jeffrey Alexander, "Perks for Trusteeship: Compensation Survey Reveals Who, What, How Much, and How Often," *Trustee* (April): 24-27, 1986.
18. Robert W. Lear, "Compensation for Outside Directors," *Harvard Business Review* 57 (November-December): 24, 1979.
19. MacEachern, *Hospital Organization*, p. 17.
20. Membership data, Association of University Programs in Health Administration, Arlington, VA, February 22, 1988.
21. "Doctors, Hospitals Oppose Combined DRGs," *Medical Staff News* 16, No. 1 (January): 1, 8, 1987.
22. "How Much Revenue Does a Physician Bring In?" *Hospitals* (June 5): 56, 1987.

Bibliography

Alexander, Jeffrey. "Governance in Multi-hospital Systems: An Assessment of Decision-Making Responsibility." *Hospital & Health Services Administration* (March/April):9-20, 1985.

American Hospital Association Committee on Hospital Governing Boards. "On Involving Physicians in Hospital Governance." *Trustee* 31 (April):38, 1978.

Barrett, Diana. *Multihospital Systems: The Process of Development.* Cambridge, MA: Oelgeschlager, 1980.

Bean, Joseph, Jr. and Rene Laliberty. *Decentralizing Hospital Management: A Manual for Supervisors.* Reading, MA: Addison-Wesley, 1980.

Berger, Sally. "CEOs May Become Outside Trustees." *Modern Healthcare* (January): 164, 166, 1984.

Berry, David E. and Jon W. Seavey. "Reiteration of Problem Definition in Health Services Administration." *Hospital & Health Services Administration* 29, No. 2 (March-April):56-70, 1984.

Bennett, Addison C. *Improving Management Performance in Health Care Institutions: A Total Systems Approach.* Chicago: American Hospital Association, 1978.

Bice, Michael O. "Corporate Cultures and Business Strategy: A Health Management Company Perspective." *Hospital & Health Services Administration* 29, No. 4 (July-August): 64-78, 1984.

Blanton, Wyndham B., Jr. "A Physician Looks at Board-Medical Staff Relationships." *Trustee* 32 (June):28-30, 1979.

_____. "Negotiating Differences Between Medical Staff and Administration." *Trustee* 34 (December):23, 1981.

Brooks, Deal Chandler and Michael A. Morrisey. "Credentialing: Say Good-bye to the 'Rubber Stamp.'" *Hospitals* (June 1):50-52, 1985.

Brown, David L. "Guidelines Can Resolve Turf Battles Between Local and Corporate Boards." *Trustee* 33 (October): 26, 1983.

Brown, Montague. "Changing Role of Administrator in Multiple-Hospital Systems." *Hospital & Health Services Administration* 23 (Fall):6-19, 1978.

Brown, Montague and Barbara P. McCool. *Multi-hospital Systems: Strategies for Organization and Management.* Rockville, MD: Aspen Systems, 1979.

Carper, William B. "Longitudinal Analysis of the Problems of Hospital Administrators." *Hospital & Health Services Administration* 27 (May-June): 82-95, 1982.

Chandler, Robert L. "Filling Empty Board Seats." *Hospital & Health Services Administration* 25 (Winter):69-85, 1980.

Collins, Thomas M. "Nonphysician Practitioners in Hospitals." *Trustee* (November): 19, 1981.

Countryman, Kathleen and Alexandra Gekas. *Development and Implementation of a Patient's Bill of Rights in Hospitals.* Chicago: American Hospital Association, 1980.

Cunningham, Robert M., Jr. *Asking and Giving: A Report on Hospital Philanthropy.* Chicago: American Hospital Association, 1980.

Derzon, Robert A., Roger B. LeCompte, and Lawrence S. Lewin. "Hospitals Say Yes to Contract Management." *Trustee* 34 (July):33-36, 1981.

Dolan, Thomas C. and Gayle C. Lane. "The Regulation of Health Care Delivery." *Medical Group Management* 27 (January-February):22-24, 1980.

Drucker, Peter F. "The Coming of the New Organization." *Harvard Business Review* (January-February):45-53, 1988.

Duval, Merlin K. "Nonprofit Multihospital Systems." *Health Matrix* (Spring):22-25, 1985.

Eisenberg, John M. "The Internist as Gatekeeper." *Annals of Internal Medicine* 102, No. 4 (April):537-543, 1985.

Fifer, William R. "Beyond Peer Review: The Medical Staff Role in the Price-Competitive Hospital." *QRB* (September): 262-268, 1984.

Fisher, Bruce and Dean Grant. "A New Organizational Model: Breaking the Three-Legged Stool." *Hospital Financial Management* 34 (July):38-40, 1980.

Flynn, James R. "Treating the Impaired Physician: The Hospital's Role." *Hospital Progress* 61 (March):44-47, 1980.

Fried, Jules M. "Corporate Restructuring: What, When, Where, Why, and How." *Trustee* 35 (June):19-23, 1985.

Gentile, Benedice J. and Marilyn Mannisto. "Trustee Survey: Trends in Board Committee Structure." Trustee 35 (November): 32-34, 1985.

Georgopoulos, Basil S., ed. *Organization Research on Health Institutions.* Ann Arbor: The University of Michigan Institute for Social Research, 1972.

Gerber, Lawrence. "A Sampling of Joint Venture Opportunities for Hospitals and Physicians." *Trustee* 35 (May):38+, 1985.

Griffith, John R. "A Proposal for New Hospital Performance Measures." *Hospital & Health Services Administration* 23 (Spring):60-84, 1978.

Hackler, Eugene T. "Hospital Trustees' Fiduciary Responsibilities: An Emerging Tripartite Distinction." *Washburn Law Journal* 15, No. 3:422-434, 1976.

Harrison, Fernande P. "Consider Values-Based Management." *Health Management Forum* (Autumn):4-17, 1985.

Henry, William F. and Vernon E. Weckwerth. "When Corporate Executives Serve as Trustees." *Trustee* 34 (November):29-32, 1981.

Hofmann, Paul B. "Establishing Standards of Institutional Performance." *Hospital Progress* 57 (February):50-53, 1976.

Hollowell, Edward E. "The Disruptive Physician: Handle With Care." *Trustee* 31 (June):11-17, 1978.

Hughes, Robert G., et al. "Hospitals and Physicians: An Organizational Model for a Changing Healthcare Environment." *Hospital & Health Services Administration* 29 (November-December): 7-20, 1984.

Johnson, Everett A. "Managing Physician-Directed Departments." *Hospital & Health Services Administration* 24 (Summer):96-101, 1979.

Johnson, Richard L. "Reorganizing the Organization: New Roles Lie Ahead." *Healthcare Executive* 1, No. 7 (November/ December):41-43, 1986.

_____. "Roles of CEOs, Boards are Changing in Not-for-Profits." *Hospitals* (December 1):84-85, 1984.

Kaufman, Kenneth, et al. "The Effects of Board Composition and Structure on Hospital Performance." *Hospital & Health Services Administration* 24 (Winter):37-62, 1979.

Kessenick, Laurence W. and John E. Peer. "Physicians' Access to the Hospital: An Overview." *University of San Francisco Law Review* 14 (Fall):43-75, 1979.

Kovner, Anthony R. "Improving Community Hospital Board Performance." *Medical Care* 16 (February):35, 1976.

Livingston, Carlyle O. "Changing Corporate Structures—From Reorganization to Mergers." *Topics in Health Care Financing* (Fall): 38-46, 1984.

Longest, Beaufort B., Jr. *Management Practices for the Health Professional.* Reston, VA: Reston Publications, 1976.

_____. "Trustees and Administrator: A Plan for Sharing Responsibility." *Hospital Forum* 23 (April-May):8-11, 1980.

Massachusetts Hospital Association Task Force on Management Contracts. "A Management Contract for Your CEO?" *Trustee* 32 (December):40-41, 1979.

Moore, Terence F. and Bernard E. Lorimer. "The Matrix Organization in Business & Health Care Institutions." *Hospital and Health Services Administration.* 21 (Fall):26-34, 1976.

Moore, W. Barry. "Survey Shows CEOs' Priorities Are Changing." *Hospitals* (December):71-77, 1984.

Morrisey, Michael A. and Deal Chandler Brooks. "The Expanding Medical Staff: Nonphysician Practitioners." *Hospitals* (August 1):58-59, 1985.

_____. "Physician Influence in Hospitals: An Update." *Hospitals* (September 1):86-87, 89, 1985.

Morrisey, Michael A., et al. "More Hospitals Compensate Physicians for Administrative Role: Survey." *Trustee* 37 (January):39-44, 1984.

Morse, George and Robert Morse. *Protecting the Health Care Facility.* Baltimore: Williams & Wilkins, 1973.

Moses, Richard P. "Rating Your CEO: A Guide to Effective Evaluation." *Trustee* 39 (October):11-14, 1986.

Nigosian, Gregory J. "Board Operating Practices Subject of AHA Survey." *Hospitals* (November 16):81-90, 1980.

Noie, Nancie E., et al. "Those Changing Medical Staffs: Survey Shows Some SurprisingTrends." *Trustee* 35 (December): 24-26, 1983.

Noll, Harlan. "How to Shape Incentive Plans for the Hospital's Top Executives." *Trustee* 35 (August):16+, 1983.

Perey, Bernard J. "The Role of the Physician Manager." *Health Management Forum* 5, No. 3 (Autumn):48-55, 1984.

Prybil, Lawrence D. "A Closer Look: Bringing Board and CEO Performance into Sharper Focus." *Trustee* 31 (April):28, 1978.

_____. "In the 1980s: Smaller Boards, Stricter Standards of Conduct." *Trustee* 33 (January):31-32, 1980.

Rehm, John L. and Jeffrey Alexander. "Perks for Trusteeship: Compensation Survey Reveals Who, What, How Much, and How Often." *Trustee* 39 (April):24-27, 1986.

Ritvo, Roger A. "Adaption to Environmental Change: The Board's Role." *Hospital & Health Services Administration* 25 (Winter):23-37, 1980.

Rosenberg, Charles E. *The Care of Strangers: The Rise of America's Hospital System*. New York: Basic Books, 1987.

Ruelas, Enrique and Peggy Leatt. "The Roles of Physician-Executives in Hospitals: A Framework for Management Education." *The Journal of Health Administration Education* 3, No. 2 (Spring): 151-169, 1985.

Schulz, Rockwell and Alton Johnson. *Management of Hospitals*. 2nd ed. New York: McGraw-Hill, 1983.

Schuster, Jay R. "Successful Hospitals Pay for Performance." *Hospitals* (March): 86-88, 1985.

Sherman, V. Clayton. "Six Cardinal Rules to Help Boards Solve Top Management Problems." *Trustee* 36 (October):40+, 1983.

Shields, Thomas C. "Guidelines for Reviewing Applications for Privileges." *Hospital Medical Staff* 9 (September):11-17, 1980.

Shortell, Stephen M. "Can Corporate Culture Enhance Productivity?" *Health Management Quarterly* (Fall):10-16, 1984.

_____. "The Costs and Benefits of Closer Group Practice-Hospital Relationships." *Medical Group Management* 9 (September):11-17, 1980.

_____. "High-Performing Health Care Organizations: Guidelines for the Pursuit of Excellence." *Hospital & Health Services Administration* 30 (July-August):7-35, 1985.

_____. "The Medical Staff of the Future: Replanting the Garden." *Frontiers of Health Services Management* 1, No. 3 (February):3-48, 1985.

Shortell, Stephen M. and Thomas E. Getzen. "Measuring Hospital Medical Staff Organizational Structure." *Health Services Research* 14 (Summer):97-110, 1979.

Simendinger, Earl A. and William Pasmore. "Developing Partnerships Between Physicians and Healthcare Executives." *Hospital & Health Services Administration* 29 (November-December):21-35, 1984.

Starkweather, David. *Hospital Mergers in the Making*. Ann Arbor, MI: Health Administration Press, 1980.

Steinwald, Bruce. "Hospital-Based Physicians: Current Issues and Descriptive Evidence." *Health Care Financing Review* 2 (Summer): 63-75, 1980.

Stensrud, Robert. "The New Generation of Executive Performance Research: Its Implications for Healthcare." *Hospital & Health Services Administration* 31 (May-June):22-33, 1986.

Talbot, G. Douglas and Earl B. Benson. "Impaired Physicians: The Dilemma of Identification." *Postgraduate Medicine* (December):56+, 1980.

Teich, Jeffrey. "How to Bring the Impaired Physician to Treatment." *The Hospital Medical Staff* (September):18-24, 1982.

Terenzio, J.V. "The Hospital Medical Staff Physician in Hospital Management." *Acta Hospitalia* 19 (Autumn):197-218, 1979.

Trivedi, Vandan M. and Walton M. Hancock. "A Tripartite Approach to Hospital Census Management." *Hospital & Health Services Administration* 26 (Special I):8-25, 1981.

Troyer, Glenn and Steven Salman. "How Boards Can Meet Their Quality Assurance Responsibilities." *Trustee* 34 (June):33-38, 1981.

Vladeck, Bruce C. "Health Administration and the Crisis in Health Care." *The Journal of Health Administration Education* 3, No. 4 (Fall):427-438, 1985.

Warden, Gail. "Board Self-Assessment: Changing the Governing Structure to Meet Changing Times." *Trustee* 31 (March):37-40, 1978.

Weil, Thomas P. "The Changing Relationship Between Physicians and the Hospital CEO." *Trustee* 40 (February):15-18, 1987.

Wentz, Walter J. and Terence F. Moore. "Administrative Success: Key Ingredients." *Hospital & Health Services Administration* 26 (Special II):85-93, 1981.

Wheeler, John R.C., Thomas M. Wickizer, and Stephen M. Shortell. "Hospital-Physician Vertical Integration." *Hospital & Health Services Administration* 26 (March-April):67-80, 1986.

White, Stephen L. *Managing Health and Human Service Programs: A Guide for Managers*. New York: Free Press, 1981.

Organization

Selection 1, "The Hospital as an Organization" by Basil S. Georgopoulos and Floyd C. Mann, is a classic in the field. It provides an overview of the acute care hospital in the context of management theory. Distinguishing features of that very complex organization are highlighted, and interactions are identified. An early leader in hospital administration, the late Ray E. Brown, wrote selection 2, "Strictures and Structures," in which he described some philosophical problems associated with hospital organization and management. His observations are insightful and give cause to consider aspects beyond managerial activities.

Selection 3, "Revisiting 'The Wobbly Three Legged Stool,' " was written by Richard L. Johnson, who develops the concept that coordination at the level required to manage contemporary hospitals cannot be obtained in the traditional triad commonly found in hospitals. Johnson recommends adopting the corporate model, but warns that it must be adapted to hospital use. The last article in this section is selection 4, "Integrated Systems: The Good, the Bad, the Ugly" by John Knox Singleton and C. Michael French. In it the authors describe the advantages of integrated health care systems, and why some succeed and others fail.

1

The Hospital as an Organization

Basil S. Georgopoulos and Floyd C. Mann

Basil S. Georgopoulos, Ph.D., is Program Director of the Survey Research Center, and Professor of Psychology, The University of Michigan, Ann Arbor.

Floyd C. Mann, Ph.D., is Director and Professor, Advanced Urban Study Institute, University of Colorado, Denver.

The community general hospital is an organization that mobilizes the skills and efforts of a number of widely divergent groups of professional, semiprofessional, and nonprofessional personnel to provide a highly personalized service to individual patients. Like other large-scale organizations, it is established and designed to pursue certain objectives through collaborative activity. The chief objective of the hospital is, of course, to provide adequate care and treatment to its patients (within the limits of present-day technical-medical knowledge, and knowledge of organizing human activity effectively, as well as within limits that may be imposed by the relative scarcity of appropriate organizational resources or by extraorganizational forces). Its principal product is medical, surgical, and nursing service to the patient, and its central concern is the life and health of the patient. A hospital may, of course, have additional objectives, including its own maintenance and survival, organizational stability and growth, financial solvency, medical and nursing education and research, and various employee-related objectives. But, all of these are subsidiary to the key objective of service to the patient, which constitutes the basic organizing principle that underlies all activities in the community general hospital.

There is little ambiguity, if any, about the main organizational objective of the community general hospital. Unlike many organizations, the hospital is able to make the role it performs in the larger community psychologically meaningful to its members. And most of its members try to give unstintingly of their energies to perform the tasks assigned to them. Many doctors and nurses look upon their profession as a sacred calling. Others find working in the hospital deeply satisfying of needs that they cannot easily express in words. They see the hospital as a nonprofit institution dedicated to works of mercy, and they sense their mission in life to give of themselves in order to help others. Immediate personal comfort and satisfactions, and even material rewards, are defined by most members as less important than giving good care to the patient and meeting a higher order of obligation to mankind. Serious conflicts regarding material rewards, such as those found in organizations where profit is the chief motive, are virtually nonexistent in the hospital. For all these reasons, motivating organizational members toward the objectives of the organization is much less of a problem in the hospital by comparison to other large-scale organizations. The goals of individual members and the objectives of the organization are considerably more congruent in the case of the hospital.

Extensive Division of Labor

To do its work, the hospital relies upon an extensive division of labor among its members, upon a complex organizational structure which encompasses many different departments, staffs, offices, and positions, and upon an elaborate system of coordination of tasks, functions, and social interaction.

Work in the hospital is greatly differentiated and specialized, and of a highly interactional character. It is carried out by a large number of cooperating people whose backgrounds, education, training, skills, and functions are as diverse and heterogeneous as can be found in any of the most complex organizations in existence. And much of the work is not only specialized but also performed by highly trained professionals—the doctors—who require the collaboration, assistance, and services of many other professional and nonprofessional personnel. In addition to the medical staff, which itself is highly specialized and departmentalized, there is the nursing staff, which includes graduate professional nurses in various supervisory and nonsupervisory positions, practical nurses, and untrained nurses' aides. In addition to the nursing staff and the medical staff, which are the two largest groups in the community general hospital, there are the hospital administrator and a number of administrative-supervisory personnel who head various departments of services (e.g., nursing, dietary, admissions, maintenance, pharmacy, medical records, housekeeping, laundry) and are in charge of the employees in these departments. There are also a number of medical technologists and technicians who work in the laboratory and X-ray departments of the hospital, as well as a number of miscellaneous clerical and secretarial personnel. And apart from all these staffs and professional-occupational groups, there is a board of trustees which has the overall formal responsibility for the organization, and which consists of a number of prominent people from the outside community. The trustees offer their services to the hospital without remuneration and are not employees of the organization. In short, professionalization and specialization are two of the hallmarks of the hospital.

High Interdependence of Services

Because of this extensive division of labor and accompanying specialization of work, practically every person working in the hospital depends upon some other person or persons for the performance of his own organizational role. Specialists and professionals can perform their functions only when a considerable array of supportive personnel and auxiliary services is put at their disposal at all times. Doctors, nurses, and others in the hospital do not, and cannot, function separately or independently of one another. Their work is mutually supplementary, interlocking, and interdependent. In turn, such a high interdependence requires that the various specialized functions and activities of the many departments, groups, and individual members of the organization be sufficiently coordinated, if the organization is to function effectively and attain its objectives. Consequently, the hospital has developed a rather intricate and elaborate system of internal coordination. Without coordination, concerted effort on the part of its different members and continuity in organizational operations could not be ensured.

It is also interesting and important to note here that, unlike industrial and other large-scale organizations, the hospital relies very heavily on the skills, motivations, and behaviors of its members for the attainment and maintenance of adequate coordination. The flow of work is too variable and irregular to permit coordination through mechanical standardization. And the product of the organization—patient care—is itself individualized rather than uniform or invariant. Because the work is neither mechanized nor uniform or standardized, and because it cannot be planned in advance with the automatic precision of an assembly line, the organization must depend a good deal upon its various members to make the day-to-day adjustments which the situation may demand, but which cannot possibly be completely detailed or prescribed by formal organizational rules and regulations. This is all the more essential, moreover, if one takes into account the fact that the patient, who is the center of all activity in the hospital, is a transient rather than a stable element in the system—in the short-stay hospital, he comes and goes very rapidly.

Hospitals: Authoritarian-Democratic?

Fundamentally, then, the hospital is a human rather than a machine system. And even though it may possess elaborate and impressive-looking equipment, or a great variety of physical and material facilities, it has no integrated mechanical-physical systems for the handling and processing of its work. The patient is not a chunk of raw material that passively goes through an ordered progression of machines and assembly-line operators. At every stage of his short stay in the hospital, he is mainly dependent upon his interaction with the people who are entrusted with his care, and upon the skills, actions, and interactions of these different people. All of these factors necessitate heavy reliance upon the members of the organization to coordinate their activities on a voluntary, informal, and expedient basis.

Paradoxical as it may seem, however, the hospital is also a highly formal, quasi-bureaucratic organization which, like all task-oriented organizations, relies a great deal upon formal policies, formal written rules and regulations, and formal authority for controlling much of the behavior and work relationships of its members. The emphasis on formal organizational mechanisms and procedures and on directive rather than "democratic" controls, along with a number of other factors, gives the hospital its much talked about "authoritarian" character, which manifests itself in relatively sharp patterns of superordination-subordination, in expectations of strict discipline and obedience, and in distinct status differences among organizational members.

Maintaining Authoritarianism

The authoritarian character of the hospital is partly the result of historical forces having their origins at a time when professionalization and specialization were at a primordial stage, and when nursing, medicine, and the hospital were all closely associated with the work of religious orders and military institutions. The absence of substantial professionalization and specialization characteristic of hospital personnel at those times, along with the emphasis of religious and military institutions on social arrangements in which the occupant of every position in the organization presumably knew "his place," and kept to his place by strictly adhering to specified rights, duties, and obligations, had much to do with the hospital's adopting a strict hierarchical and authoritarian system of work arrangements. But, the advent of professionalization and specialization, the gradual independence of hospitals from religious and military institutions, and the impact of an increasingly secular culture have greatly reduced the authoritarian character of the hospital. As Lentz has noted, within the last 50 years the hospital has undergone marked changes, dropping some of its authoritarian and paternalistic characteristics and taking on those of a bureaucratic, functionally rational organization.

Today's community general hospital, however, still has some of its traditional authoritarian characteristics along with its emphasis on rational organization. Moreover, it is unlikely that it will rid itself of all authoritarianism in the near future. There are several major counterforces at work, in this connection. First, there is the fact that the hospital constantly deals with critical matters of life and death—matters which place a heavy burden of both secular and moral responsibility on the organization and its members. When human life is at stake, there is little tolerance for error or negligence. And, if error and negligence can be prevented by adherence to strict formal rules and quasi-authoritarian discipline, such rules are important to have and obedience cannot very well be questioned (although blind obedience is mitigated because the hospital increasingly relies on the expertness, judgment, and ethics of professionals who, while abhorring regimentation, are presumably capable of a good deal of self-discipline). Second, there is the great concern of the hospital for maximum efficiency and predictability of performance. In the absence of mechanically regulated workflows, this concern virtually forces the organization to use many quasi-authoritarian means of control (including rigid rules and procedures, directive supervision, rigorous discipline, etc.), in the hope of: (1) attaining some uniformity in the behavior of its members, (2) regulating their interaction and checking deviance within known limits of accountability, and (3) appraising their performance. Third, there is the temptation to adhere to traditional, familiar ways of doing things which, coupled with the lack of apparently equivalent or superior alternatives that could be employed to ensure clarity of responsibility and efficiency and predictability of performance, also serves to perpetuate organizational reliance upon customary directive means of control.[1]

History of Regimented Behavior

In brief, while historical forces might account for the origins of the authoritarian characteristics of the hospital, it is not likely that some of these characteristics would continue to persist (especially within the context of a highly secular culture) unless they were more functional than not. And this clearly appears to be the case. In the first place, as in any organization designed to mobilize resources quickly in order to meet crises and emergencies successfully, a good deal of regimented behavior is required in the hospital. Lines of authority and responsibility have to be clearly drawn, basic acceptance of authority has to be assured, and discipline has to be maintained. In the second place, the hospital is expected to be able to provide adequate care to its patients at all times, with the precision of a machine system and with minimum error, even though it is a human rather than a machine system. It is expected to perform well continuously and to produce a machinelike response toward the patient, regardless of such things as turnover, absenteeism, and feelings of friendship or hostility among its personnel, or other organizational problems that it may be experiencing. It is also expected to be responsive to the health-related needs and demands of its community, and to meet a variety of medicolegal requirements. Because of these expectations, the hospital places high premium on being able to count upon and predict the outcome of the performances of its members. And predictability of performance can be partly attained through directive, quasi-authoritarian controls which, in the absence of apparently superior alternatives, are rather tempting to the organization.

---

[1]Incidentially, the apparent unavailability of equivalent or superior organizational alternatives is partly the result of our inadequate knowledge about how best to organize and manage human activity in a situation such as that of the community general hospital, and partly the result of the inability of hospitals to utilize the findings of modern research to best advantage.

Public Demands Efficiency

Coupled with this great concern for predictability of performance, moreover, there is an increasing concern that the hospital operate as efficiently and economically as possible. As the hospital has become a resource for all members of the community, and not just the indigent and the impoverished, the public has come to expect of it the best medical and nursing services that can be offered. These services, however, are quite costly, as are the facilities, equipment, supplies, and medicines that are required. And while the public may be willing (though not necessarily able to afford) to pay for these essential costs of hospital care, it also expects the best care possible at reasonable cost or even at least cost. At the same time, it is neither willing to tolerate nor prepared to pay any costs that may result from inefficient operations, poor administration, duplication of services, waste, negligence, and the like. It expects its hospitals to reduce to a minimum or eliminate altogether costs of this latter type and to operate with maximum economy. The hospitals themselves are quite aware of these and other pressures for efficiency, and have come to place very high emphasis on greater efficiency. Great emphasis on economic efficiency, however, is not entirely compatible with the hospital's traditional humanitarian orientation and objective of best service to the patient; the "best" service is not always or necessarily the most economical. Furthermore, this concern for efficiency is resulting both in progressive rationalization of hospital operations and in the institution of more rigid controls within the organization. Such controls, incidentally, serve to maintain the remaining authoritarian characteristics of the community general hospital.

Needed: Organizational Coordination

But, efficiency of operations and predictability of performance in the hospital could not possibly be attained only through directive and quasi-authoritarian controls. In fact, if carried to extremes, such controls would in the long run be inimical both to efficiency and to predictability. Efficiency and predictability of performance are also, and perhaps primarily, attained through a number of other factors, which are essential to effective organizational functioning. Probably the most prominent of these factors in the case of the community general hospital are organizational coordination and professionalization.

Because of the high degrees of specialization and functional interdependence found in the hospital, coordination of skills, tasks, and activities is indispensable to effective organizational performance and its predictability. The different specialized, but interacting and interdependent, parts of the organization must fit well together; they must not work at cross purposes or in their own separate directions. If the organization is to attain its objectives, its different parts and members must function according to each other's needs and expectations of the total organization. In short, they must be well coordinated. But, as we have already pointed out, the hospital is dependent very greatly upon the motivations and voluntary, informal adjustments of its members for the attainment and maintenance of good coordination. Formal organizational plans, rules, regulations, and controls may ensure some minimum coordination, but of themselves are incapable of producing adequate coordination, for only a fraction of all the coordinative activities required in this organization can be programed in advance.

The Subject of Professionalization

The other relevant factor that we wish to consider here, in addition to coordination, is that of professionalization — professionalization being one of the major distinctive features of the community general hospital. The majority of those who hold the principal therapeutic and nontherapeutic positions in the hospital are trained as professionals. The doctors, through their training, have been schooled in certain professional obligations, ethics, and standards of appropriate behavior, and have acquired a number of common attitudes, shared values, and mutual understandings about their work and work relations with others. The same is true about the registered nurses. Other groups in the organization are also on the road to professionalization: the administrators, the medical librarians, the medical technologists, the dietitians, and others in paramedical positions.

Complementary Expectations

This high degree of professionalization among those entrusted with the care of the patient has developed along lines of rational, functional specialization, and has had the effect of inculcating many complementary expectations and common norms and values in the members of the principal groups of the hospital — values, expectations, and norms that are essential to the integration of the organization. These include the norms of giving good care, devotion to duty, loyalty, selflessness and altruism, discipline, and hard work. This normative structure underpins the formal rational structure of the organization, and enables the hospital to attain a level of coordination and integration that could never be accomplished through administrative edict, through hierarchical directives, or through explicitly formulated and carefully specified organizational plans and impersonal rules, regulations, and procedures. However, increased professionalization and specialization have also had the effect of sharpening some of the status differences among the people working in the hospital — and sharp status distinctions bespeak of some authoritarianism.

Among other things, increased professionalization in the hospital has helped guarantee that certain minimum levels of competence and skill would exist in the organization, thus having a direct impact upon performance and organizational effectiveness. Similarly, professionalization and specialization have contributed to greater public confidence in the hospital, and to a wider acceptance of the hospital as a resource for the health needs of all people, for high professionalization and specialization imply expertness and knowledge. Increased professionalization has undoubtedly resulted in improved patient care and, in so doing, it has also raised the expectations of the public for both high-quality care and high efficiency in hospital operations. More and more of us go to the hospital for our various health needs nowadays but, because of improved service, we stay there for a shorter and shorter period of time. In the last 30 years, the average length of stay for adult patients in general hospitals has decreased by about a third, from 12.6 to 8.6 days — making it increasingly appropriate to refer to the community general hospital as the short-stay hospital.

No Single Line of Authority

Another of the distinctive characteristics of the community general hospital, closely related to professionalization and specialization, is the absence of a single line of authority in the organization. This feature has already been the subject of considerable discussion by Smith and others, but is important enough to warrant some brief observations here. Essentially, authority in the hospital is shared (not equally) by the board of trustees, the doctors, and the administrator — the three centers of power in the organization — and, to some extent, also by the director of nursing. In the hospital, authority does not emanate from a single source and does not flow along a single line of command as it does in most formal organizations.

A formal organizational chart of the hospital shows the board of trustees as having ultimate authority and overall responsibility for the institution. The board delegates the day-to-day management of the organization to the hospital administrator. In turn, the administrator delegates authority to the heads of the various nonmedical departments (including the director of nursing, who also wields a different kind of authority that originates in her professional expertness). The heads of these departments, in turn, have varying degrees of authority over the affairs of their respective departments and personnel. In the formal organizational chart, the medical staff, its officers, and its members are not shown as having any direct-line responsibility; they are outside of the lay-administrative line of authority. Yet, as is well known both within and outside the hospital, the doctors exercise substantial influence throughout the hospital structure at nearly all organizational levels, enjoy very high autonomy in their work, and have a good deal of professional authority over others in the organization. Over the nursing staff and over the patients, their professional authority is dominant. And although the board of trustees is in theory shown as the ultimate source of authority, the board actually has very limited *de facto* authority over the medical staff. Partly because the doctors are not employees of the hospital (they are "guests" who are granted practice privileges), partly because they enjoy high status and great prestige, partly because they have almost supreme authority in professional-medical matters, and partly for other reasons, they are subject to very little lay-organizational authority.

The Difficulties That Arise

Professionals in staff capacities in business corporations—lawyers, doctors, accountants, and others—have little or no authority to be involved in the activities of the line; they mainly serve as consultants and advisors. But this is not so in the case of the hospital. The absence of a single line of authority in the hospital, of course, creates various administrative and operational problems, as well as psychological problems having to do with the relative power and influence on organizational functioning on the part of doctors, trustees, administrators, and others. For one thing, it makes formal organizational coordination rather difficult. For another thing, it allows for instances in which it is not clear where authority, responsibility, and accountability reside. Similarly, it allows for a situation wherein a large number of organizational members, particularly members of the nursing staff, must be responsible to and take orders not only from their supervisors but also from the doctors. The lay authority and the professional authority to which nurses are subject, of course, are not always consistent. The absence of a single line of authority also makes for difficulties in communication, difficulties in the area of discipline, and difficulties in resolving problems that may be resolved through cooperative efforts on the part of both the lay-administrative and medical-professional sides. Frequently, the administrator, feeling that the responsibility for the overall management of the organization is his, and feeling that doctors through their power and pressures interfere in the discharge of his responsibilities, is motivated or actively attempts to circumvent the medical staff on various matters, and this, too, is apt to lead to problems. (The doctors, in turn, are likely to try to circumvent the administrator.) For the same reasons, the administrator is likely to be prone toward more and more bureaucratization in the hospital. And increased bureaucratization of organizational operations is likely to be fought and resented by the doctors, for it eventually means a reduction in their influence.

Delicate Balance of Power

In general, multiple lines of authority require the maintenance of a very delicate balance of power in the organization—a balance of power that is rather precarious. On the positive side, multiple lines of authority may serve as a system of "checks and balances," which may prevent other kinds of possible problems, such as organizational inflexibility and authoritarianism, or may serve to lighten the burden of responsibility in situations where responsibility may be too great for any single group or individual to shoulder. Regardless of the advantages and disadvantages of a system of multiple lines of authority, such a system is an integral part of the community general hospital. Not only is it an integral part, moreover, but also a part that is virtually inevitable for an organization such as this. This is because much of the work in the hospital is performed by influential professionals and not by low-status workers, and because of the high degrees of both professionalization and specialization characteristic of the organization. As Parsons has aptly observed, "The multiplication of technical fields, and their differentiation from each other. . .leads to an essential element of decentralization in the organizations which must employ them." For this reason, he goes on to explain that, unlike business and military organizations, "A university cannot be organized mainly on a 'line' principle. . . ." In this respect, the community general hospital is very similar to a university. (Hospitals and universities have a number of other interesting characteristics in common, but here we are interested only in hospitals.)

In summary, the community general hospital is an extremely complex social organization that differs from business and other large-scale organizations on a number of important characteristics. Among its main distinguishing characteristics, the following are worth reemphasizing:

Main Distinguishing Characteristics

1. The main objective of the organization is to render personalized service—care and treatment—to individual patients, rather than the manufacture of some uniform material object. And the economic value of the organization's products and objectives is secondary to their social and humanitarian value.

2. By comparison to industrial organizations, the hospital is much more directly dependent upon, and responsive to, its surrounding community, and its work is much more closely integrated with the needs and demands of its consumers and potential customers. To the hospital and its members, the patients' needs are always of supreme and paramount importance. Moreover, there is high agreement about the principal objective of the hospital among the members of the organization, and the personal needs and goals of the different members conflict little with the objectives of the organization.

3. The demands of much of the work at the hospital are of an emergency nature and nondeferrable. They place a heavy burden of both secular-functional and moral responsibility upon the organization and its members. Correspondingly, the organization shows great concern for clarity of responsibility and accountability among its different members, and very little tolerance for either ambiguity or error.

4. The nature and volume of work are variable and diverse, and subject to relatively little standardization. The hospital cannot lend itself to mass production techniques, to assembly-line operations, or to automated functioning. It is a human rather than a machine system, with all the attributes this entails. Both the raw materials and end products of the organization are human. And, being human, they participate actively in the production process, thus having a good deal of control over it.

5. The principal workers in the hospital—doctors and nurses—are professionals, and this entails various administrative and operational problems for the organization.

6. By comparison to industrial organizations, the hospital has relatively little control over its workload and over many of its key members. In particular, it has little direct control over the doctors and over the patients—two of its most essential components. In the short-stay hospital, the patients are not only a very heterogeneous and very transient group, but are also, mainly and ultimately, in the hands of their doctors, who are not employees of the organization.

7. The administrator has much less authority, power, and discretion than his managerial counterparts in industry because the hospital is not and cannot very well be organized on the basis of a single line of authority. The simultaneous presence of lay, professional, and mixed lay-professional lines of authority in the hospital creates a number of administrative and other problems, which business organizations are largely spared.

8. The hospital is a formal, quasi-bureaucratic, and quasi-authoritarian organization which, like most organizations of this kind, relies greatly on conventional hierarchical work arrangements and on rather rigid impersonal rules, regulations, and procedures. But, more importantly, it is a highly departmentalized, highly professionalized, and highly specialized organization that could not possibly function effectively without relying heavily for its internal coordination on the motivations, actions, self-discipline, and voluntary, informal adjustments of its many members. Coordination of efforts and activities in the hospital is indispensable to organizational functioning, because the work is of a highly interactional character—the activities of organizational members are highly interlocking and interdependent, and the various members can perform their role only by working in close association with each other.

9. The hospital shows a very great concern for efficiency and predictability of performance among its members and for overall organizational effectiveness.

10. Finally, the community general hospital is an organization which is important to us all, and which is becoming increasingly important. Several basic social trends tend to ensure this: the accelerating accumulation of new medical knowledge, new medical, surgical, and nursing procedures, and new drugs and medicines; rising levels of family income in the nation; increased use of the general hospital for numerous different diseases and health needs; and a growing demand by the general public for the best possible quality of medical-surgical and nursing care.

It has been the purpose of this section to introduce the reader to some of the key characteristics and organizational problems of the community general hospital. The characteristics and problems discussed above, along with many others to be dealt with throughout the book, show how complicated an organization the hospital is, and lead one to suspect that increased under-standing of such problems and characteristics might help ease some of the management difficulties and perhaps also improve the organizational effec-tiveness of our hospitals.

2

Strictures and Structures

Ray E. Brown

The late Ray E. Brown was Executive Vice President of the McGaw Medical Center of Northwestern University.

The governance of the American hospital has always been elusive, amorphous, and confusing. Bewildered students of management have been able to find no theories to fit the apparently headless enterprise and have dismissed the situation as an enigma in much the same manner as aerodynamics engineers have treated the notion of the bumblebee flying. Hospitals had to coordinate too many diverse parts and divergent interests to remain organizationally inexplicable, however, and so they invented their own explanation. Because hospitals weren't anxious to admit to the organizational anomaly of a headless enterprise—and even less anxious to face up to the confrontation of the interests at contest by establishing a clear-cut hierarchical structure—they retreated to the other end of the anatomical scale and created the concept of the multilegged organization. Thus was born the presently existing organizational model with no avowed head but three proclaimed legs—trustees, administrator, and medical staff. This organizational arrangement has served the same purpose as the Soviet troika by ensuring an uneasy standoff between the three principal contenders for organizational authority. But it provided capabilities more for legwork than headwork. It also was magnificently designed to ensure that the hospital could move in three different ways without going in any direction.

The awkward and fragmented governance arrangement of the hospital is an inheritance from its past. The hospital was originally conceived as an agency dedicated to doing good rather than well. It was little more than a home away from home for the sick poor. The physicians didn't need the hospital in the beginning and the hospital didn't need management. Money was almost the sole problem of the early hospital and it was not a serious one. The persons who put up the needed sums of money thereby solved the major problem. These persons were the trustees, and they sat alone in the gover-

Reprinted by permission from *Hospitals,* Vol. 44, No. 16, August 16, 1970. Copyright 1970, American Hospital Association.

nance saddle because they were responsible for the saddlebags. That arrangement was natural and appropriate and it still persists in many welfare agencies whose purpose is assistance rather than operations. Sitting on top was neither too difficult nor too threatening to others as long as hospital trustees were sitting largely on their own funds.

Some Changes Made

Scientific medicine changed the seat on which hospital trustees were sitting, however. Scientific medicine changed the nature and the traditions of hospitals and brought both the doctor and his private patients into the hospital. The hospital became the depository of the community's medical resources and, with that change, the hospital trustee began sitting on the doctor's professional and economic prerequisites. At the same time, the hospital trustee started sitting on the hospital patients' funds rather than his own. He also began sitting on top of a complex, expensive, and multipurpose operating enterprise. All this produced a need for management in large doses. It also spelled dependency for a very independent medical profession and it necessitated operational disengagement by deeply engaged hospital trustees.

The present model of fragmented, divergent, and indecisive governance of the hospital represents a stalemate between the aspirations, the fears, and the needs of the three principal participants in that governance. It is more a result of compromise than of organizational logic. In a real way it can be described as a product of organizational treaty rather than organizational treatise.

Not Too Damaging

The accommodation arrangement under which hospitals have been governed for the past half century was not too damaging to hospital effectiveness. In some ways it was highly effective. If one discounts the frustration experienced by the participants, and the occasional abortive upheaval that has occurred in a few hospitals, the individual hospital has fared well. Reviewing this apparent paradox, one sees several reasons for it. Foremost is the rapid growth in utilization and support that hospitals have experienced. It is hard to go wrong when everything is going right. Also, the momentum of growth helps an enterprise run away from its deficiencies and run over its problems. In another vein, the very rapidity of change along all environmental fronts has served to both lay the dust over hospital miscues and lay the path for them to follow. Perhaps most importantly, the expertness in brinkmanship developed by all three components of the hospital governance triad enabled the hospital to hold together and to maintain a course. Perceptivity regarding how far one can go in bucking the crew or the tide preserves sufficient order to keep things moving. In the case of the hospital, this has meant a large unity of effort, instead of large dissension, despite the diffusion of authority.

Changing Circumstances

The governance by sufferance that has characterized the hospital to date is now being challenged by changing circumstances and by other claimants to a piece of the governance. Running hospitals to suit the compromised notions of trustees, administrators, and doctors is being attacked on both organizational grounds and on public policy grounds. There is mounting concern and criticism from various groups and organizations that hospitals are not running well nor running in the right direction.

The concerns and criticisms reflect in part the changing circumstances in which hospitals find themselves. Inflation, medical advances, and increasing utilization have caused hospital costs to rise precipitously and have raised questions regarding the operating efficiency and quality of hospital management. Third-party payers are now picking up most of the tab for the hospital, meaning that hospital costs and hospital programs are concerns of the paying public—whether through private sector or governmental third parties. Social policy, now committed to adequate medical and hospital care for all members of the population, denotes governmental responsibility to redeem this commitment. At the same time, those to whom the commitment was made are asserting a right to help determine how the commitment will be met. So, the long-standing obscurity in the governance of the hospital is further clouded by the strong claims of third parties, government, and organized community groups to have an input in that governance.

It is not simply a question of adding the new claimants as legs to a three-legged entity. The present three legs have themselves become restive because of the criticism and the threats of the new claimants. Each entity is asking for a clearer definition of its role and a better structured mode of role expression. A multitude of court decisions and a host of private and governmental approval and regulatory agencies are making similar demands.

As hospitals become more expensive, involved, and committed, the need for restructuring of their governance becomes imperative. The demand for this will grow increasingly loud and incessant by all parties at interest. The organizational model that is developed must provide strength in both program determination and in operations. It also must afford a proper amount and mode of input into the governance process from each of the interest groups. Most of all, the governance must be designed to coalesce rather than to checkmate the diverse interests represented. The present governance arrangement provides an easy means for everyone to say "no" and very little means for the hospital to say "yes." The central position hospitals now have in the total medical care program of the community requires positive leadership on the part of the hospital. This does not mean that it is supposed to be easy prey for all claims made on its program or resources. It does mean that if it is to program effectively, and operate efficiently, it must have an effective governance arrangement for making up its mind and carrying out its decisions.

3

Revisiting "The Wobbly Three Legged Stool"

Richard L. Johnson

Richard L. Johnson, M.B.A., is President of Tribrook Group, Inc., Oakbrook, Illinois, and formerly Assistant Director of the American Hospital Association.

In "The Wobbly Three Legged Stool" published in *Trustee* in May 1976[1] the theme that the typical organizational structure of a hospital would not be adequate in the future because of the growing interrelationships among physicians, hospital executives and hospital trustees was developed. It was pointed out that regulatory agencies and the decisions coming out of the judicial system were continually increasing the hospital's accountability to the public and that under these circumstances what was needed was a single, unified organizational structure. Numerous examples illustrated that the coordinating function is now central to a well-balanced, soundly conceived hospital. While not specifically citing the model he had in mind the author was obviously exploring the advantages that seem to be found in what has become known in health care circles as the corporate organizational model employed by American industry.

During the last three years the author's thinking on this subject was being refined as he observed hospitals and mentally tried to fit them into the model. Gradually, an appreciation of both the similarities and dissimilarities of its use in the typical hospital was gained. The results led to the conclusion that the model can, at best, be only a loose fit. The following explains why.

Adopting the Corporate Model in the Hospital

Recognizing that the wobbly three legged stool was sadly in need of being mended, the suggested remedy has been the development of a unified organizational structure where the medical staff, governing board and ad-

Reprinted with permission of Aspen Publishers, Inc., from *Health Care Management Review*, 1979.

ministration act as part of the whole, and not as separate entities. This notion has been gaining acceptance in hospital administrative circles and has been increasingly known as the corporate structure. To those of us who have had this idea, it has become a meaningful step toward developing an organizational response to coping with external pressures that have been mounting at a faster rate than could be accommodated by the traditional organization of the hospital.

Since hospitals are complex management enterprises, it has been easy to suggest adopting the familiar corporate model in the operation of a hospital. It seems eminently clear that what has served American industry so well would obviously be suited to an industry that has increasingly become a major technological type of business. Toward this end, hospital administrators have become "presidents" and associate administrators have become "executive vice-presidents." Measured in terms of their responsibilities and complexities of assignments, hospital executives can readily be understood as being equivalent to senior executives, ergo, the titles should be the same. And if the chief executive becomes a "president," then the person leading the governing board should henceforth be named "chairman of the board."

To carry this logic one step further, those who manage major functional components such as nursing, medical affairs and finance are titled "vice-president" or, in the case of finance, "treasurer," with the controller reporting to the treasurer. To this level is now being added a "vice-president" or "director of marketing" as hospitals come to recognize that they are offering their services in a competitive marketplace.

In conjunction with these internal rearrangements, governing boards are being exhorted to more closely examine their meaning and contribution to the ongoing activities of the hospital. Their contributions are no longer being measured by their donations and gifts to the hospital, but rather by how much of what they do contributes to organizational effectiveness. It is the quality of the decisions they reach in determining the guiding policies that is the crucial ingredient of their contribution.

From the line of reasoning just unfolded, the conclusion should be reached that those hospitals that have gone furthest in developing the corporate structure will act and behave in a manner similar to their industrial counterparts. Boards of trustees of hospitals can be expected to handle matters in a fashion akin to a corporate board of directors, both spending approximately the same amount of time on the discharge of their responsibilities.

Yet if this be true, why do hospital trustees in this setting still act differently than do corporate directors? Is there something that has not been taken fully into account that makes governance in a hospital different than in industry? If so, what are these differences?

Hospital Versus Industry Governance

Accountability of Governance

As a starter, it might be useful to examine the legal and philosophical bases of hospital trustees and corporate directors. Industry is typically an economic enterprise with social overtones. The hospital, on the other hand, is a social enterprise with deepening economic overtones. This is recognized in the use of the term *trustee*. Trustees are individuals who are legally responsible for activities they do not own or have an economic interest in, but who are accountable to the public for the conduct of the affairs of the institution. This is different from a corporate director who has direct accountability to the shareholders and bondholders of the corporation.

The difference is profound and has ramifications that are felt throughout the organization and the way in which it operates. Corporate accountability to shareholders is measurable in terms of earnings per share and dividends paid. In addition, directors typically own anywhere from a few hundred shares to several hundred thousand shares of the corporation so they have a direct stake in seeing to it that the focus of the enterprise remains primarily financial. At the end of each year when the results are in, the shareholders, the investment analysts and the stock exchanges have a fair indication of how well they performed their duties as directors.

But when these same people sit down as hospital trustees, they do not behave in the same way as when they slide into their directors' chairs in the board room of the corporation. Is this because the nature of the beast is different, or is it because tradition has become so deeply ingrained that it affects individual board behavior? Perhaps it is both, to some degree. Where an industry has its historical roots in the donation of time to causes, as personified by religious groups who dedicate their lives, or in the donation of money for philanthropic reasons, the degree of accountability of governance changes.

Degree of Accountability

In the case of the for-profit corporation, if the year-end results have been financially better than had been anticipated, the board of directors recognizes senior management performance correspondingly by the amount of bonuses they approve. If, to the contrary, the results are subpar, bonuses are reduced and the operations are reviewed in an effort to determine if management failed or if what occurred was beyond their control. The customers who purchased the products of the corporation are presumed to be eminently satisfied if the profit and loss statement shows a large net profit on the bottom line.

But hospital trustees of nonprofit institutions find themselves in a different situation for a variety of reasons. As representatives of the community providing a public service, they use the year-end results of the profit and loss statement only to ascertain whether the hospital was in the red or black. If in the red, they become very concerned, unless the hospital has a tradition of losing money on its operating expenses and covering it with nonoperating revenues, such as from endowments or tax revenues. If in the black, they are interested in assuring themselves that the surplus from the year's operation is modest and will remain that way. As corporate directors, they would think the larger the black number, the more favorable the results, but not so in the hospital; it would be regarded by trustees as taking advantage of the public. In either case, a black figure or a red figure, the senior management would likely be largely unaffected by the financial results, unlike what would occur in the for-profit world. Thus, an executive in a nonprofit hospital treads a very thin financial line, not too much profit, nor too much red ink, but rather a bottom line that approximates a zero balance for the year's effort. Since there are no shareholders to be concerned about who are seeking to maximize the return on their investment, there is no direct pressure on management to provide a year-end surplus. In fact, trustees most often see their role as requiring them to protect the public which means they are as interested in the lowest possible surplus as are all other members of the community. They view their responsibilities from this perspective and give primary concern to it, so long as the hospital is not going broke.

Often, this does not square with the perception of trained administrators who see themselves as being as fiscally responsible as other corporate executives in the community. They may expect that this kind of ability should be highly regarded by their trustees. To the administrators it is a way of demonstrating fiscal competency in carrying out their complex managerial responsibilities. They buttress their thoughts by recalling prior experiences of their own or of other hospitals of which they are knowledgeable where the hospital had a staggering debt, was far behind on its accounts payable or could not get a certified audit, and the administrator or a professional colleague had taken over as chief executive and within a period of two to three years had brought the institution from a verge of bankruptcy to a solid financial condition. It then comes as a shock to find out a couple of years later when other kinds of problems have arisen that the governing board fails, in the administrator's opinion, to remember what conditions had been like and to appreciate the administrator's role in reestablishing fiscal solvency.

Administrators clearly see the interrelationship of fiscal matters to operating problems and are aware that if the wrong course of action is selected by the governing board in dealing with a current problem, the result could be a reversal in the financial state of affairs. They are unlikely to appreciate that the board is willing to take this risk believing that they would not let this situation recur and they therefore can deal with the current problem without being unduly concerned about its potential fiscal implications in the future. At the base of the trustee position is adherence to the concept of a hospital being a social enterprise with economic overtones, but these are only overtones and are regarded as such by them.

Differing Views of the Medical Staff

Because of both education and experience, hospital chief executives often view the medical staff in a different light than do trustees. They see the organized medical staff as part of the hospital operating structure. From long exposure they know they have to deal with this component with caution and great sensitivity, even though they may really see the staff as part of the management responsibility. Often they would like to deal with it in a manner akin to which they handle all of the other operating departments. While they recognize they have to treat them in a way that differs from other management people, they nevertheless may fail to understand why this is so, even though they appreciate that it must be so.

From their eyes, the governing board usually sees the medical staff as an anomaly not found in other forms of enterprise. They acknowledge that physicians have to meet certain standards for admission to the medical staff, but once having been met, they quickly come to see physicians as surrogate customers who must be treated in a manner reflecting this kind of relationship. Consequently, when physicians express displeasure with administrators, governing boards listen carefully and are inclined to be responsive. If physician dissatisfaction reaches the point where staff members adopt a collective position, such as requesting the board to terminate the chief executive, experience indicates that the board is more often than not going to accede to this position.

In such situations, there is little likelihood that fairness, weighing of administrative performance over time, or determining the validity of the medical staff's position is apt to occur. In many cases the board accepts the medical staff's recommendation without carefully and critically examining the issue. This occurs for several reasons, all intertwined in the thought process of trustees.

Trustees recognize a hospital as a medical care institution; as a community activity; as a place where minimum standards for professional performance are enforced; where physicians make free choice of whether or not to use the facilities; and where the operating departments headed by the administrator provide the support systems that permit these other activities to occur. They do not typically see the hospital chief executive as the person who leads and inspires the medical staff. In this sense, chief executives in a hospital are different than their counterparts in industry. In industry chief executives are clearly responsible and accountable for providing leadership and for pushing toward higher and higher goals and using corporate resources for attaining them. They are expected to be out in front, to challenge the organization to achieve increased performance. There are no boundary markers limiting their abilities, as long as they achieve the results in an economically sound manner. Growth in assets, net profits, units produced and share of market are applauded.

Not so in voluntary nonprofit hospitals. Even though chief executives in the hospital have all the attributes of their counterparts in industry, they are constrained in applying them in the hospital setting. They are heads of a support system, one that is expected to do its job efficiently and responsively to medical care interests. They are expected to see to it that the adopted professional standards are enforced; they are not expected or permitted to raise these standards, they can only encourage its being accomplished. They are not free to consult with the medical staff, receive their advice and then make their decisions; they must secure their approval before implementation.

Even though hospital executives are every bit as accomplished as their industry counterparts and as versatile in their managerial skills, the role they find themselves in prevents them from exercising these skills to the same degree. They cannot get out too far in front of the medical staff. If they acquire too much influence in the community, if they push to develop a multihospital system at a rapid rate, if they control the medical staff too directly, if they achieve too large a surplus on the bottom line, if, in other words they behave as aggressive, brilliant, hard-working executives, they run the strong risk of courting organizational disaster for themselves. If the medical staff feels threatened by the hospital executive's performance, this feeling often originates from their belief that the executive is in charge of the support activities of the hospital, not of the entire hospital itself, and that their role of dispensing medical care is the one to be protected. They will act on this belief when threatened.

Physician Independence

Physicians see themselves in two ways with regard to their professional activities. They accept, though sometimes grudgingly, that they are part of a larger system of medical care when using the hospital and are willing to participate in the medical staff activities, accepting the need to abide by the adopted professional standards of the institution. In their office practice they view themselves as individual entrepreneurs, solely responsible to themselves for the diagnosis and treatment of patients. They believe the same degree of skill should be applied in either setting. Thus, when seeing patients in the hospital they believe they should be left alone to do as they see fit, so long as their own personal standards of performance exceed those required by the institution. They view the hospital as providing resources on a demand basis that are needed by them for treating patients. They do not see the hospital as a control mechanism that decides for them their hours, work schedule, income or professional direction. Any steps taken by the hospital that physicians interpret as being even remotely control mechanisms are usually met with rather sharp reminders about physician independence. For example, physicians inform either board members or administrators that they are free to take their patients to other hospitals and may well do so if matters are not righted to their satisfaction. This kind of statement is often heard when trying situations develop in a hospital. Administrators often view such statements as a threat that is akin to blackmail, while physicians see them quite differently. To physicians the statements represent the exercise of a right they have maintained as customers—they can take their business elsewhere as a matter of personal freedom.

Disparity Between the Hospital's Societal Role and Physician Attitudes

The dilemma existing today is that the hospital is now a large, heavily capitalized technological enterprise operating in an increasingly complex social setting, but with attitudinal viewpoints on the part of both trustees and physicians that do not square with the dynamics and flexibility required for survival.

Increasingly, hospital chief executives are going to find themselves in the position of the messenger who brought tidings of bad news to the king and was rewarded for his efforts by being decapitated.

Physicians are apt to be a source of real difficulty in the next few years. By the very nature of their profession, they can be expected to be proponents of the status quo with respect to the role of the hospital. The fact that the health care system is under siege by the Department of Health and Human Services, reimbursement agencies, state rate review commissions and health systems agencies is not of immediate concern to most physicians unless it directly affects the services and equipment they use in their own clinical activities. Since many of them see the hospital as a support system for their own decision making, they may have difficulty understanding why housekeeping, maintenance, personnel, public relations, etc., cannot continue to receive fewer and fewer funds in order to protect the clinical services of the hospital, even when overall reimbursement is being restricted. Lacking organizational exposure to the need for balance among operational activities they may be prone to arrive at conclusions that experienced health care managers recognize as something less than desirable.

In addition, the frustration level of physicians increases with each passing year as they find their lives hemmed in, in ways over which they have little control. They are faced with higher rentals for office space, higher malpractice premiums, the necessity for providing fringe benefits for their office staff, more paper work on insurance forms, increased scrutiny of their fees, greater accountability for their clinical decisions in the hospital and a public who doubts their services are worth the prices charged; they increasingly feel the need for returning the compliment. Unable to counter the economic pressures and increased infringements on their own way of doing things, physicians may come to regard the hospital as the place where they will make their final stand to protect their professional rights. This means that the role of the physician in the hospital and the organizational relationship of the medical staff to the governing board and administration are sacrosanct and must remain in the future as they have in the past. Even though the government is forcing the hospital to become the control point of the health care delivery system, typical physicians, finding themselves increasingly threatened, determine not to let it happen in the hospital where they view their role as being of considerable economic importance, thus providing them with the leverage to protect their interests and attitudes.

Given the disparity between a changing societal role for the hospital and an inflexibility of physician attitudes, there is bound to be an increasing number of terminations of chief executives in hospitals in the next decade. This will not be ameliorated by going to the corporate structure with increased authority for this position. In terms of the external environment, this should occur if the hospital is to protect itself from increasing government control, but in terms of attitudes of physicians, the timing could not be worse. And since governing boards recognize physicians as surrogate customers, they will be careful not to adopt policies that alienate a sensitive medical staff.

Under the existing circumstances, prudent hospital chief executives should seek employment contracts from their governing boards. In the highly charged social environment that now surrounds the general community hospital, senior executives need to appreciate that they are going to be regarded with increased suspicion by the medical staff, and changes in organizational structure or policies that were easily accomplished a few years ago may become rallying issues for medical staffs out to protect their traditional turf. Fair play, honesty of intent, and desirability of proposed change are not sufficient reasons to protect chief executives in such a climate. What worked a few years ago as a way of accomplishing organizational change may not be relied upon in today's world. Logic, a sensing of the future, an approved long-range plan; none of these may be persuasive to a threatened medical profession. Yet, these represent the tools of management for coping with organizational problems. Given a period when the external factors dictate change and rapid decision making but where they must be made in an environment dominated by a desire to maintain the status quo, the chances of survival of chief executives may be questionable, even though they are competent and well trained. Under such circumstances, chief executives need greater protection than has been necessary in the past. A contract will not prevent the unrest, it merely recognizes that risks are now greater and it provides a measure of protection in this uncertain climate.

To push for a single unified structure with all major functions reporting through the chief executive is not likely to be greeted with enthusiasm by today's medical staff. Chester I. Barnard, writing in 1939 in the *Functions of an Executive*, put his finger on the reason why it cannot be easily accomplished. He pointed out that an executive's authority can be exercised only to the extent that those over whom he or she is exercising it accept his or her right to do so. Medical staffs usually deny that this right exists for administrators. In fact, in many hospitals they deny it exists even for another physician who may be in an administrative position, such as a full-time chief of staff or medical director. From the standpoint of organizational theory it seems like a good idea to have the medical staff activities led by a person who can be held accountable in the real sense of the concept. Yet, such may not be the case today. The requirement is now on leadership rather than authority, on sensitivity rather than control, and on persuasion as the preferred administrative skills. Even though a single, unified, top-level structure is certainly desirable, it seems to be unachievable for the majority of hospitals because of prevailing physician attitudes.

Revamping the Corporate Structure

Rather than striving to totally adopt the corporate structure, it now seems that some adaptations of it need to be made that recognize the uniqueness of the hospital. At the level of governance, it needs to be recognized that board members of hospitals have a degree of commitment that differs from that of outside directors of corporations. They willingly devote more time to board meetings, committee meetings, ceremonial functions, education sessions and trips on behalf of the institution. Involved trustees may invest from 500 to 1,000 hours while by contrast an outside corporate director may annually spend 50 to 100 hours.

The difference is not due to hospital management being weaker than industry management; rather it springs from the public accountability responsibility that makes a trustee different from a director. It is likely in the future that the corporate director will become more like the hospital trustee, rather than the other way around. Recently 68 leaders of business, labor, education, legal and accounting professions met at Harrison, New York, under the auspices of the American Assembly, an affiliate of Columbia University, to discuss how the private corporation should be governed. The 54th assembly stressed the need for nongovernment oversight of corporate activities, and self-regulation.

The group reached a number of significant conclusions about corporate governance, including:

1. Profit and social responsibility are compatible.

2. Corporations can and should improve their responsiveness to emerging social and ethical questions.

3. Boards have a primary role in interpreting society's expectations and standards for management and should not reflect the views and interests of a corporation management.

4. The majority of board members should come from outside corporate management, and those representatives doing a significant amount of business with the corporation should not count as independent directors.

5. There should be a separation of function between chairman of the board and the chief executive officer.

6. Corporations should hold open meetings with public groups to discuss social issues.

7. Public issue committees should be established.

8. Self-regulation of an industry should be encouraged, but to prevent self-serving it should be subject to consumer review to set standards, and to monitor compliance.

9. Corporate boards should recognize the value of a well-informed public.

Blending Interests

On balance, the American Assembly recommended that corporate governance should represent a careful compromise between those seeking to preserve corporate autonomy and efficiency, and public groups seeking to control or guide corporate power to constructive social ends. Corporate policy should be a blend between inside and outside interests, and while providing for greater public participation, it should not include worker representation as is found in European style corporations.

The goals that were outlined strike a responsive chord among hospitals. Industry is moving toward this end by becoming less restrictive. Hospitals need to move to the same ground but from the other direction of having been too liberal on the side of too much community interest. Both groups need to blend community interests with those of corporate goals. It is a delicate balance that is not easily achieved. For hospitals, the ability to cope with increasing government regulations dictates governing boards of a modest size cognizant that speedy decision making is a requirement in the evolving government-hospital relationship, but with an appreciation that community interests should not be shut out from having a voice in the development of policy.

Caution should be exercised in restructuring the governance of hospitals. To blindly adopt the corporate structure as it is today may well lead to undesirable results for hospitals. What is required is to pick and choose among those aspects of that model that will permit the hospital to carry on its role in society without compromising the public's interest in health care.

It is true, as pointed out in "The Wobbly Three Legged Stool," that patient care has come to dominate the hospital. It is also true that coordination of administration, medical staff and governance is a necessity. But the accomplishment of this coordination is not to be found in adopting the corporate model in its entirety. There is no neat and tidy organizational structure that will satisfactorily serve the interests of the three legs of the stool. Physicians can be expected to be increasingly demanding of the institution and when threatened will lash out to protect their turf as they see it. Governing boards will continue to listen carefully to physicians, and administrators will be subject to increasing demands as they attempt to bridge between diverse interests that subject them to heightened organizational pressures. As many experienced hospital executives view their roles, they are aptly describing their situation when they say that the fun has been taken out of their profession. They are caught in a pressure cooker where the heat keeps getting hotter and hotter.

Given such circumstances, the temptation has to be strong to avoid rocking the hospital boat by a chief executive. Or, the other alternative is to look to another industry where outstanding managerial talents will be recognized and appreciated. Many will consider this latter possibility, but when they do they will learn that the so-called transferability of management skill from one industry to another is really not a viable option. Each industry tends to be parochial about what kind of background is suitable for top-level responsibility. Very few hospital executives who become disillusioned about their own field are going to find positions in other industries; it just does not happen any more frequently than business executives entering the ranks of hospital administrator.

Involving Medical Staff in Revamping Organizational Structure

The revamping of the hospital organizational structure to the corporate model is not going to be accepted by physicians if it requires them to be accountable to the chief executive, even if through a medical director or chief of staff. The concept of a single, unified structure, given the prevailing attitudes of the medical profession, is a workable idea only as long as the decisions reached by the hospital do not trample over strongly held concerns of the more vocal members of the staff. In order to minimize this risk, policy development needs to involve appropriate physicians along the way from the first steps up to final approval by the governing board. The result may be no better and might not be as sound as if the administrative staff decided what to do, but once having determined policy, acceptance among the medical staff will be greater and the chance of successful implementation enhanced.

This is of particular importance for the near-term future until such time as physicians understand what additional constraints are to be placed on them and come to realize that they are not the doing of the hospital but are from external factors. Until that time internal tensions will increase, and as they grow the decision-making process dealing with shifts in programs, services and organizational structure will have to be slowed down to the speed with which medical staff acquiescence can be gained.

In those decision-making areas that are usually not of concern to physicians (such as compliance with civil rights, methods of financing long-term debt, real estate or zoning problems, retroactive Medicare adjustments and processing of certificates-of-need), rapid decision making can be accomplished if the governing board is properly sized and structured. To this extent the governing board can function like a corporate board without involving its membership in details of the operation.

The original thoughts of the "The Wobbly Three Legged Stool" still have merit. Some points may be underscored more heavily; others may be modified; but the original conclusion about the need for achieving coordination among all functions of the hospital still stands. The corporate model is a loose fit and represents a direction to go rather than a prototype to be used, as is, by a hospital.

Note

1. Johnson, R. L. "The Wobbly Three Legged Stool." *Trustee* (May 1976).

4

Integrated Systems: The Good, the Bad, the Ugly

John Knox Singleton and C. Michael French

John Knox Singleton is President of the Fairfax Hospital Association, Springfield, Virginia.

C. Michael French is Executive Vice President and Chief Operating Officer of the Fairfax Hospital Association, Springfield, Virginia.

Fairfax Hospital Association is a fully integrated multihospital system located in northern Virginia, across the Potomac River from Washington, DC. Our annual revenues are in excess of $300 million.

Today, just about everyone is involved developing integrated systems— from for-profits like HCA and Humana to not-for-profit groups like Fairfax. Even smaller hospitals are coming together for ventures involving DME, urgent care, and long-term care. The only exception is most state and local public hospitals.

Characteristics of an Integrated System

The future is in integrated healthcare systems. What are their distinctive characteristics, especially those illustrated by Fairfax?

- Multiple hospitals cover broad geographic market areas.

- Systems offer a spectrum of care—from intensive care, to self-care, to prevention.

- The physician serves as both a care-giver and a system director or manager. The physician is the system's quarterback.

- Services are organized to achieve two goals: effectiveness and efficiency.

Why Some Systems Fail

Despite their lofty goals, many of these systems fail. Why?

- Physicians are sometimes excluded from decision making.

- Systems may only cover a single community or geographic area.

- Organizations in the system lack common financial systems or inter-unit financial incentives. Until you can tie assets together, you won't have a fully integrated system.

- There is an absence of common management direction or governance.

There are both pros and cons for pursuing an integrated healthcare system, and healthcare executives need to examine both before they take their first steps.

Advantages

- Ability to sell a complete product line.

- Effectiveness through system management.

- Improved access to capital.

- Diversification of business risk.

The most attractive benefit for organizations has been the potential for lower costs through economies of scale, achieved through:

— research and development

— new product development

— shared management services: management engineering, reimbursement specialists, risk management, etc.

— shared support services: information systems, laundry, materials management, food service, etc.

— marketing and sales.

Also a plus: redirection of patients. Fairfax, for example, is currently developing eight urgent care centers to direct primary care patients to our four hospitals.

Problems and Pitfalls

But there are problems and pitfalls in integrated healthcare systems, and healthcare executives must be aware of them:

- Loss of control over individual product, service line, or marketing strategies.
- Communication requirements and costs.

Fairfax acquired a stand-alone hospital, and one of the most common complaints heard from the executive was, "All we do is go to meetings." This is a typical downside management response to integration.

- More complex and expensive management information systems.
- Slower management ability to act.

In a single hospital, healthcare executives can sometimes make decisions, but in an integrated system, the executive is no longer the final decisionmaker. Acting quickly is difficult particularly in ventures involving physicians or new businesses.

- Loss of management focus and emphasis on the local product.

In an integrated system, it's easy to stray from the basic business of hospitals.

- The loss of flexibility in pooled debt financing.

You may have to refinance debt based on the good of the whole rather than the good of the individual hospital.

- Responsibility for the operating losses of others.

Many integrated systems have significant tertiary facilities and several smaller, primary care hospitals. Large hospitals often complain they support corporate overhead and losses from other hospitals.

- Sharing development or support costs that don't benefit other operating units.

Part of the problem is the fundamental schizophrenia of integrated healthcare systems:

- Discipline and control vs. flexibility and speed.

We want the ability to have control over our hospitals, but in the process, we often slow down decision-making.

- Minimizing risk vs. bias for action and a sense of urgency.

Boards decide to enter a system to minimize their risks. But after joining, they can transfer the responsibility for their organization's most pressing problems to the new entity.

- Economies of scale vs. the cost of coordination.

Many services benefit from economies of scale: a shared laundry, collection agency, marketing. But in a system, the advantages don't appear across the board. After a thorough investigation, Fairfax realized that centralizing data processing was more effective because the costs of coordinating a decentralized system were greater than the economies of scale.

- Greater financial strength vs. financial flexibility.
- Matrix management and corporate support vs. accountability and responsibility for results.

Corporate support people, like the vice president of human resources, may go to individual hospitals to implement a wage and benefit program, but the administrator will still be held accountable.

- Physicians' desires for financial security vs. physicians' fear of control.

Doctors want to associate with winners and successful hospitals. But the more successful you become, the more frightened they become of you. To make physicians part of the solution, Fairfax has responded with a medical affairs council and also a large board of 30 members, with nine physicians.

Figures of Speech

Integrated systems often offer us confusing semantics. Fortunately, creative solutions exist.

- "We want to be part of a system, but the board doesn't want to surrender its authority." Fairfax recently acquired a small home health agency through a merger with a larger agency. To preserve autonomy, we placed one board member from the smaller agency on the larger agency's board. The solution was effective.

- "We're from the corporate office and here to solve your operations' problems." In reality, the corporate office doesn't solve operations' problems; only line operation's people do.

- "I'm making your committee responsible for that problem." Committees don't solve problems; people do.

In addition, many oxymorons characterize integrated systems:

- Well-informed, nonthreatened medical staffs.

- Nonparochial boards of trustees.

- Fast-acting, well-disciplined, multihospital systems. If your system is well-disciplined, you might not be acting fast enough.

Pitfall Avoidance

What can organizations do? How can they learn from the lessons of Fairfax?

- Don't assume that all functions are sensitive to economies of scale. Consider centralization only for those functions that offer substantial savings.

- Don't get into the business of centralizing operations like finance.

Fairfax is now in the process of decentralizing finance after discovering that coordination costs were far in excess of economies of scale.

Remember, you can't hold a healthcare executive accountable for account receivables if he lacks responsibility for that function. His perfect out will always be, "That's corporate responsibility; it's not my problem."

- Pinpoint responsibility for results on line management; not a staff person.

People at the corporate level, including vice presidents for marketing or human resources, are coordinators and consultants – not doers. They have no direct responsibility for implementing results.

- Don't lose sight of the cash cows; focus on the 20/80 rule of management effort. Remember, the basic business of hospitals is taking care of inpatients.

- Discipline is more important than flexibility.

Integrated systems have value and benefit only if parts of the system behave more advantageously together than they would apart.

- Put someone in control; make sure it's you. Stay in charge of an integrated healthcare system or it will slip away from you very quickly.

- Differentiate between different levels and types of risk.

Be sure that low risk ventures get pushed down in the organization. High risk ventures can cost you your job, so give them plenty of attention. At Fairfax, several physician joint ventures and alternative delivery systems are located in the corporate office. Only one person is responsible for each function. So, if a venture goes bad, one person—not a room of 20 managers—is approached for a remedy.

- Don't underestimate the inability of most hospital people to manage new, unregulated businesses.

There's little transference from hospital administrative talent to business line development. When Fairfax entered the urgent care market, we located an experienced urgent care manager to run the business, not a hospital administrator. Unfortunately, diversification efforts often fail because they are overmanaged or burdened with overhead.

- Don't try to manage human resources in small businesses like you do in large ones.

Fairfax grew from three to eight urgent care centers in six months, creating a payroll of 300 people. Make sure that the manager of the diversification can handle both growth and new and emerging personnel issues. Don't count on corporate human resources people to intervene in crisis situations.

- Small or developing operating units need more flexibility and decentralized authority than larger ones.

When you start a new business, give the operations person substantial latitude. Without the authority to respond quickly, they may never get that new business off the ground.

- Functional organizations are better at achieving efficiency and economies of scale. Product or market-driven organizations are better at improving effectiveness. Effectiveness (i.e., quality) is more important than efficiency (i.e., price).

Governance

The first article in this section is "Managing Change Through Values." In selection 5, John P. Brozovich discusses the importance of an organizational philosophy and describes the means by which a value system can be identified and established. In selection 6, "Have Boards Refocused Governance Functions?" Frederick H. Kerr describes and analyzes data about changes in hospital governing bodies.

Selection 7, written by Stanley Sloan, is entitled "Executive Performance." In it the author describes the role of governing body members in evaluating performance of the hospital's senior management and suggests some means by which it can be done. In selection 8, "Appraising Performance at the Top," Richard L. Johnson addresses the issue of evaluating performance of governing body members. The author makes it clear how difficult, but critical, this activity is.

5

Managing Change Through Values

John P. Brozovich

John P. Brozovich, FACHE, is Chief Executive Officer and President of Operations, Bon Secours Health System, Columbia, Maryland.

Today's healthcare executives have three options for managing change. They can adapt and allow the external environment to take control. They can cope, compromise, and meet the environment 50/50. Or they can adopt what Dr. Leland Kaiser has called the "design strategy."

Design is the healthiest and most productive of all three approaches to healthcare management. In embracing design, healthcare executives are saying, "I will decide what's important to me. I will determine what my values are, and then I will act on my environment. I will create a culture and climate in which people will respond positively to what I do."

Fundamental to the design strategy is the concept of values. Healthcare organizations have always practiced and promoted values—from competence and compassion to innovation and cost-consciousness. Such values—whether practiced by organizations or individuals—are enduring beliefs on which people act by preference. In addition, values translate into conduct. By observing how employees behave, healthcare executives can usually identify values. Of course, the reverse it also true. Employees make judgments about executive values by observing hundreds of actions and gestures.

A Values Culture

The introduction of a values culture into Appleton Medical Center, Appleton, WI, during 1980 and 1984 was based on a review of the Disney organization. "How could 34,000 employees be so consistently positive and friendly?" we asked. We discovered two basic answers: The Disney organization possessed clear values and guidelines, and it selected employees who met expectations and fulfilled organizational values.

But how could we integrate the lessons of Disney into a two-hospital Wisconsin town? The objective was to bring together *everyone* in the Appleton organization. The strategy was Leland Kaiser's ecosystem design model.

Values generation is a consensual process in which members decide—as a group—the values they will choose on which to build the organization's future. Values are then translated into goals. Goals are translated into programs. Programs are coordinated with patient and staff concerns. Finally, evaluation takes place, providing feedback for another annual cycle of the process.

The values articulation process involves asking a series of questions:

- Is the value clearly defined?
- Is there a clear strategic target?
- Is there a policy statement that reflects the value?
- Is there a detailed action plan?
- Is there a budget for this value-based program?
- Is there a measurable result?

Implementing the Process

Over a period of six months, the Appleton organization crystallized seven basic values:

1. To be compassionate (cultivate a caring atmosphere).
2. To give quality service (strive to maintain competence).
3. To be fair (maintain fairness in all transactions).
4. To practice integrity (be a promise-keeping institution).
5. To encourage personal growth.
6. To encourage creativity within the organization.
7. To be financially responsible (promote organizational efficiency).

To explain these values to individual employees, management held a values-day seminar and developed a special poster. For each value, we developed a positive statement: "We're fair." "We care." "We're competent." "We're growing." "We're honest." "We're efficient." "We're innovative."

The first values-poster subject was a 20-year nurse employee in the outpatient department who was noted for her compassionate behavior. She was a role model for others. In the vocabulary of corporate cultures, she was a hero. And what do you do with heroes? You celebrate them, letting people know that heroes are important, essential, and appreciated in the organization.

Employees like her appeared on photographic murals in the cafeteria. The values poster was placed in every department of the hospital. But, we realized that simply hanging a poster wasn't enough. We met with the employees on every shift to talk about Appleton's values. "This is what we as a leadership group hold sacred, but we want your input. If there are values that aren't there but should be, let us know," we said.

Mainstreaming

From 1980 to 1982, everyone at Appleton came to know these values. Values permeated every discussion and staff meeting. They became the terms in which we discussed programs, services, products, and people. When a manager submitted a proposal for approval, it was tested against organizational values. "Will this project bring out the compassionate value? Will it promote technical competency? Will it be innovative enough for this highly competitive environment?" We "mainstreamed" our values into the decision making process.

One of the strongest tributes to the values process came from a manager who said to me, "I had to make a decision the other day, so I put all seven values up there and tried to think of what you would do."

A first-line manager was beginning to think how executive management made its decisions. The benefit was clear: We had solidarity in decision making and organizational cohesiveness, and both emanated from a shared-value structure.

There are other rewards that come from the integration of a values process. Once an organization articulates its values, it drives out employees who don't really fit. The consistent use of values also affects upfront human resources decisions, including the employee selection process. At Appleton, we learned several lessons from Disney:

- Find out peoples' values *before* they come into the organization.

- Strive for a "values match" or a "cultural fit."

- Realize that if employees don't share similar values, they are unhappy and less productive.

- Identify people who will "resonate" with the organization. The result will be reduced time for monitoring and supervision, and more time for innovation and creativity.

Recognition

On the executive level, a design team met regularly to discuss organizational innovations. Gradually the values process became the driving force of the MBO tradition. At monthly meetings of the total management group, we reviewed objectives and recognized people who were responsible for their success.

At Employee of the Month ceremonies, we celebrated employees selected for excellence based on the values. In housekeeping, an employee was selected because with her handmade gifts and special surprises she embodied the value of compassion. In plant operations, a ten-year employee met all the requirements to practice his trade and was celebrated as a testament to the organizational value of personal growth and development. Throughout the organization, the spotlight was clearly on individuals.

But the process didn't always involve celebration. We also emphasized value opposites such as not sanctioning incompetence. If employees faltered, they were given several opportunities to improve. But when it came time for a decision, the organization chose to articulate the value of fairness and remove incompetent employees.

All of Appleton's work in values relates to designing a positive organizational culture of which healthcare executives are the lead architects. Management style is the driving force behind the culture. Healthcare executives must choose their leadership attitude and posture. But what are their options?

They can choose one of the following three notions: "I am the force." "I am the force, but I'll give you a little part of it." Or, "You are the force. You have the power. You can get things done in this organization. You don't need me unless you hit a roadblock."

We chose and promoted the third style. We gave our employees the power to create and modify their work environment and, in the process, transform the organization.

The Values Future

Executive management values will shape the healthcare system, whether we want them to or not. Prior to the prospective payment era, our values included quality service, a compassionate manner, fairness, integrity, assurance of appropriate staff training, and economic abundance.

Why? In the past, healthcare was favored by the government through third-party reimbursement. Healthcare executives identified what they *thought* patients wanted, and then they delivered it. But contrary to our illusion of being open at all times to very comer, we rarely did market research to find out our customers' real needs.

Today, healthcare executives must cope with different, more troubling realities. We will still provide quality service — and we hope it will be compassionate. We will continue to be fair with our employees, our community, governing board, and physicians. We will keep our promises and provide for staff growth. We will sustain economic abundance.

What may change is our cluster of market values. Instead of concern over third-party payment, we must ensure customers a competitive price. We must move from conservative, low-risk postures and position ourselves as aggressive risk takers. Instead of continuing to be provider driven, we must be consumer driven, looking to market research for an accurate reading of client needs.

No matter what values emerge for healthcare organizations in the 1990s, healthcare executives will have a pivotal role to play—engineering the values articulation process and ensuring that it permeates the entire organization, functioning as the force behind organizational change and innovation.

6

Have Boards Refocused Governance Functions?

Frederick H. Kerr

Frederick H. Kerr is President of St. Luke's Hospital, Maumee, Ohio.

Today, hospital trusteeship is shifting from an "association" to an "enterprise" model of governance—that is, from being purely an honor in exchange for support of the institution to the type of responsibility associated with corporate directorship. Like businesses, if hospitals are to effectively cope with competition, they must make timely policy level decisions. If the governing body is so large that the executive committee becomes the de facto board, frustration tends to replace confidence and decision-making is impeded.

Board Size and the Enterprise Model

If the best interests of the corporation are to be served, there must be a high level of communication, trust, and confidence between board members, the board and the medical staff, and the board and management. These positive attitudes are best achieved when the board is small enough to focus its policy and oversight roles.

Although historical comparisons are not available, data from a 1985 survey of chief executive officers of Ohio hospitals suggest that hospitals may be moving to the smaller board size we advocated in 1983. Eighty-one percent of the hospitals surveyed have boards of 20 members or less, only 4 percent have more than 30 members, and the median board size is 15 members. Based on the day-to-day experiences of chief executives, hospitals should have between 7 and 17 board members. Because the average size board in the survey is 15, it appears that most hospitals today are right on target (see Fig. 6-1).

The CEO respondents also were asked what changes they would make in board size if they owned the hospital. Only 8 percent indicate that they would

Reprinted by permission from *Trustee*, Vol. 38, No. 11, November 1985, pp. 17-20. Copyright 1985, American Hospital Publishing, Inc.

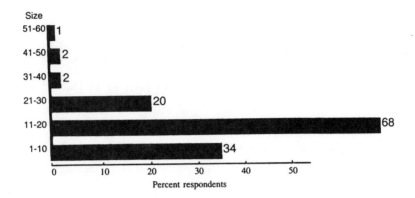

Figure 6-1. Board Size.

opt for more members while 40 percent desire fewer members. In the case of those CEOs in favor of more board members, the median board size is seven. Among the CEOs who are in favor of fewer board members, the median board size is 17.

Board Committee Structures

One might expect a hospital that has moved to more businesslike approaches to use fewer committees and to select subject matter that has a governance and policy focus. The typical board, according to the survey, has five committees: finance (80 percent of respondents), executive (70 percent), planning (61 percent), human resources or personnel (45 percent), and joint conference (43 percent).

A strong nominating committee, especially when it becomes an agent for evaluating the performance of the board and its members, can strengthen any board. However, the survey revealed that only 28 percent of the boards have any kind of nominating committee. Likewise, only 9 percent of the reporting hospitals use an audit committee—something many authorities consider essential to protect the objectivity of governance. Moreover, only 7 percent of the surveyed boards have an ethics or values committee—a finding that flies in the face of the fact that some of the most important policy questions in any hospital concern ethical decisions and the relation of patient care policies to the values of the sponsoring entity. It is also interesting to note that the joint conference committee has, in a minority of cases, become a method for liaison between the board and the medical staff. This suggests that the CEO is playing a stronger role in this important aspect of hospital affairs.

The data also show that the number of committees is related to board size: the fewer the board members, the fewer the number of committees. Yet, the survey shows that the functions of board committees tend to remain traditional in nature rather than keeping pace with the board role in a complex, competitive enterprise. As a result, boards may find the assistance of outside expertise very helpful in obtaining the fullest possible value from its committee structure.

Hospital CEOs' Roles and Authority

It was noted in the earlier article that many hospitals believed they were moving to a corporate type of structure simply by changing the title of the chief executive from administrator to president. Titles help to communicate the substance of a role and they are important in organizations such as hospitals where function is not obvious and is often contested. Correctly understood, the CEO position serves as the agent of the board; the member to whom authority is delegated to organize its information, carry out its policies, and to lead the development and operation of the corporation. When governance is refocused along enterprise lines, trustees grant full authority to the CEO, because the board can only be as effective as its primary agent. The survey attempted to assess the extent of that understanding by asking about CEO titles, degree of authority, and level of participation with the board.

At least in Ohio, *president* has become the most commonly used CEO title and the title, *administrator*, is now used in less than one-third of responding hospitals (see Fig. 6-2). That change can significantly help internal and external publics to understand the role of hospital CEOs. Moreover, some hospitals are beginning to use the CEO title most commonly used in industry: *chairman of the board*. This change suggests that some CEOs are overtly moving into positions of board leadership, which is consistent with the strategic and external role of the CEO in larger hospitals where operational responsibilities are frequently delegated to a chief operating officer.

When respondents were asked if the corporate bylaws designate their position as that of chief executive, 90 percent of the responses were affirmative. In addition, 2 percent held the title, *president*, which, under applicable Ohio law, is defined as the CEO. Because Ohio corporations must have a president, it is safe to conclude that in 8 percent of the surveyed hospitals there is a discrepancy between corporate documents and practice in the important area of executive authority.

Several questions on the survey dealt with limitations on CEO authority—that is, what actions require board approval? Three-fourths of the CEOs state that they can appoint vice-presidents without board approval, but 35 percent state that board approval is required for key executive salaries. In the case of business contracts, 36 percent of the respondents report that board approval is required, but only 14 percent state that there is a dollar limit (most frequently, $10,000) on their authority to obligate the organization

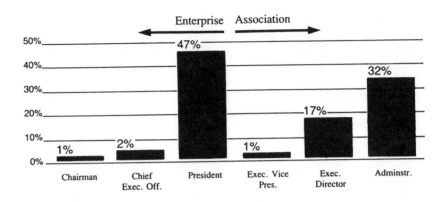

Figure 6-2. CEO Titles.

for expense items. Respondents indicate that boards more frequently authorize the CEO to obligate up to approved budget levels or rely on the judgment of the CEO to bring unusual items to it for approval. On the other hand, there are dollar limitations (most frequently, $5,000) on the authority of CEOs to obligate for capital investments in 74 percent of hospitals. Perhaps custom or history explains why such tight limits are commonly placed on hospital CEOs in the case of capital spending, while very broad authority is commonly granted for expense in general. When board approval is required for appointing key managers and for determining individual salaries (as opposed to salary ranges or incentive plan structures), the CEO's freedom of action can be more severely limited than boards realize.

As defined above, the concept of the CEO is that of a *trustee in residence*, and it demands that the CEO be a part of the board. It suggests that the CEO should have voting privileges on both the board and its committees (with the possible exception of the audit committee). However, our survey found that only 40 percent of the CEOs are voting members of the board and its committees. Another 29 percent have seats on the board, but no voting privileges.

The CEO, Board, and Medical Staff

Medical staffs expect direct access to the board and its various members, as well as seats on the board for selected physicians. Many thoughtful boards have encouraged such communication and participation while insisting that the CEO needs to be the key link between the two groups for purposes of continuity and coordination. When a vice-president for medical affairs is added to the management team, that physician can perform most of the coordination work for the CEO. From an executive standpoint, the ideal arrangement is to have medical staff participation at the board level and management participation on the various committees of the medical staff. The Joint Commission on Accreditation of Hospitals (JCAH) requires some input from various employed professionals in certain staff functions, but the key medical staff decisions for the CEO take place at the medical staff executive level and in the credentials committee. Attendance is one thing, but few medical staffs have welcomed full CEO participation. The survey found that while most CEOs are members of key medical staff committees, few have voting privileges (see Fig. 6-3). In 1 percent of the hospitals the CEO does not attend meetings of the executive committee, and 17 percent of the CEOs do not participate in meetings of the credentials committee.

A Potential Trap: Elected Officers

During recent years, the courts have clarified that both the governing board and individual trustees have accountabilities that are sometimes enforced through tort laws. The enterprise model of governance offers the advantage of placing corporate obligations in the hands of those who actually do the work and who understand the details of that obligation. Many hospitals have overlooked the advantages of this arrangement, particularly in respect to the offices of secretary and treasurer of the board.

These offices are associated with specific accountabilities regarding corporate records and assets. The outside board member who is elected to hold such an office, but lets an employee do the actual work, may assume unknown

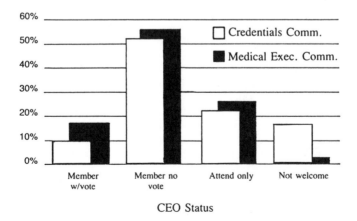

Figure 6-3. CEO Participation on Medical Staff Committee.

obligations that far overshadow the honor the title bestows. Such a contradiction also limits the legal authority of the management personnel performing the duties, thereby putting their acts in question. Therefore, the holding of office must be tied to the performance of the function.

We asked about these offices in the survey and identified a significant problem. In the case of 83 percent of the responding hospitals, a board member is elected to serve as secretary, but only 17 percent of them actually take notes and write the minutes. Similarly, in the 9 percent of hospitals where the CEO or another administrative employee holds the title, it is still the secretary to the CEO who does the actual work. In the 7 percent of hospitals where the general counsel or the secretary to the CEO hold the office of corporate secretary, those individuals almost always do their own work.

Obviously, the potential for liability is even greater when the individual accountable for the custody of funds is not performing treasury functions. The chief financial officer (CFO) is the logical choice for this position or, in a larger hospital, one of the CFO's subordinates. Yet, in 74 percent of the reporting hospitals, a board member is elected to serve as treasurer. Only 18 percent of respondents report that the CFO is the treasurer and 7 percent of hospitals state that the office is held by someone else or that it is not a hospital function. In view of the potential for avoiding problems, these data suggest that established practices relating to elected offices need to receive renewed attention.

How CEOs Rate their Boards

When chief executives were asked to rate board members' ability to function as informed policymakers for the hospital, the responses were encouraging. Twenty-five percent of the CEOs state that their board's performance is excellent, 56 percent indicate that it is good, 18 percent state that it is poor, and less than 1 percent state that it is unacceptable.

However, the survey also shows that a significant number of CEOs (28 percent) would make substantial changes in board membership if they owned the hospital. That response suggests that CEOs believe a number of boards could be improved through membership changes even though the boards are doing a good or excellent job.

One of the CEOs' primary concerns about the board is whether its members understand the appropriate role and function of the chief executive, for that determines how effective management can be. In the survey, 76 percent of the CEOs indicate that their boards understand that role, while 24 percent either do not or are undecided. One can speculate that the move to the enterprise model has raised CEOs' expectations about their own role to a higher level than that demanded by boards.

These data also suggest that there could be better communication between many boards and chief executives concerning roles, expectations, and the documents (i.e., state regulations, bylaws, and JCAH standards) that concern governing boards and management. The fact that CEOs believe that physicians tend to lag behind in their understanding of the executive role (31 percent) is not surprising. That fact probably leads to more stress for CEOs and more crisis situations in hospitals today than any other factor. If the board and management are not communicating well, there is little hope of bringing physicians to a common level of understanding. Survey results suggest that most hospitals have achieved such communication, but because the issue is of such central importance, the 25 percent of respondents who do *not* represent a major problem.

Conclusions

Hospital boards are moving toward the enterprise model and away from traditional arrangements that were based on association thinking. That change seems to be leading to smaller boards and fewer committees. It also is producing a new type of chief executive who has a role and authority that more closely resembles that of the business CEO than was true in the past.

At the same time, data reported here suggest that certain modifications to be expected from such a change have not occurred. For instance, board committees have remained traditional in function; CEO authority still lags behind the level typically found in most business corporations, particularly in terms of key appointments and capital investment; and hospitals are still following traditional patterns for designating corporate officers, such as the treasurer and secretary. Moreover, CEOs believe that boards are performing well, but that many could be improved.

7

Executive Performance

Stanley Sloan

Stanley Sloan, Ph.D., is Senior Principal of Hay Management Consultants, Atlanta.

One of the most sensitive and difficult tasks confronting today's health care trustee is evaluating the performance of the organization's top management. Most trustees recognize that making global, subjective judgments is woefully inadequate and ill-advised. Indeed, many CEOs as well as trustees have serious questions and reservations about the effectiveness with which top management performance is evaluated and linked to compensation decisions. If the board wants to obtain an adequate return on investment in executive compensation, the following questions and reservations must be addressed.

Who should evaluate the performance of the CEO?
Using the entire board for this purpose is often as unsatisfactory as using only one trustee. Consequently, an increasing number of boards are using the compensation committee or personnel committee to evaluate the CEO's performance. In cases where those committees do not exist, members of the executive committee sometimes fill this role.

What preparations should be required of the committee?
Before any action is taken, committee members need to agree on the criteria for performance evaluation and the respective roles of the committee and the full board. The board chairman often serves as the committee chairman. The committee frequently presents its conclusions, along with a salary recommendation, to either the executive committee or the full board.

Should the committee evaluate the performance of other top executives reporting to the CEO?
The overall institution's performance certainly reflects the executive team's results, but the CEO is in a better position than the board to appraise the performance of subordinates. Moreover, boards that evaluate the entire

Reprinted by permission from *Trustee*, Vol. 38, No. 11, November 1985, pp. 12, 14, and 15. Copyright 1985, American Hospital Publishing, Inc.

executive staff tend to dilute the authority and accountability of the CEO. Therefore, the CEO should evaluate reporting executives and determine or recommend salary increases for them.

How formal should the process be?
The process should be structured to provide a clear, systematic basis to consistently evaluate performance each year. On the other hand, if the process is overly formal and detailed, its administrative requirements may interfere with desired dialogue and feedback between the board and the CEO. Also, dislike of the paperwork may outweigh perceived benefits.

At the very least, the compensation committee and the CEO should agree on areas of accountability, the relative priority of those areas, and specific ways performance will be measured in each of them, including performance standards. In the final analysis, the process must be one that the board and the CEO feel comfortable with.

How often should reviews occur?
The board should formally review CEO performance at least annually. In addition, the compensation committee and the CEO should meet informally on a quarterly basis to enable the CEO to get feedback and to take corrective action in a timely manner. These discussions should be a natural adjunct to the quarterly financial review.

How should executive performance be measured?
There is wide diversity in the approaches used to measure executive performance. A specific format that is suitable to one organization may be inappropriate for another. However, most successful executive performance management systems require a consensus between a board-designated committee and the CEO on the following items:

- Specific accountabilities. Frequently, specific CEO accountabilities or key results are required in operational management, financial management, personnel management, public relations, patient care, special projects (anticipated and unanticipated), and planning.

- Relative priorities. Priorities frequently are assigned in the form of word designations (e.g., primary vs. secondary results) or percentage weightings for each area of accountability.

- Performance measures. It is critical that the committee and the CEO agree on the specific indexes to be used for measuring performance for each area of accountability. The choice of measures also must reflect consideration for the type and complexity of the organization and its business strategy and structure. For example, many health care organizations are either reorganizing or being acquired by holding companies that may consist of special for-profit units, key not-for-profit hospital units, and special not-for-profit adjuncts. In such cases, it is important to distinguish between corporate, unit, department, and individual position measures.

Some illustrative corporate indexes include operating ratios, cost containment, program development, staff development, organizational development, cash flow management, patient satisfaction, community/social responsibility, and the generation of capital funds.

At the operating unit level, some of the same measures can be used in a modified form. Moreover, other measures are also useful, such as actual vs. budgeted results per unit and productivity (e.g., occupancy, average length of stay, revenue per patient day, expense per discharge, FTEs per adjusted discharge, accreditation, and staff qualifications). Corporate and unit measures form a frame of reference for developing indexes for specific departments and individuals.

How should performance standards be developed?

The CEO should reach a consensus with board members on the differences between various levels of planned performance relative to agreed-upon measures. For example, one CEO of a major corporate health care holding company identified several measures within the area of operational management. One of those measures was financial budget compliance. This CEO currently is using a percentage variance (plus or minus 5 percent) from the fiscal year expense budget, adjusted for activity level, as the fully proficient performance standard. He is also measuring corporate resources utilization with a similar performance standard variance from the corporate net income goal, adjusted for utilization.

For some accountability areas, qualitative standards may be even more meaningful than quantitative ones. For example, one CEO measures the degree to which the corporation complies with relevant laws by establishing this standard: no significant violation cited by external agencies.

Sometimes, an indirect, qualitative patient care standard is used, such as "full JCAH accreditation or other appropriate certification of facilities 100 percent of the time; results of all major inspections reported to the board within 30 days of JCAH report, and timely reports to board on the correction of deficiencies."

Performance standards should be meaningful for an executive's particular position and the position's potential effect on the organization. The standards also should be realistic and yet challenging, useful as a practical guide to the desired type and level of results, and designed with due consideration for internal resources and constraints, as well as external factors.

What should the committee measure and document?

It is usually sufficient to specify about six to eight key accountability areas with one or two measures of performance for each area, including related standards for measuring results. A plan and the necessary resources for fulfilling it should support each performance standard.

Why should there be a relationship between the organization's business planning process and the executive evaluation process?

For the best results, the executive performance planning, measurement, and evaluation process should be directly linked to the organization's business strategy. Executive performance planning enables the board and the CEO to forecast and monitor results in ways that proactively make the right things happen, rather than passively reflecting on a CEO's accomplishments or failures.

The CEO can use the process as a team building tool in support of the strategic business plan. The dialogue generated helps executives identify issues, questions, and problems that need to be addressed to achieve the institution's objectives. Properly conducted executive group sessions can be invaluable for developing commitments between executives to achieve those objectives. Team building should become an integral part of the overall process to ensure that individual executives do not emphasize achieving their own results to the detriment of other executives or organizational units.

Bibliography

Sloan, S. "Executive Compensation," *Trustee* 39:2, Feb. 1985.

Berger, L. "New Initiatives for the Compensation Committee," *Directors and Boards*, Winter 1985, Special Supplement: Compensation Committees.

Umbdenstock, R. and Hageman, W. *Hospital Corporate Leadership: The Board and Chief Executive Officer Relationship*. Chicago: American Hospital Publishing, Inc., 1984.

Witt Associates Inc. *Executive Compensation Committee*. Free booklet available from Communication Services, Witt Associates Inc., 724 Enterprise Dr., Oak Brook, IL 60521.

Hay Management Consultants. "Managing the Enterprise—Accountabilities of the CEO." *Management Memo*. No. 305, 1977.

Hay Management Consultants. "Rousseau Revisited—Agreement for Performance." *Management Memo*. No. 286, 1975.

8

Appraising Performance
at the Top

Richard L. Johnson

Richard L. Johnson, M.B.A., is President of the Tribrook Group, Inc., Oakbrook, Illinois.

Thanks to the shift from a limited to a pervasive form of government, desirous of rigidly limiting the health field, there is bound to be increasing interest by the Pied Piper of Washington in performance criteria, consequences and controls. Like it or not, performance appraisal takes on new meanings in such an environment. Walter Lippmann defined it as "the sickness of an over-governed society." Nevertheless, it is a reality with a new twist.

Heretofore, performance appraisal meant a system of formal or informal ways of judging managerial performance — the employee was judged by a supervisor, who in turn was judged by the department director, who was judged by the administrator, who was judged by the governing board, who was judged by no one. The board itself is now being judged by this over-governed society through a plethora of measuring mechanisms.

Not only government but also the Joint Commission on Accreditation of Hospitals (JCAH) has developed an interest in the governing authority, its composition and the kinds of information it regularly receives.[1] The courts have increased their interest and are holding governing boards accountable for everything that goes on in the hospital.

Meanwhile, DHHS has its Medicare auditors, OSHA has its interests in physical safety standards, and the environmentalists have their share of clout. At the state level there is a growing number of review boards and the regional health services agencies who are mandated to determine the future of hospitals. All are looking at the hospital through their own set of interests, invoking their own criteria, controls and consequences to see if institutional performance measures up. Under such circumstances, traditional performance appraisal systems stop short of what is now needed.

Reprinted by permission from *Hospital & Health Services Administration,* Fall 1978, pages 36-47. Copyright 1978 by the Foundation of the American College of Healthcare Executives. All rights reserved.

The Need for CEO Board Appraisal

At the top, performance appraisal is needed as well as the traditional managerial review that has become part of a progressive organization. Measuring the performance of the chief executive and the governing board is a different process but should be made standard operating procedure for hospitals. Not to do so is to court unexpected public disclosure and possible embarrassment as a result of one of the outside agencies' interests in the hospital. Governing board members of hospitals that have experienced unexpected newspaper publicity over conflict of interest are attuned to the need of careful board appraisal as a result of the public bath.

Before focusing on trustee appraisal, a quick look at the nature of governance sets the stage. Governance is a collective process that is slow and deliberative, the objective being to develop the best guidelines possible for the operation of the institution. It requires that the majority of the participants be in agreement before a policy can be adopted. Conceptually, the governing board role stresses:

- A grasp of the societal forces at work in the institution.

- The application of the highest obtainable levels of judgment in shaping the role of the institution in response to the societal forces.

- A preference for cool, deliberative approaches in shaping the role of the institution.

- The use of objectivity in the decision-making process, recognizing, however, that individual board members must be sensitive to the feelings and concerns of others and giving consideration to these nonquantifiable aspects.

- A willingness on the part of each participant to maintain an open mind on each issue until all of the data, opinions and conversations have been heard.

In addition to the nature of governance, the role of the board has also changed. Clearly, the primary responsibility for the modern hospital's governing board is no longer fund raising. On a scale of importance, quality of patient care, third-party reimbursement, decisions of comprehensive health planning agencies, interest rates, bank loans and share of the market are all of greater importance than fund raising.

Evaluating Board Members

Inherently, performance appraisal at the board level must be treated differently than managerial appraisal. The purpose of an organizational structure is to pinpoint responsibility and accountability for performance so that the individual manager can be measured. At the board level, the purpose of the structure is to provide a mechanism for deliberate group action in a way that minimizes the impact of individual performance.

Yet to measure the board only in a collective manner denies that any real differences can exist between individuals' board performance. Any board watcher knows there is often a wide range of levels of performance, that there are effective board members as well as ineffective ones. Yet individual performance cannot be treated as separate and apart from the collective actions of the board.

For example, it would be unrealistic to say that X has demonstrated outstanding performance as a board member while the hospital files for bankruptcy. The two simply cannot be totally divorced, yet neither can they be totally integrated. The measurement of board performance must, therefore, involve two elements that are *equally important*, the quality and timeliness of board decisions (the output) and the degree of participation (the input) by all of the members of the board. Both elements are required for a satisfactory rating of performance.

For instance, let us suppose that a review of the decisions made by a governing board during the last ten years leads to the conclusion that, on balance, the decisions were timely, imaginative, forward looking, and have led to a hospital regarded as outstanding. Also assume that the board has 28 members and is dominated by a brilliant, dedicated chairperson who hasn't bothered to use the board structure, except to ratify decisions. Under such circumstances, what conclusion is reached about the performance of the board Certainly, the public and the institution haven't suffered, overall performance has been superlative and might well have been something less under other forms of leadership. Yet, as the organizational structure was designed, it failed to work as planned. On that score, under appraisal it would show up as a glaring weakness. It was a deliberative body where 27 members failed to carry their share of the load. The fact that one was outstanding in individual performance does not offset 27 failures.

Criticism Needed in Face of Outside Scrutiny

There is a tendency in the health field not to be too critical of individual board performance on the basis that these are persons giving of themselves for community service and it is unsportsmanlike to measure them by the same rules that apply to corporate directors. Yet as times change and boards come under scrutiny by outside forces with prescribed detailed standards, it is going to be difficult for a trustee to get off the hook for poor performance on the grounds that this was a voluntary community activity engaged in out of the goodness of one's heart. While true, it is unlikely to be sufficient grounds for defending a hospital caught in a substantial lawsuit, or in justifying its course of action to the many governmental officials charged with securing compliance with their regulations.

If there is acceptance of the concept that the governing board is a deliberative body whose members are expected to influence the shaping of the policy decisions reached, then it follows that the size of the board allows each trustee/director the opportunity to contribute to the discussion of policy adoption. When finally acted upon, his or her vote should reflect individual conclusions. If this be the case then there must be an opportunity and sufficient time allowed for *all* of the board members to provide input. When governing boards grow in numbers to 15, 20, 30 or even 75, it is reasonably clear that inputs are bound to be strictly limited in the interest of concluding a meeting. As simple and straightforward as this seems, many boards still carry on with the charade of using a small group for making decisions and talking as if all the board members of a large board are effectively making contributions to the development of policy.

Board Executive Committees

Many an administrator or a board member defends a large-sized board on the grounds that the executive committee is really where the decisions are made. I can think of no instance in my years of dealing with all sizes, shapes and forms of hospitals where a large board existed without an executive committee that met more frequently than the board and in actual fact operated as a *de facto* board. The truth of the matter isn't even honestly dealt with in hospital bylaws. Typically the section dealing with the executive committee spells out its size and composition of membership and states that it shall meet between regularly scheduled meetings of the governing board to act on matters requiring immediate attention.

Yet every member of the board who is not on the executive committee understands that at board meetings he or she is not to seriously question the decisions of the executive committee as they are dutifully reported by a spokesperson of the executive committee, who on discussing the decisions reached, usually prefaces remarks in such a way that indicates these decisions were reached on behalf of the nonparticipating trustees to lessen their onerous burdens as board members. With institutional performance increasingly being scrutinized by Big Brother, there is going to come a time when nonparticipating trustees will recognize the perils of playing such roles.

Measurement of board performance includes answering the question, "Does the governing board carry out its functions in the way in which the organizational structure, as defined in the bylaws, requires?" Answered openly and honestly, large boards simply cannot stand up under such scrutiny. Inevitably they are dominated either by a single trustee or a handful of trustees who in a real sense call all the shots.

This sham is usually aided and abetted by the chief executive who goes along because it reduces the amount of time spent with individual trustees. As the individual charged with managing the hospital, the CEO knows that the more time spent on governance, the less time available for operating matters. This time factor encourages the CEO to build personal relationships with this inner circle to insure the adoption of his or her recommendations. Playing up the importance of this small decision-making group reinforces the gap between the inner group and the rest of the trustees. Thus, the chief executive becomes part of the conspiracy that is dedicated to not operating in accordance with the responsibilities of trusteeship as defined in the bylaws.

Questions for the Board

In evaluating the performance of the governance level of a hospital with a board, two types of inquiry have to be made: the questions dealing with the inputs to policy making and the outputs in terms of appropriateness of the policies reached. The input kinds of questions to be answered are:

1. Does the board carry out its responsibilities in the organizational framework outlined in its own bylaws?

2. Have position descriptions been written and followed for board members, chairperson and CEO?

3. To what extent do all trustees exercise their responsibility for providing inputs into the decision-making process?

4. What periodic and formal review is made of the individual trustee performance?

5. What periodic and formal review is made of the performance of the chief executive?

Output questions that should be studied include:

1. From a careful review of board minutes, to what extent do they indicate the adoption of timely courses of action?

2. To what extent does the regular reporting system provide trustees with a clear picture of the quality of care being given in the hospital?

3. Do trustees receive appropriate financial information?

4. Can it be demonstrated that the board acts appropriately on the reports it receives?

5. Does the board periodically review the objectives and goals of the hospital and determine to what extent performance has met them?

There are a number of advocates for large, consumer-oriented governing boards in hospitals, believing that a broad representation of community viewpoints leads to increased responsiveness on the part of the operating organization. This may or may not be the case, but its relevance in this discussion is to point out that if it results in large boards with nonparticipating trustees, it leads away from organizational effectiveness, not towards it. It must be remembered that consumer-dominated boards are usually not of a common mind, but are made up of small enclaves of quite different viewpoints to offset each other and stalemate effectiveness.

What the Role of Board Appraisal Entails

If the questions outlined are to be used, who applies them? If a committee of physicians answers them it is certain that some questions will be weighed more than others. Likewise, administrators and trustees will see them through their own set of experiences and insights. How, then, to bring about measurement of trustee performance?

Basically there are only two approaches to this kind of performance review, either externally by an outside organization or from within. An outside group would lack real familiarity with the hospital and its problems with the almost certain result of a superficial analysis and conclusions, which leaves internal review as the only practical road to follow.

Since overall governing board performance is the collective result of individual trustee activities, evaluation of each one on an annual basis would seem to be in keeping with sound organizational practice. Medical staffs are expected to review individual physician performance annually and hospital employees are reviewed at least as often. As the organizational landscape is surveyed, there is no reason to think that this shouldn't be an appropriate period for reviewing trustee performance. But who should do the measuring?

Since this review is missing in nearly all hospitals, finding a logical base for it does not infringe on past practice or tradition. Because the nominating committee is charged with recommending trustees, as well as the slate of officers at the annual meeting of a hospital corporation, it is the most suitable for undertaking this task as an extension of its existing responsibilities. As the definition of the functions of a nominating committee is reviewed in hospital bylaws, it becomes obvious that a careful and thorough review of each trustee's performance annually would be an invaluable asset in determining whether or not to reappoint for another term. Written reviews by such a committee would be a first step in bringing about a minimum standard of performance for all trustees.

The value of a properly structured performance appraisal of governance is that it balances the output factors with the input ones. All too often it seems to be forgotten that organizational structures are simply mechanisms for accomplishing the hospital's goals and objectives. Structure is a means to an end and not an end unto itself. Often forgotten is that more than half of the hospitals in this country have very small boards or, like the largest system of hospitals, the Veterans Administration, have no governing boards at all. It is only after the goals and objectives have been determined that the appropriate organizational structure can be realistically determined. When hospitals have to rely on philanthropic funds for covering annual operating deficits and for the majority of capital funds, it is easy to justify large boards of potential donors. As accountability for hospital performance is mandated, trustees will come to appreciate that large governing boards are as obsolete as large luxury automobiles. As nonfunctioning trustees find the heat in the kitchen to be uncomfortable they will leave governing boards. Those that remain will be fewer in numbers but will be tougher and more demanding of administrative performance. This will change the dimensions of the chief executive's role as it relates to both the governing board and the internal operations.

Need New Approach

Traditionally, the hospital CEO has been a manipulator who carefully orchestrated the board, never bringing up sensitive subjects before carefully laying a foundation for such a discussion. The strategies employed depended upon having a keen ear for emotional traps and a nose for timing to lead them to a desired decision. So long as there were no serious constraints on the time element, board decisions could be delayed for months or years until board attitudes were successfully harmonized.

Today, this key to board strategy no longer can be freely used. The time that is available to respond to the pressures of outside forces cannot be stretched to meet the needs of board strategy. Because of the complexity of the problems now being dealt with at the governance level and the speed with which they have to be resolved, the chief executive simply must bring up unpleasant situations and problems and avoid straddling the fence on difficult issues. Circumstances demand that the truth be spoken, whether or not board members are ready to hear bad news. The focus of measuring chief executive performance has shifted away from the skills of manipulation to those of administrative courage. Facing reality is a basic requirement, though the temptation remains strong to avoid this approach because it may lead to difficulties and jeopardize relationships.

Many CEOs tend to believe that formal performance appraisals apply to the rest of management but not to themselves, thinking that the test for the chief executive is overall institutional performance as presented in the monthly board statistics and the recommendations at such meetings. This is similar to the college football coach who, when asked why his salary is higher than members of the academic faculty, responded that he is the only person in the university having his performance reviewed at weekly intervals in the fall before 50,000 people. Certainly it is true that there is a continuing informal review that goes on through casual comments among individual board members before and after meetings. Occasionally a board chairman may drop a remark to the chief executive about performance on a particular matter, but it is rare to find an organized feedback system.

Inexperienced chief executives often ask key board members, "How am I doing?" But those with more experience usually come to believe they are sensitive enough to be able to read and interpret board thinking and modify their own behavior accordingly. While there is a small number that possess this ability, my observations lead me to conclude that those that possess this skill are far fewer in number than those who believe it of themselves.

What the Role of CEO Entails

The chief executive is in a unique organizational position as the bridge between the deliberative and the operational sides of the hospital. More than a manager, the CEO is also a trustee, either in name or in a de facto way. Not only does the CEO possess more information about the hospital and the health industry than anyone else at the board table, but he or she also is the only one who has the authority to direct the activities of all those employed in the institution. This makes it particularly difficult to accept a formal performance review. Even the best health care executives fall into the trap of believing they should be evaluating their management staff and trustee performance while they will shun one for themselves.

Several years ago I naively thought that a chief executive should sit down periodically with trustees and be willing to review their individual performances as well as having his or hers reviewed simultaneously. I know from experience that this won't work. It is too much to expect the chief executive to be candid and frank about individual trustee performance. The CEO is likely to phrase remarks so carefully that they lose impact. Telling it straight from the shoulder to a trustee is not reasonable even though chief executives frequently rate trustee performance informally with key subordinates. I've come to the conclusion that hospital executives dissect trustee performance far more often than do trustees concern themselves with administrative performance.

The purpose of a formal appraisal system for the chief executive is the same as for other subordinate managers — to bring about modifications in behavior. Unlike some others, I do not believe that performance appraisal and a review of salary can be treated separately. Together they act to reinforce each other with respect to modifying behavior. It is the application of a penalty or a reward system which should financially recognize good performance more than poor performance.

A Difficult Process

Measuring the performance of the chief executive is more complex in hospitals than in other kinds of industry because of that organizational facet known as the medical staff. In a very real sense, physicians lie outside the control of the chief executive. As the unabashed critics of hospital activities they are often vocal in their feelings about administration to individual trustees, who in turn have no real basis for judging the validity of their criticisms. Not being part of the medical staff and spending only a few hours per month in the hospital board room, trustees lack any basis for judging for themselves the extent to which the administrator has failed to deal appropriately with matters of patient care.

From a financial reporting standpoint there is also an unusual degree of complexity in determining the chief executive's capability. Most trustees do not conceptually understand how cost reimbursement differs from a pricing system, such as they may use in their own businesses, though they accept the fact that there are real differences. Because they do not feel comfortable about it, they are often unsure of how to measure the competence of the chief executive on financial matters.

The net result of these differences is to make it difficult to apply definitive yardsticks of performance. This does not mean that formal evaluations of performance cannot be made. Rather than the typical performance appraisal a different format for reviewing chief executive performance is indicated. Basically it should be a peer review, taking place at stated intervals in a manner that can best be described as a loosely structured meeting with as much room as possible for candid, honest and open discussions among key governing board members and their chief executive. Such a conversation assumes a confidence in this person and therefore should be directed in a positive direction towards improvement. Obviously, if confidence is lacking the conversation will, and should, take on an entirely different tone. Sugar-coating major performance deficiencies leads only to more problems. Straightforward discussion is a necessity under such circumstances. It may not be pleasant, but it can prevent reaching the point of no return where the only solution is for the chief executive to move on to another hospital.

The difficulty with performance appraisal is that it often gets in the way of social relationships. Many of the actions between a chief executive and board members are carried on in a semi-social situation. Board meetings may be preceded by a dinner with the chief executive acting as host. Or, the chief executive may meet several trustees for lunch on varying dates throughout the month to discuss individual matters. Chief executives usually see themselves as in the same peer group as trustees with the result that this pattern of social interaction acts as a real deterrent to the kind of objectivity needed in the annual or semi-annual performance appraisal.

Because performance appraisal at its heart is criticism, thoughtful people, be they trustees or administrative personnel, do not take easily to the use of this organizational tool. Improperly applied it can be destructive even though it was meant to be helpful. Somerset Maugham in his book *Of Human Bondage* understood the feelings of everyone who has been subjected to performance appraisal when he said, "People ask your criticism, but they only want praise."

Note

1. *Recommendations on Standards to the Joint Commission on Accreditation of Hospitals.* (Chicago: American College of Hospital Administrators, 1974).

The CEO and
Senior Management

Wendell Trent examines how different management as practiced in health care institutions is when compared to other American business endeavors in selection 9, "Some Unique Aspects of Healthcare Management." This theme is continued by Peggy Leatt and Bruce Fried in selection 10, "Organizational Designs and CEOs," in which the authors describe various designs to structure and change an organization to achieve optimal effectiveness.

In selection 11, "Evaluating the Performance of the Chief Executive Officer," James D. Harvey develops criteria and measures of accountability to evaluate the performance of the CEO. This critical task gets far too little attention from governing bodies and senior managers generally. "The Lessons of a Profession" are discussed by Everett A. Johnson in selection 12. This is a classic article in which the author provides insights on the many special relationships of managers in the hospital environment.

9

Some Unique Aspects of Healthcare Management

Wendell C. Trent

Wendell C. Trent, FACHE, is Administrator of Lawrence County Memorial Hospital, Lawrenceville, Illinois.

Management is management is management seems to be a prevalent belief among management scholars. Common threads, roles, and functions are accepted as generic executive roles. Planning, organizing, directing, controlling, and coordinating are common denominator management roles regardless of time, place, or function. Throughout history, management has performed these basic functions; the future will probably be little different.

From this perspective, a kinship transcends management functions, a kinship blind to geographical and cultural boundaries and insensitive to time, place, or industry. The first recognition of this universality of management function is generally attributed to Henri Fayol. The universality of these management functions, however, is not completely applicable to hospital administration.

Evolution and Roles of Hospital Administration

The 1918 Hospital Standardization Program initiated by the American College of Surgeons became the stimulus that eventually culminated in the ascendancy of lay administrators over physician directors.[1] Later, the American College of Surgeons' "Minimum Standards" document (now the JCAH) ". . . required the chief executive officer to have some experience in management."[2] A committee of the American Hospital Association in 1913 noted the desirability of university training for hospital administrators, and, in 1922, a Rockefeller Foundation study recommended that university courses be ". . . offered for the training of hospital administrators."[3]

Hospital administration thus gradually evolved into a profession, one comprised of elements of management science, but that functioned in a management environment uniquely different from that of other professions. This article attempts to establish this premise.

Administrative Functions

The Commission on Health Education defines the function of healthcare management as planning, organizing, directing, controlling, coordinating, and evaluating resources and procedures by which needs and demands for health and medical care are met by the provision of services to individual clients, organizations, and communities.

Many people, forces, and factors determine the role and function of the healthcare manager: physicians, trustees, medical care professionals, scientific and professional societies, professional schools, news media, society, and the manager's own self-image.

The American Hospital Association (AHA) in its guideline, the "Role and Functions of Hospital Executive Management" perceives the ". . . chief executive officer as the leader of the executive management team who provides the management expertise for ensuring that the hospital's philosophy is adhered to and that its mission, goals and objectives are achieved."[4] The CEO must not only ". . . manage the internal affairs of the organization, but also . . . be aware of conditions, events, and issues that affect the community's health status."[5]

That responsibility, according to the AHA, requires political consciousness, involvement, and acumen. Functioning as an agent for change, the CEO must take risks and accept accountability. Similar to the expectations of executives in other industries and business, the AHA paper suggests the CEO should serve as the catalyst, facilitator, coordinator, and communicator to ensure that strategies to meet goals and objectives are developed and that programs are carried out and evaluated.

Many roles and functions of the hospital CEO, then, do not differ markedly from role expectations for executives in other professional endeavors.

Hospital Management is Different

Despite these similarities in role, function, and responsibility, management *is* different in hospitals. Many reasons exist for this phenomenon:

- The profession is relatively young; it is still growing and establishing itself.

- Healthcare management is not yet widely recognized as a profession by the American public.

- Healthcare executive management has previously been subordinate to physician domination.

- Performance requirements, until recently, have probably not been as exacting as those in industry.

- Because of the duality of command and tradition, hospital administration has been relatively devoid of the authority and control inherent in comparable executive positions in business.

Recent changes and demands are quickly altering these characteristics, however.

Duality of Hospital Command

According to Letourneau, "there should be only one chief executive of the hospital."[6] In practice, one CEO is usually responsible for the hospital's operation to the board of trustees. It is not unique, however, for members of the medical staff to represent physicians at board meetings or to actually be board members. In reality, the administrator may be subordinate to the medical staff (as board members) when he is titularly responsible to the board for certain overviewing functions of the medical staff.

In medical areas, particularly, the position is necessarily subordinate to physician direction; in many professional and technical areas, the administrator must rely heavily on these specialists.

Many patient-care services are under the medical direction of physicians, while the professional staffs provide administrative and professional direction. These are physicians who may or may not be employees of the institution in which they practice and who have varying degrees of loyalty to the hospital. They exercise significant medical and administrative direction. The CEO may be the titular head of the organization; however, substantial aspects of management are clearly outside his control. This is not necessarily negative, but is rather a statement of the uniqueness of the healthcare management environment.

The net effect of these differences translates into greater management complexity and a tendency to overprotect the hospital from an increasingly litigious patient population. As more sophisticated patient-care technology becomes available, medical professionals feel obligated to make that technology available to patients.

Healthcare management is characterized by an intensity of concern, a depth of dedication, and a degree of professional commitment whose intensities are unique to our profession. One of the obvious results of this uniqueness is greater healthcare costs. Our collective professional characteristics tend to exacerbate the growing problem of healthcare expenses.

Restrained Authority

Letourneau writes that ". . . neither the governing body nor the administrator of the hospital may exercise control over the professional judgment of the practicing physicians."[7] In some settings, the "professional judgment" of the physician, as perceived by the administrator, is given wider latitude and credibility than his own.

Letourneau writes that the administrator and board have a legal duty to protect the patient against incompetent physicians. The administrator, usually untrained and inexperienced in medical affairs, rarely observes the "ministrations" of doctors. His knowledge of medical/professional work performance and competence is usually indirect.

These characteristics perhaps originally served as the basis for the extensive involvement of physicians in hospital management, although board responsibility may not have then been as clearly established as today. Those conditions clearly argue for physician involvement in hospital management and for the continuation of command duality. Such extensive consumer involvement in management is probably unique to healthcare.

Stark writes that the ". . . health services administrator is seen as an individual with a limited scope of responsibility, usually restricted to technical and more routine tasks within an institution or agency. He lacks an entrepreneurial image altogether. In some critical aspects of on-going institutional life, he is excluded or instructed to refrain from any direct interference or involvement. The historical pattern has been that the administrator in health affairs has developed as a caretaker."[8]

Stark also writes that trustee perceptions of hospital administrators range from "housekeeper" to "office boy," unless the administrator happens to have an M.D. after his name. Then, Stark observes, the physician is generally thought to be misusing his talent on administrative work. The weakly perceived role of the chief executive officer is another unique, but fast-changing, aspect of our profession.

Involvement in Macrosystems

The Commission on Health Education observes that when national solutions for healthcare system problems are offered, administrators are not usually among those involved.

The Commission writes that administrators "seem to be viewed as neither crucial nor essential to the system's functioning."[9] The commission notes that, "Rather than assuming a leadership or controlling stance, . . . administrators appear to be manipulating, and are being manipulated, by physicians."[10] Evidence strongly suggests that today's administrators are involved to a greater degree in establishing healthcare policy, and as the profession is strengthened, the relative degree of involvement of CEOs in macrosystem design will most likely expand.

Administrative Reticence

Earlier, this article stated that hospital administration was a profession of great managerial complexity. The Commission for Health Education substantiates this and notes that the *complexity of demands* on those in administrative positions creates barriers. Administrators are accountable to institutional owners, the community, consumers, resources, regulatory bodies, and third-party payment agencies. They are also responsible to the board of trustees, the medical staff, hospital employees, and various personal and professional standards.

"Juggling these sets of accountabilities," the Commission states, "without significant recognition as leaders and decision makers, does not ease the administrator's daily tasks."[11] Administrators are responsible to many interests that influence hospitals.

Eliot Friedson describes the nature of physician dominance as a "barrier to other healthcare professionals' performance."[12] Sheinbach writes that ". . . many administrators and other health professionals have traditionally played a subservient role to the clinician because they simply did not assume the prerogative and authority which go with the professional responsibility and positions."[13]

The Report of the Commission on Education for Health Administration, like Letourneau, concludes that a unique feature of the medical care industry is the degree to which its services must be "individualized." It concludes that healthcare must be customized for each client.

Customizing in business and industry are uncommon; mass production is the rule. Should we be searching for mass production techniques in hospital healthcare? The Commission states that the health and medical care industry is the most highly professionalized "industry" in our society.

Environmental Change

Rapid changes in the hospital environment exert substantive influences on hospital administration:

- These changes include corporate restructuring

- Facility mergers, acquisitions, or affiliations

- The "for profits"

- The complexity of management

- Changing reimbursement that dictates greater effectiveness and efficiency of human resources.

Charles M. Ewell, Ph.D., states, "Fundamental changes in hospital management during the past five years are having an enormous impact on hospital administrators' career development, compensation, and job continuity."[14] He identifies the shift from generalist to specialist and concludes that these changes will alter the manner in which graduate schools train administrators. Ewell questions whether the generalist can keep up with the specialist administrator.

Healthcare Partners

Richard L. Johnson of TriBrook Management Consultants notes that one of the first surprises encountered by the neophyte hospital administrator is that of the medical staff's attitude toward management. "The beginner believes that since they are both striving in their respective ways toward the same goals, they are partners," Johnson writes. It comes as a shock to learn that physicians see it differently."[15]

He notes that some administrators never overcome resultant hostilities and spend a career making sure that physicians lose as many organizational battles as possible. Others appreciate the necessity for never taking the medical staff for granted. This intra-professional rivalry is not unique to the medical profession.

Johnson writes that the administrator is the organization man and the physician is the entrepreneur. Bureaucrats and entrepreneurs frequently clash. Perhaps it is not so much the *person* of the administrator but rather that of his *position* that causes the clash.

"Medical staffs usually deny that [authority] exists for chief executives of hospital, [and] in many hospitals they even deny [that] it exists for another physician who may be in an administrative position, such as a medical director," Johnson observes.[16]

Some physicians think of the hospital as a support system for their own decision making. With the problem of long-term debt, "the hospital executive has difficulty reconciling physician attitudes with the imperative of meeting his debt service requirements, coordinating of diverse talents, and of responding to a variety of external community pressures, while at the same time providing a future course for the institution," Johnson writes.

The hospital's largest consumer, committed to the best possible care for his patient, is pitted against an administration forced by today's hospital environment to control or even eliminate certain expenses. These differences in position, both honestly and professionally motivated, exacerbate medical-professional-administrative tension. Healthcare structure promotes system stress, and combined with other system quantities, ensures that healthcare costs will be difficult to control.

Despite these differences in perspective, hospital management is expected to cooperate with its customers: physicians. Johnson writes that the chief executive is expected to cooperate with the medical staff. This causes a great deal of organizational uncertainty because of the peculiar relationship of the medical staff in the organizational structure. The administrator may find himself in a dilemma, he notes, in that the governing board expects him to be vigilant about the quality of patient care, but at the same time expects him to cooperate with the medical staff.

Such cooperation is not always possible. Johnson states that even though he does what senior executives in other industries do, operating on the basis of second and third-hand information and statistical reports, these sources are often not regarded as valid by physicians. The administrator's dilemma is that he can neither claim clinical competence with nor direct authority over the medical staff. Many hospital boards place greater reliance on medical staff input than on the reports of hospital administration. This is one of the unusual aspects of hospital management.

Hospital bylaws mandating the CEO's cooperation with the medical staff result in significant organizational uncertainty for the administrator because of the unusual relationship of physicians within that organizational structure. Ultimately, the administrator finds himself increasingly boxed in, without any way out, because he has no end product measurements he can turn to that reflect the overall results of organizational performance. The end result of this dilemma is that the administrator may conclude that he should get along by going along, Johnson writes.

In many respects, representing and acting for the hospital, administration can only obliquely influence the medical staff. The administrator would like to work with the medical staff in the manner in which he deals with other operating departments, but recognizes that physicians must be treated differently. When physicians express displeasure toward the administrator, to or through the governing board, the board listens carefully and is inclined to be responsive. "If this dissatisfaction reaches the point where a collective position of staff members is adopted, such as requesting that the board terminate the chief executive, experience indicates that the board is more often than not going to accede to this request.[17]

In such situations, he observes, there is little likelihood that fairness, weighing of administrative performance over time, or determining the validity of the medical staff's position is apt to occur. Boards, Johnson writes, do not typically see the CEO as the person who leads and inspires the medical staff. In this respect, the hospital CEO role is different from that of his counterpart in industry, another unique aspect of our profession.

In industry, the CEO is responsible for providing leadership and establishing higher goals and using corporate resources for attaining them. Business CEOs are expected to be out front, challenging greater performance, not confined to boundaries that limit their abilities as long as efficient and effective results are achieved.

In hospitals, Johnson writes, the CEO is expected to do his job efficiently and responsively to medical-care interests. The CEO is expected to assure that professional standards are enforced (he is not expected and usually not permitted to raise these standards) and can only encourage their being accomplished. The hospital CEO may be as accomplished and versatile as his industrial counterpart; however, the role he finds himself in prevents him from exercising product management skills common in business and industry. If business CEOs were forced to competitively operate in a hospital executive's role in affecting changes, it is doubtful that many firms could survive long. A hospital CEO, then, is not a CEO in the usual sense; he is uniquely restricted in how he may accomplish results.

Ingrid K. Kuhl, in the research work, "The Executive Role in Health Service Delivery Organizations," concludes that medical-care policy formulation "is generally resistent to bureaucratic intervention which hospital executives may institute. Hospital executives are often preempted from using strategies associated with problem solving, bargaining and persuasion in this area of decision making."[18]

Kuhl further writes that, "Where decisions call for problem solving processes, hospital executives are not likely to be viewed by the medical staff as having a legitimate claim to participate."[19] Since the goals and interests of hospital executives are often at variance with those of the staff, she says, CEOs are not likely to be successful in attempting to persuade the staff to act in accordance with their point of view.

Central Direction and Management

In assessing the uniqueness of hospital management, Basil J. F. Mott, Ph.D., observes that hospitals are not "centrally directed and managed organizations in the usual sense."[20] Historically, he writes, hospitals have *not* been organizations whose trustees and administrators decided the organizational mission, or brought together and managed the resources required to carry out their decisions, and the output of a hospital is not something that boards of trustees and management can determine or control to ensure organizational efficiency, as do their counterparts in other organizations."[21]

This is substantially different from industry. "Each physician, on a case-by-case basis, decided whom he will admit, what services his patients will receive, and when they will be discharged. In no other type of organization are the work load and the type of work performed so much beyond the control of management or even of the professionals who do the work,"[22] he writes.

Mott declares that physicians often perceive administrative policies and decisions as interfering with their professional prerogatives, noting that many other health professionals have a built-in "anti-administrative bias."

"Because their income is not [usually] controlled by the hospital," Mott says, "they are not subject to the most powerful control that management traditionally exercises over personnel in organizations."[23]

For these reasons, Mott concludes that hospital costs are more difficult to control than expenses in other organizations. The basis of this problem is that the principal work of hospitals, the provision of medical care, is outside the direct control of administrative management.

He states that arguments for maintaining and improving the quality of healthcare have an advantage over arguments to hold down expenses, because quality can rarely be determined objectively.

Summary

From these perspectives, then, evidence substantiates that hospital administration does differ significantly from management as it is traditionally considered. For many reasons, this study has not attempted to compare the profession of hospital administration to specific roles in other industries. That task would be too broad, and such comparisons would likely reveal that executive roles in each industry were uniquely different.

Healthcare is changing, and changing quickly. HMOs, PPOs, DRGs, and other changes in reimbursement are mandating change in the healthcare system, forcing greater resource efficiency and effectiveness. These and other changes yet to come will raise the level of medical-administrative-professional tension and conflict. This will ultimately result in healthcare management that is more similar to the management in other endeavors.

Notes

1. Letourneau, *The Hospital Administrator* (Starling Publications, Chicago, 1969), p. 6.
2. *Ibid.*
3. *Ibid.*
4. "Role & Function of Hospital Executive Management" (American Hospital Association, Chicago, 1982).
5. *Ibid.*
6. Letourneau, *The Hospital Administrator* p. 16.
7. *Ibid.* p. 52.
8. *Education for Health Administration*, Vol. 1, p. 38.
9. *Ibid.* p. 39.
10. *Ibid.* p. 40.
11. *Ibid.* p. 48.
12. *Ibid.* p. 49.
13. *Ibid.*

14. Charles Ewell, Ph.D., "Changes in Hospital Management Demand Special Administrator," *Modern Healthcare* (March, 1982) p. 90.
15. R.L. Johnson, "The Managers & The Medical Staff" (Tribook, Inc., Oak Brook, Illinois, 1982), p. 1.
16. *Ibid.* p. 4.
17. *Ibid.* p. 5.
18. Ingrid K. Kuhl, *The Executive Role in Health Service Delivery Organizations* (AUPHA, Washington, 1977), p. 52.
19. *Ibid.* p. 53.
20. Basil J.F. Mott, Ph.D., "Is The Hospital Beyond Our Understanding?" *Trustee* (Vol. 34, No. 4, April, 1981): pg. 21.
21. *Ibid.*
22. *Ibid.*
23. *Ibid.*

10

Organizational Designs and CEOs

Peggy Leatt and Bruce Fried

Peggy Leatt, Ph.D., is Professor and Chairman, Department of Health Administration, University of Toronto.

Bruce Fried, Ph.D. is Assistant Professor, Department of Health Administration, University of Toronto.

Organizational design involves constructing and changing an organizational structure to achieve optimal effectiveness;[1] this includes decisions about allocation of authority, responsibility, information flow and reward systems.[2] In other words, organizational design determines who has formal power in the organization, who has authority to make particular decisions, and how information is communicated.

In most health care organizations, decisions about organizational structure traditionally have been made in an informal and somewhat *ad hoc* manner. Design is often a reactive process with minor changes made in the organization chart as individuals leave or enter the organization. It is rare that a health care organization engages in a systematic and proactive assessment of the total organization with consideration given to the range of possible alternative organizational models. Yet fragmented episodic approaches to organizational structure are likely to have unanticipated ripple effects on other parts and frequently lead to incomplete organizational designs, inefficiencies, and compromised performance.

Organizational design is a conscious deliberate process which is essential for all organizations on an ongoing basis. It has many implications for the changing roles of chief executive officers.

The Design Process

It is possible to conduct the organizational design process at several different organizational levels. For example, at a micro level, individual positions or roles and their relationships to other positions may be analyzed and redesigned. At a macro level, the design process may include analysis of the entire system of health care for a province with the identification of networks of organizations and how they might interrelate. Usually, however, the design process is limited to a single organization such as a hospital, nursing home, or primary care centre.

Organizational design is the primary responsibility of the chief executive officer and senior management team. This does not imply that senior management should complete the design task without consulting others in the organization. Recent literature suggests that participatory approaches to organizational design not only produce a model which is better tailored to the organization's needs but also may be implemented more successfully because of greater commitment by other organizational members. Outside consultants also may be used to help identify the range of models which may be appropriate; however, the final adoption of a design lies ultimately within the organization itself.

The Idea of Choice

In the early 1900s, the choice of an organizational design was not considered an issue. During this period organizational theorists, as well as management practitioners, were advocating "the one best way" to organize. For example, Frederick Taylor, a practitioner, promoted "scientific management" and Max Weber, an academic, advocated an "ideal-type" bureaucracy. As late as the 1960s, supporters of the human relations and human resource schools of thought suggested that participatory models were not only the most ethical but also essential for all organizations to be effective.

In the last decade, two critical changes in thinking have had a major impact upon decisions about organizational design. First, there has been a recognition that there is not one best way to organize which is applicable to all organizations. For example, depending upon the circumstances of an organization at a particular time, it may be quite appropriate to assume either an autocratic or a participatory model. Second, organizations have been recognized as open systems which are profoundly influenced by the environment in which they are located. Events occurring outside the organization may require changes in organizational structure as well as in the roles which individual managers assume. Related to these two changes in thinking has been an acknowledgement that in situations of high uncertainty, over-determined and static organizational designs should be avoided; flexibility must be encompassed in the design of the organization so that it can respond appropriately and efficiently to changing circumstances.

A Framework for Organizational Design

Contingency theory, which has dominated the organizational behaviour literature for the last decade, suggests that the effectiveness of an organization in enhanced if structure is matched with the contingencies with which it is faced. The most important factors to be taken into consideration in selecting an appropriate model are illustrated in Fig. 10-1.

In selecting a design which will maximize organizational performance, four aspects of the organization's context must be addressed: the external environment; the organization itself; the human resources of the organization; and the political processes.

Environmental Assessment

An analysis of the constraints and opportunities presented by the organization's environment is essential in selecting an organizational design which will accommodate future external events. Usually an environmental assessment includes the development of a series of critical questions and the collection of data to shed light on these issues. Questions which may be addressed in an environmental assessment for a Canadian health care organization are as follows.

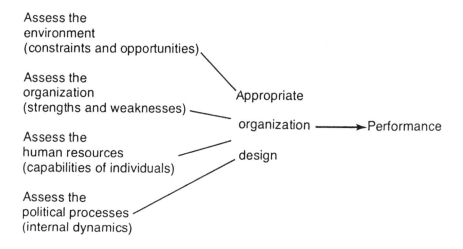

Figure 10-1. A Framework for Organizational Design. Modified from Kimberly, J.R., P. Leatt and S.M. Shortell. "Organizational design." In Shortell, S.M. and A. Kaluzny, eds. *Health Care Management: A Text in Organization Theory and Behaviour*. New York: John Wiley, 1983.

Economic/Political/Legal Conditions.

To what extent will the pressures to contain health care costs increase, remain the same or decrease?

Will the demand for health care increase, remain the same or decrease?

Will it be necessary to limit the supply of certain services? If yes, how can this be done?

Will competition for scarce dollars increase, remain the same or decrease?

What incentives will be provided for containing or reducing costs and to whom?

What effects will changes in political parties and leaders have?

How much pull will there be to privatization?

What effects will the Canada Health Act have upon health care organizations?

Demographic/Culture Conditions.

What are the key characteristics of the persons being served by the organization?

Will Canada's population increase, remain the same or decrease?

Will the geographic and cultural distribution of the Canadian population change or remain the same?

Will there be changes in the major causes of mortality and morbidity?

Will Canada's population continue to age at the same rate or an increasing rate?

New Organizational Forms.

Will the trend to move to multi-institutional arrangements (e.g., mergers and corporate structures) continue?

Will new networks of organizations develop at local levels?

Will the trend to develop alternatives to hospitalization continue through the development of health service organizations (H.S.O.s) new ambulatory care programs, primary care centres, and home care?

Will alternative funding mechanisms, such as health maintenance organizations be experimented with?

Will consumer participation in decision-making about health care increase, stay the same or decrease?

Technological Developments.

Will developments in medical technology continue at the same rate and from where will the major breakthroughs come?

Will limits be set upon expenditures for capital-intensive, high livesaving technologies? If yes, how will decisions be made?

Will technologies increasingly require the need for multidisciplinary team approaches?

What will be the most critical developments in managerial techniques?

Organizational Assessment

One of the most important steps in an organizational assessment is to review the mission of the organization and reconsider this in relation to the organization's future environment. In addition, it is essential that the goals and specific strategies developed by the organization are congruent with the constraints and opportunities presented by the environment. The quantity, quality and types of services to be provided as well as the history of the organization should be taken into consideration. Included in the analysis should be an examination of the strengths and weaknesses of the organization. It is during this process that problems with the current structure and internal processes may be identified, such as inability to anticipate problems and take corrective actions quickly, communication barriers, difficulties resulting from conflicting roles, employee turnover, and recruitment and selection problems.

Human Resources Assessment

This assessment involves evaluating the capabilities and potential of key persons in the organization. Quality of performance by persons in both senior and middle management positions is essential not only in meeting the goals of the organization but also in implementing proposed changes in organizational structure. Strategies for human resource development over the long-term may also be outlined in the assessment of human resources.

Political Process Assessment

This assessment involves a systematic analysis of the informal internal dynamics of the organization. The informal leaders and groups should be identified and analyzed particularly in terms of how they facilitate or impede the achievement of organizational goals. Informal leaders may help or hinder attempts to bring about changes in organizational structure; it would seem wise to bring such persons into the planning process at an early stage.

Although there may be some duplication in the information obtained through these four assessments, senior management will consequently be more knowledgeable and in a stronger position to select an appropriate structure if all relevant information is made available.

A Functional Model

Most persons in the health care field are familiar with a functional model where labour is divided into specific functional departments, e.g., finance, dietary, nursing, pharmacy, housekeeping, and so on (see Fig. 10-2). This arrangement is most prevalent in relatively small (100-200 beds) acute hospitals, chronic care facilities and nursing homes.

This organizational model is most useful for small organizations providing a limited range of services, and with only one main goal. The primary advantages of the functional model are that it facilitates decision-making in a centralized and hierarchical manner and career paths for departmental managers are clear.

The functional model is likely to be inappropriate when an organization is involved in major new growth or diversification. At such times, lateral coordination and decentralized decision-making are required. The functional model is also inappropriate for organizations operating in complex, dynamic environments because it cannot accommodate and process the rapid information flow generated by the environment.

A Corporate Model

There is increasing use of the term "corporate structure" in hospitals in Canada. In the world of business, this term is used to define any organization which is legally incorporated and this would include all hospitals, universities and so on. Ewell has outlined the basic characteristics of a "true" corporate structure in relation to both the form of governance and top management.[3] These are:

Governing Body.

1. There are salaried corporate executives who serve as board members and typically include a president, vice-president(s), controller, and legal counsellor.

2. There is a full-time chairman of the board who functions as the executive of the corporation (this person is usually the chief executive officer).

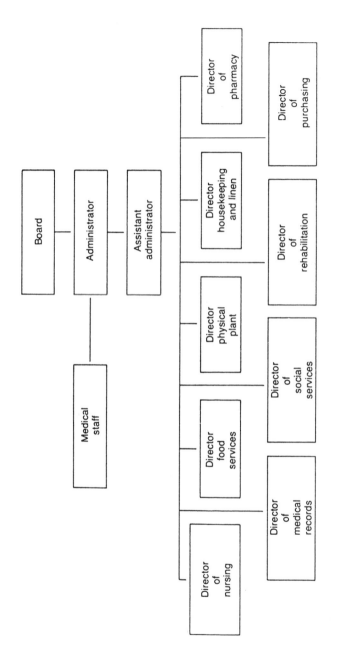

Figure 10-2. A Functional Model.

3. Board members are elected and paid a fee for attending meetings.

Top Management.

1. Chief Executive Officer, with the title of president, is a voting member of the board. He/she may also be the chairman of the board.

2. The senior management team is made up of vice-presidents including an executive vice-president.

3. There is a group of corporate staff who provide ongoing long-range support services to the vice-presidents. Typically, these staff provide support in such functional areas as human resources, public relations, data processing, legal affairs and planning.

4. There is a great emphasis on a team approach to management and decentralization of decision-making.

An example of a corporate model is shown in Fig. 10-3.

The corporate model is most useful in large, complex organizations which have several goals and which operate in changing environments. Corporate structures often develop where two or more hospitals merge. Variations of the corporate model also are used where a regional authority has overall responsibility for several health programs serving a particular geographic area.

The corporate model is less suitable for a small organization where conversion to a corporate structure would mean simply a change in titles for the senior managers: the organization would be top heavy. The model is also inappropriate if the chief executive officer is not prepared to delegate responsibility and authority to other members of the senior management team or if management team members do not possess the necessary skills to assume the delegated authority.

A Divisional Model

With the divisional model, labour is divided and divisions are created around products, services or markets. In health care organizations, these divisions usually centre around types of patients (e.g., medical, surgical, paediatric, and psychiatric) or types of programs (e.g., acute care, long-term care, ambulatory care). Each division is a semi-autonomous unit with full responsibility and accountability for its clinical and financial affairs. Accordingly, each unit has its own management team which includes representatives of administration, finance, nursing, and medicine.

The most publicized example of a divisional model in health care is the structure at The Johns Hopkins Hospital in Baltimore, Maryland. The model

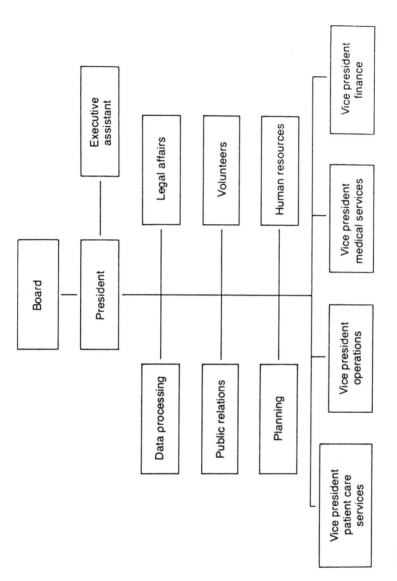

Figure 10-3. A Corporate Model.

was adopted with the aim of bringing the hospital out of a financial deficit position by placing responsibility for expenditures more directly in the hands of physicians.[4] This structure is illustrated in Fig. 10-4. In The Johns Hopkins Hospital, the units independently purchase laboratory, radiology, housekeeping, laundry, and other services from centralized departments within the hospital. If they desire, they may also purchase these services outside the hospital. Since units are allowed to use any accrued savings for their own purpose, there is a clear incentive for them to operate efficiently.

The divisional model is most appropriate for large organizations with a variety of highly specialized programs or products. It is typically seen in organizations with multiple goals where decisions need to be made by persons possessing specialized knowledge and who are close to the situation/point of decision impact. The model is most useful for organizations operating in complex, changing environments; in these situations, division heads are given authority to deal directly with selected aspects of the environment.

The divisional model has several difficulties which must be addressed by management. First, there is frequently uncertainty about the appropriate method by which the organization should be subdivided. For example, divisions may be created around traditional medical specialties such as medicine, surgery, and paediatrics, or alternatively, around newly emerging programs such as gerontology or oncology which may cut across several traditional specialties. Divisionalization may foster counter-productive interdivisional competition and may not permit needed lateral co-ordination and communication in the organization. Care must be taken to ensure that the goals of each division are in keeping with the overall mission and goals of the organization. In times of resource constraint it may also be difficult for senior management to set priorities among the divisions; lack of resources may also require more sharing of resources among divisions.

A Matrix Model

The matrix approach to organizational design was developed initially in the aerospace industry. The matrix design is characterized by a dual authority system where individuals have two or more bosses.[5] The organizational structure is usually drawn as a diamond form (see Fig. 10-5) with functional directors and program managers on the top edges of the diamond. This arrangement is intended to increase the opportunity for lateral co-ordination and communication which frequently emerge as problems in other design configurations. Functional directors (e.g., nursing, social services, medical records) are responsible for the standards of services provided by their department. Typically, functional directors bring stability and continuity to the organization and sustain the professional status of staff. Program managers (e.g., palliative care, geriatrics, oncology) have responsibility for individual multidisciplinary programs and co-ordinate team functioning. It is the responsibility of the chief executive officer to maintain balance between both sides of the matrix.

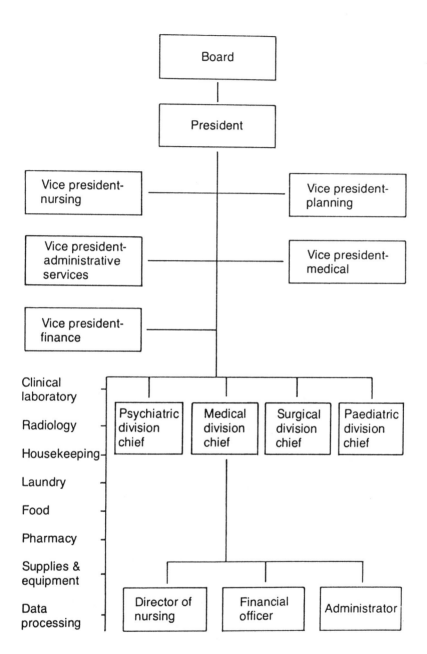

Figure 10-4. A Divisional Model.

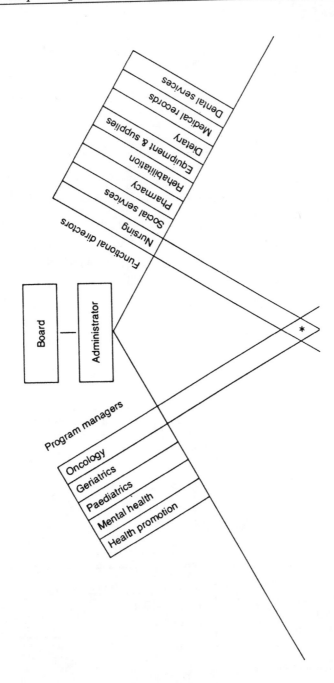

Figure 10-5. A Matrix Model.

The matrix model facilitates innovation in technology and is, therefore, most useful to organizations that work with highly specialized technologies. It is appropriate in the initiation of new programs and where multidisciplinary approaches to care are essential. At the program level, each team member contributes his/her specialized expertise to the program's objectives. One criticism of the matrix model is that it creates untenable stress for individual workers because of the "two boss" system. Also, in order for both functional directors and program managers to be held accountable for the work of subordinates, clinical and financial information systems must be organized by program as well as by department. Health care organizations, however, are accustomed to working with multiple authority lines; in fact, some experts suggest that most health care organizations have a *de facto* informal matrix structure.

A Parallel Model

The parallel model evolved from the Quality of Working Life movement as a mechanism for improving employees' work life by including them in decision-making.[6] As illustrated in Fig. 10-6, the functional arm of the structure is responsible for the relatively routine work of the organization and for maintaining stability. The parallel side consists of a series of permanent and temporary committees with a cross-section of representatives from appropriate departments on the functional side of the organization. The parallel side has responsibility for solving problems common to all or part of the organization. Committees are typically given a specific problem for analysis and are expected to make recommendations for its solution to senior management.

The parallel model is appropriate in situations where organizations are faced with critical and complex problems with no easy solutions. The model is useful when it is necessary to include a broad range of disciplines in the development of policies and procedures. Organizational performance may be improved not only by identifying solutions to difficult problems but also by the cross-fertilization of ideas which result from the interdisciplinary approach. Individual members of the organization may also grow personally from their involvement in the parallel structure and are likely to feel that they are important to their organization.

Problems may arise with the parallel model if the parallel arm of the structure begins to assume decision-making responsibilities which should remain with the functional arm. There may be differences in priorities set by each side of the structure. Also, individuals at lower levels in the organization may end up spending a great deal of time at meetings, thus interfering with their abilities to do their job.

In reality, most health care organizations have elements of a parallel model, particularly as a mechanism for involving physicians and other health professionals in forming organizational policies.

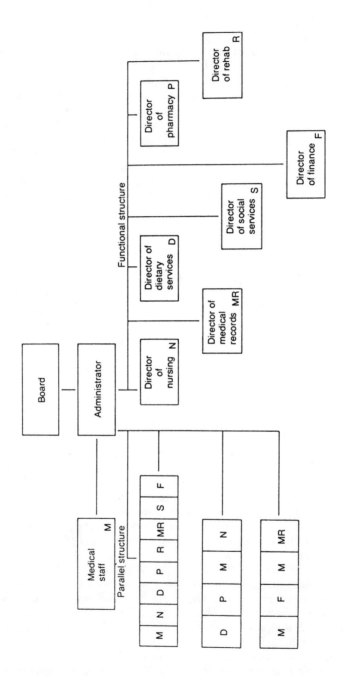

Figure 10-6. A Parallel Model.

Guidelines for Selecting Designs

As the environment facing health care organizations becomes increasingly complex and unpredictable, it is necessary for senior management to periodically assess the appropriateness of the organization's structure. It is likely that the environment of the future will require health care organizations to depart from simple traditional designs such as a functional structure and adopt more complex mixed structures. In such organizations it can be expected that most people in the organization will be accountable to more than one boss. Such arrangements will require considerable effort to clarify new roles and relationships.

The models outlined in this paper have been described in "pure" versions in order to illustrate their differences. In real organizations it may be necessary to combine one or more models to fit the needs of a particular organization at a given time. Clearly, any organizational model must facilitate problem identification and solution, information flow, and create an environment conductive to productivity; however, there is no one "best" way to meet the requirements of all situations.

Implications for Changing CEO roles

Although it is recognized that all chief executive officers in the health care system must carry out the traditional functions of management first described by Henri Fayol as planning, organizing, leading, co-ordinating and controlling, the more complex health care environment and changing organizational models will bring new dimensions and responsibilities to the chief executive officer's role.

In large complex organizations with a corporate structure the role of the chief executive officer increasingly becomes externally focused. The roles of this person become highly politicized; in this position, the chief executive officer functions as spokesman for the organization in the wider social-political-economic environment. The skills of importance relate to the person's ability to chart a future course for the organization through a complex and unpredictable political maze. The chief executive officer in these circumstances requires a broad range of public relations, negotiating, and strategic planning skills to keep the organization on target. In a corporate design, it is probably appropriate to appoint a chief operating officer to manage day-to-day internal operations of the organization.

In a divisionalized structure the role of the chief executive officer is similar to that in a corporate structure because of the size of the organization and the characteristics of the environment. However, in a divisionalized model the chief executive officer must assume added roles to ensure that individual divisions do not deviate from the mission of the total organization and that lateral communications among the divisions are maintained. Appropriate delegation of tasks is of vital importance in this regard.

The matrix and parallel models share the characteristics of utilizing two overlapping structures. Effective management of these types of organizations requires considerable flexibility about roles, relationships and lines of authority and accountability. Here, the chief executive officer is likely to experience considerable ambiguity about the roles to be assumed. A critical role of the chief executive officer, however, is to maintain balance between both sides of the organization; consequently, the role of conflict-handler is important. It is also necessary for the chief executive officer to clarify who has the authority to make decisions, particularly concerning the allocation of resources. Team building and participatory management approaches are essential with these models.

In organizations that face more stable and predictable environments, a traditional functional structure with an internally focused general manager may continue to be appropriate. The administrator will continue to make many of the major decisions for the organization and will require basic financial and human resources management skills.

Finally, in all organizational models of the future, it will be the chief executive officer's role to demonstrate ethical leadership. The decisions and problems currently facing health care managers, especially in relation to program cutbacks and retrenchment, are complex and have no simple solutions. It will be the chief executive officer's responsibility to bring relevant parties together to make decisions based on a sound philosophy which recognizes individual worth and takes into consideration society's priorities for health care.

Notes

1. Kimberly, J.R., P. Leatt and S.M. Shortell. "Organization design." In Shortell, S.M. and A. Kaluzny, eds. *Health Care Management: A text in organization theory and behavior.* 291-332. New York: John Wiley, 1983.
2. Shortell, S.M. "The medical staff of the future: replanting the garden." *Frontiers of Health Services Management* (Winter, 1985).
3. Ewell, C.M. "Organizing along corporate lines." *Hospitals* 46 (1972): 58-62.
4. Heyssel, R.M. et al. "Decentralized management in a teaching hospital." *New England Journal of Medicine* 310(22) (1984): 1477-1480.
5. Davis, S.M. and P.R. Lawrence. "The matrix diamond." *Wharton Magazine* 2(2) (1978): 19-27.
6. Stein, B.A. and R.M. Kanter. "Building the parallel organization: creating mechanisms for permanent quality of work life." *The Journal of Applied Behavioral Science* 16(3) (1980): 371-386.

11

Evaluating the Performance of the Chief Executive Officer

James D. Harvey

James D. Harvey, FACHE, is President of the Hillcrest Medical Center Foundation, Tulsa, Oklahoma.

In 1973, the American College of Hospital Administrators published a very important and potentially valuable task force report entitled *Principles of Appointment and Tenure of the Executive Officer*. Added to its usefulness as elicited in the document's title, it avers that:

> . . . formal performance review of the chief executive officer should be done annually. . . . Evaluation is a major responsibility of the board of trustees, not to be delegated by them to anyone, regardless of the resources the board may choose to employ in this process. . . . Often, it isn't done well. Experience of consulting firms called into hospitals in which the chief executive has been terminated or is under board pressure indicates that, in a high percentage of these situations, routine formal evaluation is missing entirely, or the process lacks frankness or lacks criteria to which both parties would agree.

The task force report goes on to say that the evaluation should be carried out at four levels:

1. Areawide health care status
2. Institutional success
3. Role of the chief executive officer
4. Management skills

The report points out that while evaluation of the health status of the population served by the hospital might well be related to the effectiveness of the hospital itself it is not fair to hold the chief executive officer (CEO) responsible for this aspect. It should always be considered, however, because this is the outcome sought by the individual hospital.

The institutional success level, the role of the CEO level, and the management skills level are all within the realm of chief executive evaluation, the document points out. It asserts that there are probably many ways for this process to be accomplished. It contains this one qualification: "However it is to be done, evaluating the CEO requires pre-agreement on what is to be evaluated and standards for measuring if evaluation is to be meaningful and equitable." Embodied in this mild statement are two word groups, the lack of which are the major obstacles to achieving effective evaluation. They are "pre-agreement" and "standards for measuring." Precious few hospital boards evaluate performance of the CEO by pre-agreed standards.

The ACHA, as if noting this deficiency, produced a report in October, 1976, on a pilot study on executive compensation entitled *The Position of the Hospital Chief Executive*. This document sharpened the CEO's account-abilities, e.g., those results expected of a chief executive officer in the performance of his or her duties.

Using the tenets contained in the *Principles of Appointment and Tenure of Executive Officers* and the accountabilities of the CEO as listed in *The Position of the Hospital Chief Executive*, a model emerges which can be used to develop an effective performance evaluation process.

The Position of the Hospital Chief Executive study suggests that the CEO has seven accountabilities. They fall within the following areas of activity:

1. Planning and organizing

2. Achieving hospital objectives

3. Quality of medical services

4. Allocation of resources

5. Crisis resolution

6. Compliance with regulation

7. Promotion of the hospital

Chief Executive Levels

Each accountability is written in one or two sentences. Each points out that the CEO may act within an accountability at one of three levels:

1. Chief administrative officer

2. Chief executive, tactical

3. Chief executive, strategic

This differentiation recognizes the fact that a CEO operates differently from institution to institution and implies that the governing board involves itself in the hospital in different ways. Rather than speculate as to the level a particular CEO may be involved, this article will demonstrate how measures and standards can be developed for each accountability. The type of standard used to gauge performance in fulfilling an accountability would naturally be derived from the level at which the CEO operates.

Accountability Statements

Following is a listing of each accountability statement taken from *The Position of the Hospital Chief Executive*. (The ultimate result of each statement is underlined.)

Accountability I. Planning and Organizing: Participates with the board in charting the course the hospital is to take in response to the developing needs of the community for formulating and recommending sound strategies and plans.
Comment: "Participates" and "formulating and recommending" are key words leading to "charting the course."

Accountability II. Achieving Hospital Objectives: Ensures the attainment of hospital objectives through the effective administration of the operation. This is accomplished chiefly through the selection, development and motivation of hospital personnel and the continuous review and control of their efforts.
Comment: This accountability emphasizes getting things done through people. The words "selection, development and motivation" stress this.

Accountability III. Quality of Medical Services: Responds to the community's need for quality health care services by monitoring the adequacy of the hospital's medical activities, and closely coordinating with the board and medical staff in achieving and maintaining the required standards of medical performance.
Comment: Key verbs in achieving this end result are "monitoring" and "coordinating."

Accountability IV. Allocation of Resources: Ensures the provision of health care services at prices the community can afford by the acquisition and utilization of available resources and the development of improved techniques and practices.
Comment: The action words deal with marshalling appropriate resources and operating efficiently.

Accountability V. Crisis Resolution: Fosters a smoothly functioning, efficient operation through timely and effective resolution of disturbances as they occur.
Comment: This is self-explanatory.

Accountability VI. Compliance with Regulation: Ensures compliance with all regulations governing health care delivery and the rules of accrediting bodies by continually monitoring the operation and its programs, and initiating changes where required.
Comment: The key action words are "monitoring" and "initiating changes."

Accountability VII. Promotion of the Hospital: Encourages the integration of the hospital with the community and a favorable attitude among its various publics by establishing and maintaining effective communication and public relations programs.
Comment: This emphasizes the use of communications to achieve the end result, presumably through means beyond conventional PR efforts.

The fulfillment of each of these accountabilities could never be verified if measures reflecting achievement were not articulated. This is a step where the evaluation process could easily stall. Measures should be identified and agreed upon by the CEO and the governing board. Only after this has been done should standards be attached to the measures. Measures are the yardsticks to be used in determining accomplishment of accountabilities.

As an example, the measure for the high-jump is inches/feet or meters; for the 100-yard dash the measure would be hundredths of a second. The standard for the world record holder in the high-jump is 7' 7 1/4" while the standard for the world record holder of the 100-yard dash is 0:09.1 seconds. The standard for qualifying for the Olympics in the high-jump is something less than the world record. As a matter of fact, each high-jumper has a different standard.

There may be measures that are applicable to one CEO's accountability and not to another's. Also, there are vast differences between institutions which would dictate that the standards for a CEO's job in one hospital would differ markedly in another hospital. This is why it is so important for a governing board and its incumbent chief executive officer to agree in advance about the latter's accountabilities.

Assigning Measures to Accountabilities

In developing the evaluative process, the major initiative normally should come from the incumbent CEO. If, however, a governing board is looking for a CEO and wishes to draft measures on its own to enhance its recruiting effort, consultative help probably should be sought. This will clarify the mutual expectations of the governing board and the prospective chief executive officer and can, in the future, be used as an objective means of appraising the CEO's performance.

Examples of measures which represent areas of activity in which standards could be established for the previously listed accountabilities are:

Accountability I. Planning and Organization

Possible areas of measurement:

- *Effectiveness of the planning process*
- *CEO's input to board decision-making*
- *Community's perception of needs being met*

Accountability II. Achieving Hospital Objectives

Possible area of measurement:

- *Institutional goal achievement record*

Accountability III. Quality of Medical Services

Possible areas of measurement:

- *Quality care reports and followup activity*
- *Development of new/improved patient care programs.*
- *Mix of physicians by age, clinical background, etc.*
- *Effectiveness of medical staff organization*

Accountability IV. Allocation of Resources

Possible areas of measurement:

- *Cost containment effectiveness*
- *Budget performance*
- *HAS reports, comparison with other institutions*
- *Paid liability claims against the institution*
- *New/expanded revenue sources developed*

Accountability V. Crisis Resolution

Possible areas of measurement:

- *Number of problems*
- *Number of problems resolved effectively*
- *Review of systems developed as a result of conflict*

Accountability VI. Compliance with Regulation

Possible area of measurement:

- *Regulations not complied with*

Accountability VII. Promotion of the Hospital

Possible areas of measurement:

- *Public exposure*
- *Public relations*
- *Communication efforts/effectiveness*

A Personal Accountability

The CEO should add self-accountability assuring career-long competence. If he or she does not, the governing board might impose such an accountability as protection for the institution. Such an accountability might read:

Takes a leadership role in educational programs, including participation both as a teacher and as a student, to promote career-long competence in professional pursuits.

Possible areas of management:

- *Extent of teaching responsibilities*
- *Useful educational meetings attended*
- *ACHA advancement/recertification*

One might react to such a list of measurement areas by saying, "So what?" Certainly, one can't gauge achievement of these measures any better than the accountability itself. The point is that the measures should be developed as representing the areas of activity through which the CEO successfully accomplishes the specific end result. Only then should explicit standards be developed. It is important that the standards define and clarify the extent and direction in which the chief executive should be channeling efforts. The board/CEO agreement will stipulate that through these standards the end result will be achieved. It is impossible to set standards for every ounce of energy a CEO expends. This should not be the objective. The governing board and the CEO will agree that the negotiated standards, if accomplished as agreed, would signify that the job is being done.

Setting Standards

It is desirable to settle on a standard which, in the board's and incumbent CEO's opinion, would represent fully adequate performance. This is a level of performance which reflects that the job is being done in a way the governing board wants it to be done and in the way the institution needs it to be done. At performance evaluation time, bad marks or "brownie points" can be calculated in degrees of deviation from the fully adequate performance standard.

For the seven accountabilities for which measures have previously been suggested, standards can now be developed. It must be emphasized that the standards listed below are examples only. They are written to stimulate development of appropriate standards in specific situations. Areas of measurement, likewise, are only examples.

Accountability I. Planning and Organizing

    1. Measure: Effectiveness of the Planning Process

      Suggested Fully Adequate Standard:

- *The established planning process, including long-range plan, development of program elements, institutional management and departmental goals, and budgeting is carried out in a one-year continuing cycle, which includes annual review and endorsement by the medical staff and approval of the governing board*

    2. Measure: Input to Board Decision-Making

      Suggested Fully Adequate Standards:

- *The board is not forced by external pressure to initiate or disband any program, or conversely, all new programs approved by the board are generated through the planning process*
- *Annual private poll of trustees concerning their confidence in making policy decisions is conducted, revealing 80% of the board is satisfied*

3. Measure: Community's Perception of Needs Being Met

Suggested Fully Adequate Standards:

- *Routine contributions to the hospital (provided it is a tax-exempt organization) exceed the previous year's level of contributions*
- *Impressions of the institution's response to community needs by local and state health department officials plus local and state health planners are generally positive. This feedback should be solicited by the chairman of the governing board*

Comment: Overt responses from community service agencies and city-county governments might also be appropriate to obtain. The acceptable level of positive reactions from these individuals might be measured as a percentage of total reactions if the governing board and chief executive officer desire to go that far.

Accountability II. Achieving Hospital Objectives

1. Measure: Institutional Goal Achievement Record

Suggested Fully Adequate Standards:

- *Achievement of 80% of institutional and management goals set each year*
- *Achievement of 80% of all departmental goals*

Comment: The assumption is that the goals mentioned are attached to organization subdivisions, while the program elements in the first accountability standard above deal with clinical services and programs cutting across organizational lines. A third standard might be:

- *Year-round planning cycle is adhered to by the administration*

Comment: This differs from the first standard above which emphasizes medical staff and governing board approval. This standard deals with process.

Accountability III. Quality of Medical Services

1. Measure: Quality Care Reports

Suggested Fully Adequate Standards:

- *A medical staff care report is rendered at each board meeting and each executive committee meeting*
- *Decisions made in response to problem areas identified in quality care reports are implemented within the time frame designated 80% of the time*

2. Measure: Development of New/Improved Patient Care Programs

Suggested Fully Adequate Standard:

- *Achievement of 70% of the program elements contained in the long-range plan within designated time frame*

3. Measure: Physician Mix

Suggested Fully Adequate Standards:

- *As part of the continuing planning process, a study of the mix of physicians by age, clinical background, etc., is carried out annually with specific recruitment and retention goals set as a result*
- *Goals established for recruitment and retention are accomplished in 80% of the instances within the established time frames*

4. Measure: Medical Staff Organization

Suggested Fully Adequate Standards:

- *A composite average attendance percentage of all physicians in all committees connected with medical staff activities is 60%*

Comment: This standard does not necessarily reflect effectiveness — it assumes that the more participation by physicians, the better the medical staff operates — and could be fallacious. However, it is better than nothing.

- *75% of the actions taken by the medical executive committee relate to major policy determination or changes in regulations and/or are reportable as such to the governing board*

Comment: Here, the function of the medical executive committee as a policy body as opposed to a "chowder and marching society" is emphasized. It is also good for the medical staff to understand such standards – but it's the CEO who must be facilitative.

Accountability IV. Allocation of Resources

1. Measure: Cost Containment

   Suggested Fully Adequate Standards:

   - *Cost containment goals are set for each department in the institution and are met 80% of the time*
   - *Aggregate cost containment results equal $100,000 (example only) each year*

2. Measure: Budget Performance

   Suggested Fully Adequate Standards:

   - *Budget is approved by the governing board prior to the beginning of the fiscal year*
   - *Expenses do not deviate from budget by more than 2% when adjusted for occupancy fluctuation*

Comment: Some boards may wish to establish a bottom line standard.

3. Measure: HAS Report

   Suggested Fully Adequate Standards:

   - *A comparison with HAS reports is revealed to the board on a semi-annual basis, together with appropriate analysis*
   - *By mutual consent, goals for improved performance in HAS indicators are negotiated annually by the governing board and the chief executive officer; achievement of 80% of the goals is expected*

4. Measure: New/Expanded Revenue Sources Developed

   Suggested Fully Adequate Standard:

   - *At least one new source of revenue (more than $10,000) is generated annually which does not affect the cost of patient care, but rather is recoverable from non-inpatient sources*

Comment: This kind of standard, of course, could vary considerably depending on individual circumstances.

5. Measure: Liability Claims

Suggested Fully Adequate Standard:

- *Claims experience for period under review is less than previous period*

Accountability V. Crisis Resolution

1. Measure: Number of Problems

Suggested Fully Adequate Standard:

- *No more than three internally generated problems requiring board action occur each year*

Comment: Examples are strikes, disciplinary actions on groups of employees or physicians, etc., serious problems in accounts payable in which creditors' lawsuits are brought against the institution, etc.

2. Measure: Number of Problems Resolved Effectively

Suggested Fully Adequate Standard:

- *A specific section of the CEO's annual report to the board deals with the CEO's impressions on problems facing the institution (not necessarily internally generated) which were solved effectively*

3. Measure: Review of Systems Developed to Resolve Conflict

Suggested Fully Adequate Standard:

- *In the annual report to the board, the chief executive officer reviews systems in place to resolve conflict, reports on the activities within those previously defined systems and makes comments as to their relative effectiveness by comparing statistics against previously agreed upon numbers*

Comment: Examples are grievance procedures, union contract negotiations, EEOC actions, unemployment compensation claims, worker's compensation,

OSHA penalties, counseling activities, boiler inspection reports, malpractice record, physicians' due process appeals, etc.

Accountability VI. Compliance with Regulation

1. Measure: Regulations Complied With

Suggested Fully Adequate Standards:

- *Full licensure 100% of the time*
- *JCAH accreditation maintained*
- *CEO reports to board on all inspection/accreditation reports, submits plan for followup and reports followup on a routine basis*

Comment: A fully adequate performance standard should normally require no less than full accreditation by the JCAH. There are institutions, however, where this might be impossible and a different standard would be appropriate.

Accountability VII. Promotion of the Hospital

1. Measure: Public Exposure

Suggested Fully Adequate Standards:

- *Twelve local speeches delivered by the CEO to an aggregate crowd of 1,000*
- *Six appearances by the CEO on television and radio programs*

Comment: This kind of standard, since it deals with public exposure, does not deal with the quality of exposure. Another standard might involve public exposure by other members of the hospital family. Again, the numbers are negotiable.

2. Measure: Public Reaction

Suggested Fully Adequate Standards:

- *Answers to patient questionnaires meet predetermined percentage standards*
- *Specific feedback from consumer groups and consumer surrogates with whom the hospital deals (HEW, Medicare and Medicaid, Blue Cross, etc.) indicates general satisfaction with institutional performance in specific relationships with the groups.*

Comment: The governing board and the chief executive might establish actual numbers here. It should be noted that when accountabilities are subdivided into measures and standards, subjective opinions can be made more confidently because of the narrow range covered by the standard. There's nothing wrong with someone else's opinion being used in a performance evaluation so long as it relates to a specific standard. The way someone feels is a fact, after all. A "feeling" on a narrowly framed standard is much more likely to be objective than a scatter shot opinion of a person in toto.

3. Measure: Communications Efforts and Effectiveness

Suggested Fully Adequate Standards:

- *A subjective review of internal and external communications by the development committee of the governing board is made and compared to previously established goals on written communications*
- *Response from the reader population is ascertained by:*

    a. *spontaneous feedback*
    b. *opinion poll which indicates level of satisfaction equal to a predetermined percentage*

Comment: After one or two attempts, acceptable parameters could be established. Public relations prizes awarded for the hospital's publications would be another way of measuring effectiveness, though certainly not the only, or best, way.

In connection with the author's added accountability on assuring lifelong competence, the emphasis rests on the effectiveness of the educational process undertaken in the self-development of the CEO.

Measures:

Performance as preceptor to students

Performance in lectures to groups

Participation in journal clubs and other in-house education activities

Speeches to hospital-related groups

Services on commissions and committees with health services and planning objectives

Standards should be as follows:

1. Measure: Performance as Preceptor

Suggested Fully Adequate Standard:

- *CEO is acceptable to a recognized graduate program to serve as preceptor*

2. Measure: Performance in Lectures

   Suggested Fully Adequate Standard:

   - *Group feedback — anonymous poll indicates 75% of the attendees are satisfied*

3. Measure: Participation in Journal Club and Other In-house Educational Activities

   Suggested Fully Adequate Standards:

   - *Regular participation — attends 60% of the designated meetings*
   - *Participates in six employee orientation meetings a year. Teaches hospital supervisors one six-hour course on leadership with no attendance requirements — 75% of enrollees attend 50% of the lectures*

4. Measure: Speeches to Hospital-related Groups

   Suggested Fully Adequate Standard:

   - *CEO is invited to speak to one health-related group external to own hospital during a year's time*

5. Measure: Services on Commissions and Committees

   Suggested Fully Adequate Standard:

   - *Serves on at least one such group at all times*

A Word About Goals . . .

It should be noted that achieving the end results of accountabilities meets the continuing expectations placed upon the job-holder by the governing board. Implicit in all jobs is the need to improve.

Improvement in performance of a job is accomplished through achieving goals which should not be interpreted in the same context as achievement of accountabilities. Thus, standards for specific accountabilities may well include establishment of a specific goal. For instance, if a standard stipulates that the number of days revenue in accounts receivable is 75, and the governing board and the chief executive arrive at an understanding that this could and should be improved, a specific goal to reduce that number to 60 days may be in order. Achievement of this goal would impact positively on the individual's performance for that period of time — thus more brownie points.

It should be pointed out that achievement of a goal tends to raise the standard of performance for a given accountability. This phenomenon is exemplified by athletes who are performing against standards today which, in some instances, were unattainable goals for their great grandfathers in the nineteenth century. The accepted standard today was an out-of-reach goal of yesterday. This is the nature of a system which emphasizes achievement of day-to-day end results plus goals, the latter serving to elevate the day-to-day standards in the long run.

The Process

Obviously, the entire governing board should not engage in negotiations to establish a CEO's accountabilities, measures and standards. The task should be assigned to no more than a three-person group, the chairman of the board being one. An understanding of the process is important for all involved. The same individuals should participate in the performance evaluation itself. An accounting of the process should be made to the full governing body periodically.

These guidelines are not intended to be prescriptive. Expected performance can be defined within understandable limits so that an objective performance appraisal can later be carried out. Having negotiated standards in advance allows performance of the individual concerned to be measured with ease. In itself, this process tends to improve performance. This is the object of any sort of evaluation. As the parties to the evaluative process become more sophisticated, performance at other levels might be defined, clarifying the difference between marginal and superior performance.

A definite schedule for developing the job description, accountabilities, measures and standards should be established, the board being advised, through appropriate mechanisms, on the progress being made. A continuing cycle is established so that review and salary decisions are made at predetermined dates. There should also be a time set aside to evaluate and update the CEO's accountabilities, measures and standards themselves, as distinct from the process heretofore described. This should be done separate from the evaluation.

The CEO should furnish written input concerning his or her performance to the chairman of the governing board. This would follow the format above, with the CEO simply giving the facts. Based on these facts, the evaluators on the governing board would make a determination. Misunderstandings, before and after the evaluation, can be almost totally eliminated this way. Uncertainties in the relationships between the governing board and the chief executive officer of the hospital will disappear, effectiveness will be enhanced, and mutual satisfaction will prevail.

In those rare instances where the process causes dissatisfaction, a well understood and amicable disassociation has a better chance of taking place. Whatever the outcome, understanding and acceptance based on objectivity will have resulted. The motivational rewards for all involved will be plentiful.

Notes

1. ACHA Task Force V. *Principles of Appointment and Tenure of the Executive Officers*. Chicago: American College of Hospital Administrators, 1973.

2. *The Position of the Hospital Chief Executive*. Chicago: American College of Hospital Administrators, 1976.

3. *Accountability Management Performance Appraisal Manual: Hillcrest Medical Center, April 1970*. Dallas: Edward N. Hay & Associates, 1970.

12

The Lessons of a Profession

Everett A. Johnson

Everett A. Johnson, Ph.D., is Professor and Director, Graduate Health Administration Program, Georgia State University, Atlanta.

For more than two decades hospital administrator-watching has been an order of business in my daily work. I have observed both the student and the practitioner, as worker and boss, follower and leader. These observations have spanned hospital changes from the institutional freedoms of the fifties to the disciplines and restraints of the seventies.

When prospective students for graduate programs in hospital administration ask questions about the life and work involved in the administrative profession, they want to know exactly what work is done, and what quality of life they can expect as an administrator. Too often, unasked questions in the student's mind concern happiness, contentment, fulfillment, and service. Answers to these questions, if asked, would be difficult, because they are personal. However, my twenty years of administrator-watching may be useful to potential colleagues in describing how the career hospital administrator feels.

An Administrator's World

The student first needs to understand that an administrator's world is his own. Its agonies and ecstasies are totally private. His personality is unique, singular, and beyond the complete understanding of another. He is at once both a man of silence and public utterance, of motivation and apathy, of straight-forwardness and confounding of prediction in judgment and action.

A hospital administrator is a decision-maker, a risk taker and an intellectual about the good of society. He is a person of love, concern and tenderness — a pragmatist who molds, moves, and decides other peoples' futures.

Beyond the human quality of the man, an administrator is a mixture of competence and incompetence, of great ability and skill and maddening blind spots and insensitivities. As a hospital administrator he knows much and yet very little. He is a generalist among a mass of specialists.

Reprinted by permission from *Hospital Administration,* Summer 1972, pages 9-17. Copyright 1972 by the Foundation of the American College of Healthcare Executives. All rights reserved.

He is seen by some as an earth-shaker, by others as a definer of goals or as a busybody without accomplishments. He can be both devil and saint, simultaneously or over a period of time, as well as by issue or through the relationship of perceiver to hospital.

A Variety of Expectations

A society is a potpourri of expectations. Organizations function as vehicles of expression for personal worth, for identification purposes, for masking of hidden failures with accolades of public success, and as a raison d'être for making life worth living.

A hospital serves many expectations for many people: It serves the young nurse who has not found her own niche in life and is privately working out her scheme of usefulness, the mature nurse who is complete in her family life and reaching for greater goals by serving man, the newly-certified medical specialist, sure of his skills and sense of the world, and the experienced senior physician, aware of the limits of the science of medicine and the limits of those who care about the future of medicine and its total usefulness.

Working with Trustees

Since an administrator directly serves the expectations of hospital trustees, their desires must also be measured. In working with this group, he finds pressures abounding, pushing and demanding new programs and conveniences from the hospital. He finds that administrative life is a constant series of changes, one after another—the only predictable point in his career.

On the other hand, the administrator will find that most trustees do not really desire change. Their position typically will be that if the administrator can find the money, persuade all key parties that it is a worthwhile improvement and keep all dissonant voices to a murmur then he may proceed. If the stakes begin to rise—and particularly if the change appears to be generating active opposition from the medical staff—then the administrator must adjust, delay, modify or postpone to a more appropriate time. The student will later learn that most necessary fundamental improvements in patient care have floundered on this particular shoal.

In previous times, as well as today, it has always been an article of faith with hospital administration that boards of trustees are necessary and highly useful. When the student sees local government hospitals with patronage and other political problems, he will know that they are a less workable system than one with a board of trustees. Looking at the rigidities of operation that exist in state and federal hospitals, the student similarly will be disenchanted.

Seeing Trustees' Motivations

When he sees many private hospitals with trustees continually involved in daily operations, he will be aghast. He will wonder, and wonder again, about the notion of trusteeship. As student life fades into first active administrative work the individual will need to reinforce his faith that hospital trustees typically are motivated by good intentions and seriousness of purposes. He will learn to suffer privately the understanding that dedication and intelligence are no substitute for experience, specific knowledge, and appropriate behavior.

When the new administrator experiences the hospital boardroom becoming a center ring for local power struggles, he will see how rarely patient care is a primary consideration. When the local physicians close ranks and lay it on the line, he will generally watch the local élite quickly ride off into the hills. Too often he will see the chief administrator, left at the pass to cover the retreat, get wiped out.

The fledgling administrator must learn the rationality and irrationality of an organized medical staff and its constituent parts, the physicians of the community. He will learn that whenever change occurs in a hospital, physicians will typically be slow to accept it, require personal attention to insure understanding and generally offer comments about how to spend hospital funds more profitably. Medical staffs almost never believe that new boilers are a necessity; they believe that administrative offices are mostly personal aggrandizement, that too much space goes into storage areas and that home-type ranges ought to be satisfactory in the main kitchen.

The frustrations of unreasonable opinions need to be counterbalanced with an understanding that the physician's life and interest spins around clinical concerns. His great sense of assurance and independence, his lack of awareness that medical care is now a process involving many people rather than only himself and his unwillingness to accept the expertise of administrators will block or make difficult an easy accommodation to change.

When administrative innovations aimed at improving medical affairs in hospitals are tried, the rigidities of attitude and behavior of trustees and physicians are joined. Yet, the administrator's future will be filled with one pressure after another for using the hospital to force adjustments in traditional medical practices.

Administration of a Medical Staff

Past administrator-watching has taught me that only foolish or independently wealthy chief executive officers have ever seriously believed that they could direct and administer a medical staff. Even though most administrators have been concerned seriously with medical administrative practices that abuse patients, they have been unable to do more than skirmish on the fringes of concern.

Conformity and endless continuation of these existing practices have been part of past administrative life. The unvarnished lesson, that the organizational triad of trustee, medical staff and administration is the best way to run a hospital, is a myth. It is a fair weather device that quickly buckles under a light breeze.

When trustees hire and set conditions of employment for administrators and when physicians direct the hospital's financial future by controlling patient admissions and dismissals, it is only the starry-eyed neophyte that believes all three parts are equal. In a major hospital crisis, when stakes are high and both physicians and trustees make a hospital momentarily their primary concern, administrative leverage is lost.

In situations where physicians squeeze a board of trustees, the chief executive officer learns that the usual outcome is for trustees to accede to physician pressure. Trustees do not have the daily administrative experiences which lead to understanding the nuances of hospital issues of deciding how much of a gamble can be run with some safety and the importance of alternative outcomes. When one administrator must try to hold a board of trustees in line against an assault of fifty or two-hundred and fifty physicians it is understandable for the trustees to opt for the prestige and goodwill of medicine and to ignore the reasoned judgement of their employee, the administrator.

A young hospital administrator will probably learn another lesson: only in rare circumstances does a board of trustees really exercise control for the quality of medicine practiced in the hospital. Early in his career he will discover that this is a joint operation between medical staff and hospital administration and that this state of affairs bothers physicians. Not that trustees don't understand or aren't part of the picture, but rather administrative types have a nasty habit of recognizing medical problems being swept under the rug or remembering which closets hold which skeletons.

An Administrative Dilemma

The hospital-based, full time medical staff specialist generally requires special advice for the inexperienced administrator. To wit, when one of these medical types is quite competent and has a personality like a friendly local car salesman, it is almost a guaranteed tamper-proof administrative dilemma. Older administrative heads know for sure, that if it comes down to a take it or leave it situation, the medical staff will choose to support one of their own — and the patient be damned. While trustees may get indigestion over these problems, they typically fold their tents and accede to the wishes of the medical staff rather than take the bull by the horns; and that's what an administrator is left with — a bum steer.

In the tumult of daily administrative-medical interaction, a fundamental perspective can easily be lost. The administrator should remember to respect physicians as individuals who are delightful, well-meaning, hard-working people, who carry some of the toughest loads in our society.

Too often today, progress toward improving patient welfare depends upon an unusually competent chief executive officer. When he leaves an administrative post, the drive for improvement in his institution and the skills and the acceptance he has developed necessary for accomplishing that improvement are lost. Because of the subtleties in medical staff and trustee relationships, the succeeding administrator will spend several years in developing a position strong enough to win the successes of his predecessor. The need for hospital administration to achieve a more secure status was once covered in a remark by Walter Lippmann, "The genius of a good leader is to leave behind him a situation which common sense, without the grace of genius, can deal with successfully."

Frustration is the handmaiden of hospital administrators. The daily grist of hospital operation is often shackled by stodginess and the mediocrity of its institutional setting and structure. However, the administrator's status is reflective of the practices of our times and the restraints all organizations tolerate as part of a society with multiple inter-relationships.

Use of Emotional Understanding

The prospective student for hospital administration at some point will need to sort out and develop an understanding of the basic relation between emotion and intellectual understanding and conceptualization. In many administrative activities, demands of the situation seem to contra-indicate a successful assimilation of both styles of operation. Unfortunately most nonadministrative people experience a hospital organization emotionally. They become irked when, upon asking housekeeping to move furniture or maintenance to replace a light bulb, it is not done immediately. When a nurse errs on a medication, a physician's reaction often is anger, rather than an effort to help figure out what went wrong and how it can be avoided tomorrow.

Too often, a physician, department director or other person arrives at the administrator's office door in a state of agitation, because he is reacting to some activity in the organization. These people express a sense of justice, righteousness, and an impeccable logic on their side with a ready-made conclusion that hospital operation is stupid, inept, and poorly run.

To be rational and logical at this time is to create even stronger feelings. An administrator has the dilemma of figuring out the cause of a problem, yet he must respect another person's feelings, no matter how irrational or unwarranted. He must react to those feelings without losing control of his emotions and still find a way to explain and regain their support of the organization. To have feelings and sympathy, without losing one's own emotional control, is a never-ending administrative struggle.

The Skill of Rapport with Others

At some point in an administrative career one must develop the aptitude of concealing one's own administrative skills and maintaining rapport with other people in the organization. It is not an easily developed habit.

The administrator's use of self-control and intellectual abilities to handle feelings and emotions of others assures that there will be many times when, at day's end, he will finally turn off the lights, lock the door, leave the office, and go home — low in energy and convinced that he is mad to remain in hospital administration.

Probably the most difficult administrative skill is the art of delegation. Habits, psychological needs, self-discipline, ability to work with others, and individual analytical abilities are some of the personal factors that affect one's ability to use this mode of administration. As size of organization and complexity of operation increase, an administrator's time span is outgrown in his attempt to expand his efforts centrally to control all important, and sometimes unimportant, decision-making in the hospital.

Delegation involves accepting responsibility for other people's judgment and abilities. It means the administrator's acceptance of a quality of work that may be somewhat less than his own, because he was not free to totally handle a particular matter. A lack of flexibility and difference in others' thought processes also causes an instinctive rejection of another's work.

In the world at large, adequate administrative delegation of work seems to be the rarest of skills. It is discussed in graduate programs in management, but it is largely left unpracticed. Yet, its essence is to be able to delegate in situations of much stress and confusion. Probably the only way delegation can be mastered is in the hustle and bustle of daily administrative events.

What then is the answer to a potential administrator's unspoken question: "What are reasonable expectations in a hospital administration career for happiness, contentment, fulfillment, and service?" The answer lies within another question: "What kind of life do you think you will need to live to be happy at forty years of age?"

If you seek fame or fortune, hospital administration is a poor choice. If you need a strong sense of security, a well-structured work situation and some spare time to contemplate the world at large, you should look elsewhere.

Lessons of Administrative Profession

In hospital administration, happiness is having more work than time, greater demands than ability to respond completely, and a sense of continually helping other people. Happiness is to enjoy painting a wall at home for immediate satisfaction, because instant accomplishments are almost never experienced at work. Fulfillment is knowing that at the end of a career you will have lived and served as you would have wished throughout a lifetime of work.

The lessons of this profession are never found in textbooks. To experienced hospital administrators, these caveats have been lived at one or another place and time. To trustees, physicians and friendly psychiatrists, they will appear as one person's effort to rationalize and work out totally personal struggles. It is in truth, though, a message of realism for the coming generation of hospital administrators: an invitation to join the fray—to do so with their eyes open and their minds informed about the real world in which a great profession works. It is a profession facing major problems, coping with some, failing with others—but sure of a demanding, exciting time ahead.

As hospital administrators, our issue is to move from being operators of support systems for medical care into becoming managers of medical care systems. I believe it can happen. No other health profession is more central to our developing notions about the total medical care process than today's hospital administration.

Today's Administrative Milieu

To move from today into tomorrow, hospital administrators must now accept the responsibilities and perils of leading a medical staff, trustees, hospital staff, and community that must be led before tomorrow arrives. Administrators now face a time to stand up while the house is counted. They have passed the day when boards of trustees could be looked to for local leadership, and administrators could gracefully pass the buck. Today, the buck is in the hands of hospital administration, and because it is there, sufficient leverage exists for major accomplishments.

If today's administrative milieu appears foreboding, frustrating, and turbulent, it should be remembered that the Hellespont could only be crossed by vigorous swimming.

A Gratifying Commitment

Our sense of well-being and happiness as hospital administrators in the tumult of today was said in Kahlil Gibran's *The Prophet* when he wrote about the work: "Then a ploughman said, speak to us of work. And he answered saying: work is love made visible. And if you cannot work with love but only with distaste, it is better that you should leave your work and sit at the gate of the temple and take alms of those who work with joy. For if you bake bread with indifference, you bake a bitter bread that feeds but half man's hunger. And if you grudge the crushing of the grapes, your grudge distils a poison in the wine. And if you sing though as angels, and love not the singing, you muffle man's ears to the voices of the day and the voices of the night."

Talent, commitment, and ability are needed in hospital administration. If a young person believes that it is important in life to be stretched to the toes, to strive to touch the untouchable, then join us—now, and for the days ahead. But do it with the point of view once expressed by Martin Luther, "If I rest, I rust."

Medical Staff

In selection 13, "Ten Guidelines for Success of Hospital-Physician Partnerships," Stephen M. Shortell discusses what he characterizes as the third generation of hospital-physician relationships and the challenges they pose to hospital managers and medical staff. John R. Ball addresses a critical issue in selection 14, "Credentialing Versus Performance—A New Look at Old Problems." Of all the problems that confront hospital managers, credentialing is among the most important, and the most difficult.

Kathy M. Brubaker discusses the potential benefits and synergism that could result from nursing input into physician credentialing in selection 15, "Credentialing of Medical Staff: The Nursing Department's Role." This is a role not likely to be readily accepted by the typical hospital medical staff. In selection 16, "The Hospital Medical Staff of 1994," William R. Fifer predicts 15 attributes of the medical staff of the future. Although admittedly only a forecast, it provides much food for thought.

13

Ten Guidelines for Success of Hospital-Physician Partnerships

Stephen M. Shortell

Stephen M. Shortell, Ph.D., is A.C. Buehler Distinguished Professor of Hospital and Health Services Management, Program in Hospital and Health Services Management, Kellogg Graduate School of Management, Northwestern University, Evanston, Illinois.

Cost containment pressures, increased competition and changing public expectations are spurring the rapid growth of partnerships between hospitals and physician group practices.

These partnerships are entering a third generation that poses special challenges to hospital managers and physicians. They can meet these challenges successfully, however, if they follow certain guidelines.

Three Generations

The first generation of such partnerships existed from about the 1960s through the early 1970s. They were created to build and manage physician office buildings, sometimes with the hospital subsidizing the start-up of physicians' practices. The objective was to attract competent physicians to the hospital's staff when physicians were in relatively short supply in relation to the number of hospitals desiring their services. In most cases, physicians were able to negotiate attractive deals.

The second generation of partnerships, occurring from about 1975 to the present, has involved hospital-physician sponsored ambulatory care centers, health maintenance organizations and preferred provider organizations. As the physician surplus in many specialties and locales has grown, both hospitals and physician group practices have had to fight to maintain or enhance market share. This has led to various forms of joint ventures. However, it's important to note that these have involved a relatively comprehensive range of fairly traditional healthcare services.

The third generation of partnerships, just beginning to emerge, involves more specialized relationships centering around specific market niches. Examples include home care, retirement centers, sports medicine, diagnostic imaging, renal dialysis, health promotion, birthing centers and even non-health-related activities.

New Issues

The newer forms of partnerships pose significant technical, political and cultural issues. Because hospitals are diversifying into areas in which they have little experience, the technical issues of how to do something become important. At the same time, political issues involving the allocation of power, authority, and responsibility loom large. Underlying both of these concerns is the extent to which the new ventures require departure from established norms, beliefs and traditional ways of doing business. In brief, they require creation of a new culture within which hospitals and physicians can function.

The ability to effectively deal with these technical, political and cultural issues will in large part determine the hospital's ability to sustain its competitive advantage over the long run.

Sustainability is the key factor in successful hospital-physician partnerships of the future. For most of the new diversified lines of service, the barriers to entry are relatively low. Further, these ventures primarily involve "low-tech" technology that is easily duplicated by competing organizations. The factor that is less easily duplicated is a strong hospital-physician partnership that can adapt to changing circumstances over time to maintain its early competitive advantage.

Ten Guidelines

Based on existing research, national demonstration programs and firsthand experience, here are 10 guidelines — some of which run counter to conventional wisdom — that can help promote more successful hospital-physician partnerships:

1. Centrality to Mission

The success of new hospital-physician ventures can be directly linked to the degree to which they are central to the hospital's mission and strategic plan. Where this linkage is weak, the parties involved are less likely to deal with the difficult problems that arise. For example, among 53 group practices sponsored jointly by hospitals and medical staffs and funded by the Robert

Wood Johnson Foundation, those practices seen as more central to the hospital's mission were significantly better able to sustain themselves after foundation support ended. These practices also had a more positive financial impact on hospital operations. Centrality to the hospital's mission also helps to promote synergy across programs. This can greatly increase the number of patients and consumers brought into the hospital's network.

2. Competitive Analysis

A venture is more likely to succeed if a hospital and physician group practice jointly examine the likely short-term and long-term responses of competitors. This analysis involves examining not only current competitors but also future new entrants.

An analysis of a venture's competitors should focus on current market share, financial strengths, expertise and experience, and the ability to respond rapidly to change. This analysis ought to answer six questions:

- What is the market share for our new services and who are likely competitors?

- Is the business opportunity consistent with our mission?

- What impact will it have on our capital position?

- What contribution is it likely to make toward our share of the in-patient market?

- To what extent does the opportunity enable the organization to leverage human and technical resources it already has?

- To what degree do new opportunities provide for risk sharing with participants other than management?

3. Assess Strengths

Both hospitals and physicians need to be candid in assessing their strengths and weaknesses. This should be done on both an overall basis and on an individual departmental or program-by-program basis. Areas to examine include:

- Financial health, both in terms of cash flow and capital position.

- Availability of necessary expertise and experience to launch new services. This includes the strengths and weaknesses of the institution's management development program because successful new partnerships rely heavily on communication and conflict management skills.

- The quality and relevance of existing information systems.

- Are the reward systems of the organization appropriate? Do new kinds of financial and nonfinancial incentives need to be considered? Are team or group incentives required?

- Is the current organizational structure appropriate for launching or supporting new ventures? What changes may need to be made and how easily can they be made.

- The quality and continuity of top level managers is important. Frequent leadership turnover at the top of an organization hurts new program development, particularly the organization's ability to sustain programs over time.

Specific issues relating to the medical staff also should be examined, including:

- The specialty mix of the staff. Does an appropriate balance exist between specialists and generalists?

- Age of the staff, particularly in terms of the percentage of admissions accounted for by physicians at or below the median staff age.

- Board certification and related qualifications.

- Interest and involvement in teaching activities.

- Ability to recruit and retain desired physicians.

- The quality and continuity of medical staff leadership.

- The effectiveness of the medical staff's processes and systems for decision-making.

4. Right Incentive

Among the 53 group practices mentioned above, those with built-in financial incentives for productivity were more successful than those that didn't have incentives. The incentives varied depending on the age, specialty mix and goals of the practice.

There is a need for hospitals and physicians to openly explore what each wants from the partnership—both short-term and long-term—and then design a system of rewards that best meets these needs. It's important to remember that short-term productivity and financial gains made at the expense of quality or convenience of care will damage long-term viability. This is particularly true in highly competitive and rapidly changing markets where consumers have a wide variety of services from which to choose.

It's also important for hospital administrators and physicians to understand each other's values before designing incentives.

In pragmatic terms, each party must answer the question of "What's in it for me?" While financial incentives are important, however, the more successful partnerships don't ignore the quality and convenience considerations.

5. Autonomy/Integration

Successful hospital-physician partnerships are built on both physicians' need for autonomy and the hospital's need for integration and accountability.

In healthcare, physicians' need for clinical autonomy is well recognized. But successful partnerships also require physicians to have some degree of business or managerial autonomy as well.

Physicians need to have some understanding and significant involvement in the management of the partnership with the freedom to indicate where personnel, purchasing, staffing, and budgetary policies and practices may need to be different from the hospital's experience with delivering inpatient acute care.

Many physicians have some experience in these new business areas from their own office practices. This experience needs to be recognized and drawn on.

At the same time, the hospital needs to protect its side of the investment and ensure that its objectives are met. In working with physicians this is best done not by exerting close supervisory control—as might be done with a hospital department—but through lateral relationships involving physician group leaders in high-level policy and decisionmaking activities affecting the partnership and the hospital's future.

This accomplishes four important things. First, it provides physicians with the opportunity to continually educate the hospital about the joint venture. Second, it enables physicians to learn more about the overall strategic plans of the hospital. Third, it provides an opportunity for physicians to suggest an expanded role for the joint venture in the hospital's future plans. And fourth, it provides a forum for managing conflict in a constructive fashion.

6. Information Systems

A partnership has a greater chance of succeeding when information systems are available to provide the parties involved with relevant data for making key decisions. The information needs will obviously vary for different partnerships. The most frequently needed data, however, include information on hospital admissions, visits, revenue, ancillary services used by the provider, sources of referral to and from the practice, accounts receivable, cash flow, third-party payer breakdowns, waiting time for an appointment, waiting time in a physician's office, time spent with patients, missed appointments, patient satisfaction and quality of care indicators.

Accurate and timely information provides both managers and physicians with a common base upon which differences of opinion or judgement can be more appropriately addressed. With these data, departures from desired norms can be more readily corrected. An effective information system also promotes mutual understanding.

7. Market Analysis

The claim is frequently made that the new competitive environment requires complex market analysis. This has become so much a part of the conventional wisdom that to challenge it appears foolish or heretical. Yet there is little evidence to support this assertion. For example, only a few of the 53 hospital-medical staff group practices cited earlier did any market analysis. And those that did were no more successful than those that didn't. In fact, many of the more successful practices did little formal market analysis. Other factors—such as physician leadership, physician recruitment and retention, incentives, and designing appropriate autonomy and integrating mechanisms—were more important to their success.

Market analysis is important, but it should be kept relatively simple. For example, existing data and focus groups can be very helpful tools for managers and physicians considering new ventures. It may be that as competition and change accelerate, and as experience with new markets grows, more sophisticated tools will be needed. This should be anticipated but, at the same time, it's wise to recall the old dictum that "analysis should not lead to paralysis."

Taking action also immediately "disrupts" the market that has just been analyzed and, therefore, places more of a premium on the "learning by doing" approach.

8. Compete/Collaborate

Conventional wisdom also suggests that hospitals should pursue businesses that complement medical staff interests rather than those that compete with physician services. While this may be a reasonable strategy to follow in specific areas, it fails as an overall strategy because it doesn't recognize the realities of the current competitive healthcare environment.

In the current environment, physicians and hospitals will simultaneously find themselves as collaborators and competitors. For example, a hospital may enter a joint venture with its medical staff to develop a PPO while simultaneously developing two or three freestanding emergency centers that compete with the PPO. Hospitals will have to compete with their collaborators because different market strategies are required for different market segments.

Emergicenters, for example, capture that part of the consumer population looking for quick, convenient acute care that's typically not provided by members of the hospital's medical staff outside of traditional office hours.

Emergicenters also can act as a patient referral source, not only for the hospital but also for physician members of the PPO.

Hospitals and physicians must recognize that collaboration and competition no longer are mutually exclusive. They must recognize and learn to live with both.

Further, they must develop communication and decisionmaking processes that foster trust and respect even as hospitals and physicians recognize each other as competitors.

9. Limited Involvement

One of the most cherished dictums of modern management theory is that people need to be involved in decisions that affect them. But this doesn't mean that literally everyone must be involved or that all people need to be involved to the same degree or at the same time. Thus, in forming partnerships, hospitals need not have widespread involvement of the entire medical staff.

A more effective strategy is to target subgroups with specific interests. Within these subgroups, it may be important that different levels within the medical staff organization be represented as well as different specialty and age groups. But this will largely be determined by the specific undertaking being considered.

It is also important to clarify at the beginning of a joint venture who is going to make final decisions. Will it be the hospital chief executive officer and/or hospital board, medical staff leaders, or both? Clarification at the outset will eliminate unnecessary uncertainty, politics and game-playing.

Most important is the need to keep all participants informed to maintain trust. Marketing, financial, utilization and projected quality of care data should be available to all and openly discussed by all. Assumptions should be made explicit and openly debated.

Still, the larger medical staff shouldn't be ignored. In fact, it's extremely important that this larger group be kept informed so that these physicians see the process as open and visible, have an opportunity to see in what direction the decision may be made, and have some time to give up old ways of doing things and make appropriate adjustments.

In particular, the concerns or opposition of the larger medical staff must be openly addressed and, when necessary, taken into account in the subgroup's deliberations.

But keeping the larger group informed and dealing with its concerns is different from totally involving everyone in the partnership.

10. Inefficiency's OK

Some degree of inefficiency and redundancy are associated with the most successful partnerships between hospitals and physicians.

Inefficiency goes hand-in-hand with risk-taking. It's part of the "learning by doing" approach. There's nothing wrong with this approach as long as people learn from it. The partnerships that succeed are made up of fast learners.

One way to promote learning is to build in redundancy. For example, the more successful hospital-medical staff partnerships mentioned earlier were those with dual-track information and billing systems. That is, they combined the hospital's and the physician group practice's systems. The successful partnerships also had more staff than they needed initially, done in anticipation of future demand. They had multiple promotion and advertising efforts, and often dual personnel, purchasing programs, performance appraisal systems, and budgeting policies and practices.

Such redundancy provides a set of checks and balances and greater opportunities for learning what works and what doesn't. It isn't efficient, but it is effective. Redundancy is a blessing.

The Bottom Line

One more element is needed to make a partnership successful: leadership. Among the successful partnerships studied to date, leadership was embodied in the 10 guidelines discussed above. Key individuals understood the importance of each of these requirements and were willing to depart from conventional wisdom.

The 10 guidelines help to promote the kind of experimentation, risk-taking and learning required for successful partnerships in today's environment.

They're based on current research and experience and it may be that as the third generation of hospital-physician partnerships evolves, new forms of technical, political and cultural issues will arise that challenge some of these guidelines. For now, however, following these 10 guidelines is likely to increase the probability of successful partnerships.

14

Credentialing Versus Performance — A New Look at Old Problems

John R. Ball

John R. Ball, M.D., J.D., is Associate Executive Vice President of Health and Public Policy, American College of Physicians, Washington, DC.

Hospitals and physicians have always been faced with a set of very basic issues: What services will be provided? Who will provide them? Who will decide? and How will the decisions be made?

The importance of these issues, however, has been heightened by two general trends of which health care providers are all aware. It is fairly safe to say that hospitals and physicians will continue, at least into the near future, to be beset by pressures to contain costs, and that there will be, at least until the end of this century, a surplus of physicians — and many other categories of health personnel — relative to predicted need.[1] These trends will combine to change, indeed to upset, the balance of power that has existed between physicians and hospitals for several decades. How physicians and hospitals respond to that changing balance may well affect the provision of medical services for decades.

Changes Affecting Privilege Delineation of Physicians

The term "privilege delineation" refers to the process by which individual members of a hospital staff — physicians and nonphysicians — are granted the right to perform certain activities within the hospital. Broadly, it refers both to who is a member of the staff and to what services each member may provide. Although it has been technically the responsibility of the hospital's governing board to grant staff membership and staff privileges, historically the role of the medical staff was more important and its recommendations were *de facto* rubber-stamped by the governing board. The balance of power was tilted toward physicians, and hospital privilege delineation was centered around staff needs. Cost pressures were not intense, and hospitals had little economic incentive to question medical staff recommendations for privileges. In addition, physicians were not in oversupply, and hospitals operated in a seller's market, in which the sellers were physicians. A number of factors have combined to shift the balance of power.

Legal Changes

First, a set of evolutionary legal changes has held the hospital responsible for care delivered within its walls.[2] (We tend to forget that general acceptance of this principle is less than two decades old and that until relatively recently the legal responsibility for a physician's medical care was almost solely the physician's.)

As a consequence, hospitals have begun to scrutinize more closely medical staff recommendations for privileging and to establish stricter procedures for privilege delineation. A second legal change has reflected the general and increasing litigiousness of society: hospitals have become both the symbolic and the practical battleground for the resolution of conflicts, both between physicians and nonphysician groups and among physicians themselves. The stakes in the conflict are the expensive and finite resources of the hospital and who is to have the right to use them.

Manpower Changes

Add to these legal factors a second pressure—the physician surplus—and tensions within the hospital increase even further. Based on available statistics, the physician population has increased by 40% in the last decade, and it is predicted that there will be a 30% surplus by the year 2000.[1] Equally impressive is the concomitant increase in nonphysician providers: the total number of physician assistants and nurse practitioners is predicted to increase fivefold by 1990—from 10,400 in 1976 to more than 50,000 by 1990.[1]

The physician surplus provides the context for an economic and professional tension: the trend toward subspecialization and the natural tendency of the subspecialist to preserve for the subspecialty the privilege of providing certain services (particularly those that require sophisticated technology and are reimbursed more highly) versus the opposite, and somewhat more muted, trend toward family practice and general internal medicine and the generalist's natural tendency to broaden the scope of practice. The interests of both subspecialist and generalist are increasingly at odds over clinical privileges, and lately hospitals have become the arena for the resolution of these conflicts. The similar activities of nonphysician groups in seeking access to the crucial resources of the hospital puts further pressure on the hospital's decision-making process.

Economic Concerns

Thirdly, in addition to legal and manpower pressures, the pressures brought about by health care costs and prospective payment systems are compelling. Faced with the necessity to at least break even financially, the hospital has two basic choices — increase revenues or decrease expenses. Questionable methods to increase revenue are well known: "DRG creep"; computer programs to enhance discharge diagnosis categories, thereby enhancing payment; "cream-skimming"; readmissions; and the like. Other methods include vertical or horizontal expansion, sophisticated cost allocation accounting systems, and aggressive marketing of services. Ways in which hospitals may reduce expenses are less prolific.

Although more efficient purchasing of services and materials is one logical way for a hospital to save money, there are other possible mechanisms that much more directly affect physicians. One has to do with which patients are treated in the hospital, the other with which physicians are allowed privileges in the hospital. Although the Medicare prospective payment system allows an increased payment for outlier patients, that increased payment is substantially limited. Thus, the incentive exists for the hospital to admit more ill patients and not to admit less severely ill patients within the same DRG. The mechanisms by which hospitals may affect patient admissions are, at this point, problematic, but one should not sell short the ingenuity of hospitals when survival is at stake.

The Hospital's Influence on Physician Behavior

More important for the purposes of this discussion are the steps the hospital may take to modify physician practice behavior. In this regard, the most important step the hospital has available is the refusal to grant clinical privileges or the withdrawal of clinical privileges. Both are legally within the hospital's authority and responsibility. The basis on which the hospital will decide is critical. Historically, the hospital made such decisions in response to physicians' needs. More recently, greater attention has been focused on the hospital's responsibility for the *quality* of the medical care provided by medical staff.

In the future, however, the incentive will exist for the hospital to make such decisions on an *economic* basis, granting privileges to physicians and to nonphysicians who are likely to practice more economically and withdrawing privileges and staff membership from physicians who practice uneconomically (i.e., those who overutilize services). Because of the hospital's incentive to weigh economic issues when making credentialing decisions and the increasing supply of physicians, the balance of power between the hospital and the physician is shifting. This, in effect, makes the hospital the buyer in a buyer's market. Thus, economics as well as professional competence will be influencing physician practice behavior in the hospital as never before.

Privilege Delineation

Based on information from a survey of the policies of national medical specialty societies performed by the American Medical Association in early 1982[3,4] and a 1983 survey of college governors by the American College of Physicians, it can be said that most hospitals view privilege delineation conceptually the same way. Most use the same general process when delineating privileges, and most encounter the same basic set of problems. All medical specialty society policies and most hospitals make it clear that to have clinical privileges presupposes medical staff membership. To some extent (for example, under the new Joint Commission on Accreditation of Hospitals [JCAH] standards) this requirement is changing,[5] but it is important to note that, in practice, admission to the medical staff is a prerequisite to attaining clinical privileges and that physician groups clearly believe in a significant correlation between privileges and staff membership.

Clinical privileges, then, are just that—privileges, rather than rights. Licensure conveys the *right* to practice. It does not mandate a *duty* on behalf of the hospital to allow practice within it. Thus, the privilege of practicing within the hospital and the specification of what services the practitioner may perform are privileges granted by the hospital on the basis of established criteria, applied in each individual case.

Process of Delineating Privileges

Privilege delineation is conceptually (and often, practically) a two-step process: admission to the medical staff and granting of the right to perform certain services within the hospital. The information that individual applicants must supply, although generally similar, differs for each of the two steps. For admission to the medical staff, the following information is usually the minimum required.

- Education and training;

- Experience;

- References (regarding competence and character);

- License (current);

- Professional memberships; and

- Possible other relevant information (e.g., malpractice actions, licensure revocation, loss of privileges elsewhere).

The granting of specific privileges usually requires that the applicant give evidence of competence in the management of disease or in the performance of procedures. That evidence may be in the form of board eligibility or certification, specific training, case reports, or letters from previous chiefs of training programs or medical staffs. What should be emphasized is that the granting of staff membership and the granting of clinical privileges are different. In granting staff membership, the hospital today seeks to assure itself that the practitioner is legally able to practice and is neither immoral nor *incompetent*. In granting clinical privileges, the hospital seeks to ensure that the practitioner is *competent* to practice or at least to perform specified services.

The procedure for delineating privileges is relatively uniform across hospitals and involves review of an applicant's request by one or more clinical departments, review of the department's recommendations by the medical staff credentials committee, and granting of privileges by the hospital's governing body. Note that the medical staff *recommends* and the governing body *grants* privileges—based, in large measure, of course, on the recommendation of the medical staff.

Once privileges are granted, the practitioner undergoes a period of provisional status, lasting from three months to two years, during which his or her performance is monitored. The monitoring is usually the responsibility of the chief of service. Although the policies of medical specialty organizations and of hospitals emphasize the importance of monitoring during the provisional period, in practice the degree of monitoring varies greatly.

Theoretically, renewal of clinical privileges potentially requires more evidence of competence than the initial grant, because consideration is given to such additional factors as the practitioner's participation in medical staff activities and medical education, and his or her performance. In practice, it is not usually so strict, and the renewal of privileges is likely to be recommended on less formal information than that required for the initial grant. Where performance is reviewed, that process usually consists of reviewing any written reports made during provisional status as well as the results of medical audits and informal case review. Not many hospitals, and fewer medical staffs, have complete medical staff performance data on which to base renewal of privileges, although this is likely to change in the future.

Determining Qualifications for Privileges

Having briefly touched on the concept and administrative process of privilege delineation, there remains the approach used by hospitals to determine whether an individual applicant is qualified for privileges. Here, again, it should come as no surprise that, although there are variations on the themes, there are only two general approaches: the disease-based (or procedure-based) approach (also called the "laundry list") and the categorical approach.

The disease-based approach, in which the applicant checks off those conditions he or she wishes to treat and those procedures he or she wishes to perform, has been widely criticized[6] but is still used quite commonly. Often more meticulous than necessary, this approach can be inefficient. In addition, it is subject to both errors of commission (if the physician is granted privileges for which he or she is not qualified) and errors of omission (if the physician is *not* granted privileges for which he or she is qualified). It is notable, however, that the existing polices of a substantial number of specialty societies favor the disease-based approach, perhaps because it is more likely to ensure that the practitioner is competent to perform specified services.

The categorical approach to privilege delineation requires the applicant to estimate his or her level of knowledge in an area of practice. One categorical approach might be based on degree of training. For example:

- Category 1: Provide emergency care;

- Category 2: Provide primary medical care for uncomplicated medical problems and perform minor surgery;

- Category 3: Provide medical care or major surgical procedures requiring specialized training or experience; or

- Category 4: Provide medical care or major surgery requiring subspecialized training or experience.[7]

Another categorical approach may be based on patient risk:

- Category 1: Diagnosis or treatment with minimal threat to life;

- Category 2: Major diagnosis or treatment but with no significant threat to life;

- Category 3: Major diagnosis or treatment with serious threat to life; or

- Category 4: Unusually complex or critical diagnosis or treatment with serious threat to life.[8]

This general categorical approach has itself been criticized[9] because, although it avoids the inefficiency of the laundry-list approach, it leads to the opposite problem—that is, not producing a meaningful description of the physician's clinical practice. What is missing is a set of definitions.

Because of the deficiencies of both basic approaches, many hospitals have begun to combine the two. Although some hospitals combine the most problematic aspects of each approach (that is, undefined levels applied to every diagnosis or procedure), others have been able to establish broad but well-defined categories, giving examples to clarify their meaning. This approach has some promise, because it combines both administrative efficiency with basic assurance that patients will be managed by practitioners whose skill is appropriate to the patient's condition. Nevertheless, even the combined approach is potentially problematic, because in an increasingly tight market for physicians, those who are denied certain privileges are likely to attack the legality or reasonableness of less than explicit criteria.

Problems and Predictions

The problems, as I view them, flow from three sets of conflicts — between hospitals and physicians, between physician generalists and physician specialists, and between physicians and nonphysicians.

The Hospital/Physician Conflict

Although there has always been a tenuous balance of power between hospitals and physicians, in the past the balance was tilted toward physicians for two main reasons: physicians were in relative short supply and, under cost-based or retrospective reimbursement, the physician's and hospital's economic interests did not conflict significantly and often coincided. Today the hospital is being courted as physicians attempt to become members of medical staffs that are already large, and this situation will intensify in the future. In addition, prospective payment changes the hospital's economic incentives so that it may be in conflict with the physician's economic incentive. In other words, hospitals tend to lose money for each DRG as more technology is applied, while physicians tend to gain money for each patient as more technology is applied.

What this means for privilege delineation is not fully clear, but a likely possibility is this: While physicians historically have applied for the maximum procedural privileges for which they are qualified (and will do so to an even greater degree as the number of physicians increases), hospitals have, under prospective payment, the economic incentive to award the fewest procedural privileges possible.

Add to this economically defined scenario the issue of quality, and the difficulties multiply. For the physician, the professional ethic demands that the best possible care be provided to all patients. Medical education generally teaches that to satisfy this ethical requirement, it is necessary to understand all that is known about the patient's disease process and to treat the patient in the latest, most effective way possible. For better or worse, quality is often equated with quantity.

Under prospective payment, however, the hospital has the incentive to assure only minimally acceptable quality (rather than the optimal achievable quality desired by the physician). I would argue that it is possible to decrease the number of services (thereby significantly decreasing hospital costs) without significantly reducing quality; moreover, hospitals, too, are aware of this. Health care today operates at the margin in the sense that, in many cases, it takes maximum costs to produce even minimal benefits. Hospitals know that although they have what may be perceived as conflicting dual responsibilities (i.e., minimize costs and maintain quality) they can meet both because of the greater "buffering" capacity built into quality.

To resolve the hospital/physician conflict, two steps, both of which are highly beneficial to patients, should be taken. First, hospitals and physicians need to work together to develop data on which cost-effective, medically effective choices can be made. For example, given the plethora of medical technologies and the number of clinical approaches to medical problems, which are the most effective (in terms of both clinical outcome and cost) to use? Perhaps prospective payment will finally stimulate hospitals and physicians to examine critically the real value of the medical services they provide. Second, hospitals and physicians will have to agree on which practitioners are best able to provide which services. The need for such decisions puts increasing emphasis on the availability of hospital-based practice data, which can be generated by already available but underutilized mechanisms, such as utilization review, sophisticated medical audit, and the results of other quality assurance mechanisms.

An unacceptable outcome to this conflict would, of course, be the polarization of physicians and hospitals. As the balance of power tilts toward hospitals, the hospital can begin to dictate privilege delineation and, to some extent, clinical practice. With legal authority, a powerful incentive to survive economically, and little fear that its actions will seriously compromise quality, the hospital now stands in a strong position vis-à-vis physicians. It is, of course, too early to predict the outcome, but as a bellwether, the for-profit hospitals should be worth watching.

The Physician/Physician Conflict

Although the conflict between generalists and subspecialists has been smoldering for several years, it is likely to become more acute in the future. Until the last three decades, the majority of physicians were general practitioners. In the last decade, the trend toward specialization has at least slowed, as physicians choosing to practice family medicine, general internal medicine, and pediatrics became much more numerous.[10,11] As a consequence of both the specialist-generalist flux and the physician supply, turf battles between disciplines are being fought increasingly in the hospital setting.

There is a natural tendency of physicians to expand their scope of practice, and family practitioners have been both aggressive and successful in seeking expanded clinical privileges, many of which were once the sole province of the specialist. At the same time, in part because of economic considerations, specialists are attempting to carve out exclusive domains—from intensive care units to emergency rooms to the reading of bone marrow slides—and are expanding their practices beyond specialty care into primary care. The pivotal issue for these conflicts involves the privileges that hospitals allow members of the staff, with the specialists arguing that not only are they better qualified to perform certain services, but that the generalists are not even minimally qualified to perform those services. The argument often focuses on board certification in a specialty or subspecialty as the sine qua non of qualifications; this credential, however, although often used, is considered as only one of several valid criteria by both JCAH[12] and the American Board of Medical Specialties.[13] Often the battle comes down to which group holds the economic and/or political power in the hospital, and an outcome on that basis is being increasingly and successfully challenged. Many, if not most, hospitals have chosen to tolerate the grumbles of the subspecialist rather than encourage the lawsuit of the generalist, and thus they have granted expanded privileges, rather than denying them, to the generalist.

Whether this trend will continue will depend on several factors, the most important of which are the hospital's response to prospective payment and the specialists' ability (or inability) to marshal data in support of the claim of quality. Most economic analysts claim that hospitals will make choices depending on which of their DRG case mix are economic losers and which are winners. If that be the case, different hospitals will make different choices relative to the specialist/generalist conflict. It is also possible that prospective payment will favor those groups and individuals who use fewer procedures, but the differential weighting (based on historical reimbursement) for the more technologically-intensive DRGs could reduce this possibility. As for the ability of the specialist to prove that certification in a subspecialty leads to significantly better patient outcomes, I have little optimism. It has been shown in very few cases, and in general is quite difficult to demonstrate.

What the outcome will be is hard to predict, but for the near future the generalists will probably be gaining expanded privileges, particularly if their use of hospital resources is less than that of the specialist for the same DRG. Subspecialists will continue to have only major surgery and the most complicated of procedures as their sole province.

The Physician/Nonphysician Conflict

The trend of nonphysicians (e.g., clinical psychologists, podiatrists, dentists) gaining access to the hospital is likely to increase the conflict between physician and nonphysician (e.g., psychiatrist versus clinical psychologist; orthopedist versus podiatrist; and obstetrician versus nurse midwife). The arguments will be familiar, with the physician arguing that the nonphysician is not sufficiently qualified to deliver certain hospital-based services, and the nonphysician countering with the stronger (at least for now) argument that there are few data to support the physician, that the physician is concerned about economic competition, not quality, and that the nonphysician will use fewer of the hospital's resources. Hospitals may soon be more predisposed to grant admitting privileges to nonphysicians, even to the point of divorcing admitting privileges from medical staff membership.

Comment

The hospital, with the legal authority, economic incentive, market power, and use of data on provider practice patterns, has the potential to dictate the way in which hospital-based medicine is practiced. I don't believe such an outcome would be good for patients, but, like other physicians, I don't have the data that could refute the decisions of hospital management. As physicians, our economic incentives and our professional ethic are coming back into line. Now we need to examine critically the ways in which we manage patients and determine which ones are medically effective and which are not. If we are lucky, the medically effective methods will also be cost effective, and the outcome will be a happy one for all parties — physicians, hospitals, and most importantly, patients.

Notes

1. Graduate Medical Education National Advisory Committee: *Summary Report*, vol 1, DHHS pub no. HRA 81-651. Hyattsville, MD: U.S. Department of Health and Human Services, Health Resources Administration, Sept. 30, 1980.
2. *Darling v. Charleston Community Memorial Hospital*, 211 N.E. 2d 253 (IL. 1965), cert denied, 383 U.S. 946 (1966).
3. American Medical Association (AMA): *Statements on Delineation of Hospital Privileges*. Chicago: AMA, Jan. 1982.
4. American Medical Association (AMA): *Report on Medical Staff Activities Survey of AMA Federation Members*. Chicago: AMA, Jan. 1982.
5. Joint Commission on Accreditation of Hospitals: *JCAH Perspectives*, vol 4, no. 1, Jan./Feb. 1984.
6. American College of Physicians (ACP): Delineating hospital privileges by the medical staff. *The Bulletin*, June 1975.
7. Joint Commission on Accreditation of Hospitals (JCAH): *Back to Basics: An Introduction to the Principles of Quality Assurance*. Chicago: JCAH, 1982.
8. American College of Obstetricians and Gynecologists (ACOG): *Standards for Obstetric-Gynecologic Services* (5th ed). Washington, DC: ACOG, 1982.
9. Illinois Hospital Research and Education Foundation: *Hospital Medical Staff Membership and Delineation of Clinical Privileges*. Naperville, IL: Illinois Hospital Research and Education Foundation, 1978.
10. Tarlov AR et al: National study of internal medicine manpower: III. Subspecialty fellowship training 1976-77. *Ann Intern Med* 91: 287-294, 1979.
11. Tarlov AR et al: National study of internal medicine manpower: IV. Residency and fellowship training 1977-78, 1978-79. *Ann Intern Med* 91: 295-300, 1979.
12. Joint Commission on Accreditation of Hospitals (JCAH): *Accreditation Manual for Hospitals* (1984 ed). Chicago: JCAH, 1983.
13. American Board of Medical Specialties (ABMS): *ABMS Statement on Delineation of Staff Privileges*. Evanston, IL: ABMS, Jan. 28, 1977.

15

Credentialing of Medical Staff: The Nursing Department's Role

Kathy M. Brubaker

Kathy M. Brubaker, M.S.N., R.N., is Vice President of Clinical Services, Chelsea Community Hospital, Chelsea, Michigan.

In a rapidly changing health care environment, more and more emphasis is being placed by hospitals, medical staffs, accrediting bodies, insurance carriers, and utilization review agencies on credentialing of the medical staff. An increasingly litigious society and soaring malpractice costs accentuate the need for a comprehensive, specific system for defining and validating physician clinical privileges. In addition to expertise and skill in diagnostic, therapeutic, and technical abilities, greater importance is assigned to the physician's ability to interact with the patient, family, and interdisciplinary team in preparing the patient for earlier discharge and/or transfer to home care, sub-acute, or long-term care facilities.

The nursing and medical staffs are the two key clinical disciplines responsible for the care of each patient entering and negotiating the hospital system. Knowledge and respect for one another's clinical practice increasingly are overcoming traditional turf and role battles. Nurses in a hospital setting are generally cognizant of individual physician clinical/technical skills and deviations from the standards of medical care. The Darling case of 1965 first identified nursing staff accountability for acting on this knowledge.[1]

It is in the context of the interchange between these two clinical disciplines that the nursing department role in credentialing physicians is presented as an additional means of addressing the competency of a medical staff in an increasingly complex health care system. One hospital's experience in involving the nursing staff in the medical staff credentialing process is described.

Reprinted with permission from *Nursing Management,* 18(12), December 1987, pages 45-46. Copyright 1987 by S-N Publications, Inc. All rights reserved.

Credentialing Defined

Medical staff credentialing consists of verification and assessment of physician qualifications and granting and delineation of clinical privileges. Essential for ensuring standards of quality and efficiency in patient care, the credentialing process is at the heart of the hospital/medical staff relationship.[2]

JCAH defines the process for reappointment to the medical staff and/or the removal or revision of clinical privileges. Minimally this includes gathering information concerning the physician's current license, health status, professional performance, judgment, and clinical/technical skills. While the method used is hospital-specific, there must be evidence that delineation and granting of clinical privileges is based on the individual's current demonstrated competence.

The question of whether or not a physician's personality can affect the granting of hospital privileges has been reviewed judicially as valid depending on whether or not the physician's personality was reasonably related to the welfare of patients and whether it directly jeopardized or posed a specific threat to the quality of patient care.[3] The following is quoted from an Oregon case: "Most other courts have found that the factor of ability to work smoothly with others is reasonably related to the hospital's object to ensuring patient welfare. This conclusion seems justified, for, in the modern hospital, staff members are frequently required to work together or in teams, and a member who, because of personality or otherwise, is incapable of getting along, could severely hinder the effective treatment of patients. . . ."[4]

Nursing Department Role

The Nursing Department at Chelsea Community Hospital, Chelsea, Michigan has been involved in the credentialing of medical staff for over ten years. During the credentialing process, the Vice President of Clinical Services first receives a list of medical staff members due for review. The head nurse of each department subsequently obtains input from the RN staff.

The nursing staff address a number of different factors when providing input on a physician to the Credentials Committee and Chief of the service. Attention is given to the nursing staff's perception of the physician's clinical skills and judgment. Considerable emphasis is placed on interactions with interdisciplinary team members, communication patterns with patients and families, clarity of physician orders (written and verbal), and rounding patterns. Nursing staff input is generally given in a narrative format. Both input on strengths and potential problem areas are communicated.

Communication with the medical staff leadership regarding physician practice issues is an ongoing process. Medical staff leaders, like most managers, do not want to hear of a dated or long standing issue for the first time at the time of the evaluation. It is the goal of the Nursing Department to use the formal credentialing program as a means of validating prior input, and updating the medical staff leadership on physician practice.

Chelsea Community Hospital's experience with this process has been very positive. It is our belief that documented input by the nursing staff is advantageous for both the medical staff leadership and the hospital. Through the years, nursing staff input into the medical staff credentialing process has affected the privileges of several physician members. Occasionally, the Credentials Committee has been alerted to monitor a particular physician's practice more closely. Most important, the Nursing Department input, when positive, helps validate a medical staff member's review by his peers and supports the medical staff and hospital decision to renew a physician's privileges.

Strategies

A number of considerations are important for hospitals and nursing departments wishing to introduce nursing staff input into the medical staff credentialing program. It is most important that the medical staff/nursing staff relationship be a positive one. Nursing staff input will be sought if communication patterns are positive and if nursing staff is viewed as having significant and unique information. Nursing staff leadership should begin an ongoing dialogue with the medical staff leadership regarding both successes and problems with physician members. It is our experience over time that physicians, especially medical staff leaders, will view nursing's involvement in the credentialing process as an opportunity instead of a threat.

One important strategy for setting the stage for nursing staff input into the medical staff credentialing process is for nursing leadership actively to solicit physician input into nursing staff evaluations. At Chelsea Community Hospital we have a long history of requesting physician input into head nurse as well as staff nurse evaluations. It is important in such a program to act on medical staff input and to provide continuous feedback on your responses and reactions.

Another avenue in which the nursing department at Chelsea Community Hospital has developed a close working relationship with the medical staff is involvement in physician recruitment and orientation to the hospital. In the last ten years Chelsea Community Hospital has recruited a number of primary physicians and specialty physicians to the hospital. Nursing staff have been significantly involved through attending medical recruitment workshops, participating in the formal interview process, and providing leadership in the orientation of new physicians to the hospital. It is within the context of these early interactions with physicians that the nursing staff is able to set the stage for a positive working relationship. Medical staff are made aware early of the positive relationship between nursing and medicine which has characterized the hospital. Likewise, the Nursing Department involves physician members in the selection of nurses for its leadership positions.

Paramount to successful implementation of this program within an institution is commitment to an independent, yet collaborative model of medical and nursing practice. Input into credentialing/evaluation systems gives neither nursing nor medicine the authority to govern or control the practice of the other. The challenge to nursing and medical leadership is to facilitate and participate in a collaborative practice model while acknowledging the autonomous nature of each discipline.

A comprehensive credentialing program will assure the medical staff, hospital administration and board of trustees of a competent physician staff to deliver high quality patient care in the hospital. Broad based input from medical staff committees and peers and clear documentation are essential to a sound credentialing program. Nursing staff input can significantly enhance this process.

Notes

1. *Darling v. Charleston Community Hospital*, 211 N.E. 2d 53, (Illinois, 1965).
2. Brooks, D.C. and M.A. Morrisey, "Credentialing: Say Good-bye to the 'Rubber Stamp'," *Hospitals*, 59:50-52, June, 1985.
3. Sattilaro, A.J. and J.C. Cameron, "Change Challenges Traditional Hospital Medical Staff Relationship," *Hospitals*, 55:139, 142-144, April, 1981.

4. *Ladenheim v. Union County Hospital District*, 394 N.E. 2d 770, (Illinois App., 1979), cited in "Hospital's Right to Revoke Doctor's Privileges Affirmed," Action Kit for Hospital Trustees, (May/June 1981).

16

The Hospital Medical Staff of 1994

William R. Fifer

William R. Fifer, M.D., is Clinical Professor of Medicine and Public Health, University of Minnesota, Minneapolis, and President of Clayton, Fifer Associates, Minneapolis.

Now that the year of George Orwell has arrived, the temptation to look ahead to 1994 is understandable. Recent best-selling books such as *Megatrends* remind us that innovation continually shapes our destiny and that one can predict the future best by understanding the trends and issues of the present as they forecast the future. With a bow to futurists everywhere, this article predicts 15 attributes of the hospital medical staff of 1994. Some of the predictions will come true. Some won't. We will have failed to anticipate some forces shaping our future. Even with these shortcomings, we hope to provide food for thought.

As a codicil to the predictions, let us indicate their limits. We have taken as the model in transition the medical staff of the voluntary, community, acute-care general hospital. It is clear that the same predictions will not apply equally to the inner-city public hospital, the academic health center, the isolated small rural hospital, and the specialty (psychiatric, rehabilitation) facility. We have chosen not to consider the 1994 medical staff's involvement with clinical research or health sciences education, limiting our sphere of concern to the arena of patient care.

The hospital medical staff won't be a hospital medical staff because the hospital, as we know it, will not be around in 1994. Jeff Goldsmith's insights in *Can Hospitals Survive? The New Competitive Health Care Market* remind us that the hospital industry is a "mature" one in its traditional conceptualization. The evidence for this point of view is clear: the best measure of the growth of the core inpatient services of the hospital (bed days) shows no growth in the past several years. The implications are clear, too. Hospitals must stop being "places" and become "things,"[1] must stop relying on further growth of inpatient services and must diversify their "product lines" to in-

Reprinted by permission from *The Hospital Medical Staff*, Vol. 13, No. 6, June 1984. Copyright 1984, American Hospital Publishing, Inc.

clude a whole skein of integrated health care services needed by their communities. The hospital as an organization is undergoing a profound reconceptualization—in 10 years it will not be defined as a brick edifice on the corner of Seventh and Main housing horizontal sick people.

The hospital medical staff won't be a medical staff. The evolution of medical care to health care will have progressed by 1994 to the point where a hospital will have redefined its clinical mission and developed a cadre of professional staff whose composition "fits" with its expanded realm of health services. There are some 230 species of health care professionals other than physicians (HCPOTPs) in the work force. These "allied health professionals" outnumber physicians 16 to 1. The Joint Commission on Accreditation of Hospitals (JCAH) rewrote the medical staff section of the *Accreditation Manual for Hospitals* in December 1983 to reflect the reality of HCPOTPs and to allow hospitals to grant appointments and appropriate clinical privileges to nonphysician professionals. The "medical staff " won't be only "medical" in 1994.

The hospital medical staff will be defined. Up to the present, hospitals have passively reacted to individuals who sought them out and requested appointments. By 1994 the hospital will actively derive the size and composition of a staff from its strategic planning process. The "defined staff " will be smaller, and it will contain a greater proportion of women (28 percent of today's U.S. medical students are women). Hospitals will have manpower plans, dynamic blueprints that are revised frequently, to guide an active process of recruiting and shaping the kinds and numbers of practitioners required to support their clinical missions. Please note we have chosen to describe the 1994 staff as "defined" rather than "closed."

The relationship between the individual member and the staff organization of 1994 will be pluralistic. Given the technology imperative, the core staff of hospital-based practitioners will be larger and more diverse. These members (the directors diagnostic labs, special care units, regional referral programs, and so on) will be salaried employees of the hospital. Some other members will participate in risk-sharing competitive medical plan (CMP) organizations as joint ventures with the hospital. Their relationship will be an economic one of an entrepreneurial nature. Notwithstanding, hospitals will continue to have a "voluntary attending" staff whose relationship will still be defined by a set of bylaws setting forth their prerogatives and responsibilities to the institution.

The hospital medical staff of 1994 will be an organization. Although we have given lip service to the "medical staff organization" or "organized medical staff " up to now, such an organization has not existed. Wary of the potential of group autonomy to compromise individual autonomy, the present-day medical staff prevents leadership development by one-year terms of office and has developed a redundant array of committees to ensure the preservation of participative democracy as an organizational trademark. By 1994 the organization will begin to look like an organization; it will be better internally managed by an accepted leadership with defined responsibility and accountability. There will be continuity of effort and a clear set of organizational values and objectives. Shortell's work[2] indicates that such a staff will achieve superior patient care outcomes, reinforcing the raison d'être for a medical staff organization.

The hospital medical staff of 1994 will be part of something bigger. The hospital field has moved out ahead of its medical staff counterpart in developing integrated arrangements. Thus, horizontal integration has brought about multihospital systems, hospital alliances, and widespread development of contract management of various kinds. Yet to my knowledge we have not witnessed the development of "multi-medical staff systems" as a counterpart. Hospitals are also vertically integrating a line of new services from wellness to hospice, creating network organizations that are diversified both geographically and functionally. Organizations involving physicians such as HMOs and preferred provider organizations (PPOs) are "going national" in scope and becoming publicly owned. Just as the individual physician becomes part of something bigger when he joins an individual medical staff, the medical staff of 1994 will compound that multiplication by becoming part of something bigger itself.

The hospital medical staff of 1994 will be more closely bonded to the hospital. A number of existing forces are bringing physicians and hospitals closer together: (1) the need to involve physicians in resource allocation programs ("product management") has been enhanced greatly by fixed-price (prospective) payment for Medicare beneficiaries; (2) the unaligned, solo physician is steadily losing market share to the big, heavily advertised and marketed HMOs and IPAs; and (3) the hospital, faced with a "no growth" situation with regard to inpatient revenues, is diversifying into the territory of the physician.

These forces will lead to a variety of joint ventures such as PPOs and Ellwood's MeSH organizations as described in the December 1983 issue of *Hospital Medical Staff*. Such organizations align the financial and professional incentives of both hospital and physician, thereby attempting to manage the risk and market the services of both hospitals and physicians to employers and third parties.

Will the joint venture organization replace the medical staff? Probably not. Rather, it will be superimposed on both the corporately restructured hospital and its pluralistic medical staff. Such a new organization will be powerful, however, because it is integrated. No longer will there be two sets of bylaws and fuzzy expectations and relationships.

The bond between medical staff and hospital will be "monogamous." By 1994, the present situation wherein an individual physician enjoys membership in three or four hospital staffs will have been replaced (with some exceptions) by a monogamous marriage—one doctor to one hospital. The reason for this evolution is contained in competition theory—the individual hospital attempting to strategically position itself for survival. Such strategy cannot be revealed to "the enemy," as would occur if casually aligned physicians participated in more than one strategic planning process.

The medical staff of 1994 will participate in both policy formulation and professional management within the hospital—roles that are foreign to the present staff. The present-day increase in physician membership on hospital governing boards will be enhanced by the need to involve physicians in strategic planning. At the same time, more physicians will assume "professional manager" roles involved in technology assessment, product management, and cost-effective clinical decisionmaking. The future challenge is to manage care, not simply provide care.

The medical staff of 1994 will be entrepreneurial, involved with the hospital in a variety of new business activities in the health care field. This development will cause some soul-searching, as exemplified by Relman's current concern[3] that physicians may suffer the loss of the professional ethic to the business ethic. Cunningham[4] has expressed the same concern for the hospital. Should physicians own surgicenters and emergicenters and even hospitals? These concerns will surface again and again in the '90s.

The medical staff of 1994 will be capitated, that is, paid a fixed price per month to assume the financial risks involved in the care of a defined population. The present-day mode of fixed price (incentive) payment, which transfers the financial risk to the hospital for an episode of inpatient care, will evolve to capitation payment, as in Durenberger's "voucher" proposal. In this evolution, the physician medical staff functions as "gate-keeper" or resource allocator in the system,[5] a distinctly new role for most physicians and medical staffs.

The hospital medical staff of 1994 will care for a defined population as a natural out-growth of capitation payment. Of the three major dimensions of care (quality, cost, access), two will have been solved by "population medicine": access will be ensured (albeit a directed access), and the open-endedness of reimbursement for costs or services will be replaced by closed-ended (capitation) payments.

This newly defined mandate will profoundly affect the provision of preventive care and "wellness" services. It will also contribute to redefining the medical staff as those appropriate numbers and varieties of practitioners necessary to provide comprehensive care to a defined population, an implication of which will be an increased number of primary care physicians who form the broad base of a practitioner pyramid that culminates in a single transplant surgeon at the apex.

The medical staff of 1994 will still provide good care. To be sure it may be of a different sort, given the demographics of an aging population and the many potential substitutions for an inpatient day. But the medical school "class of '94" will have discovered that there is not an inevitable trade-off between cost and quality. These physicians will probably deliver less care as traditionally measured (numbers of surgical procedures, inpatient days, and stays), but it will not be worse care. From home health to hospice, there will be substitution for core inpatient services. Technology such as intensive care and imaging will be used because it reduces overall cost while simultaneously enhancing overall quality.

The medical staff organization of 1994 will be the principal focus for collective physician function. This prediction is based on the tremendous display of interest in the development of the American Medical Association's (AMA)

Hospital Medical Staff Section, which is now being cloned at the state medical association level. Does the steady decrease in the percentage of licensed physicians who belong to the AMA contain a message? It is likely that, given the scope and rate of change in the context of medicine, the AMA and county medical associations will increasingly be unable to serve as the focus of collective physician activity. The specialty societies' unique contribution of today is the delivery of "update" CME information to the specialist, a role that home computers could easily replace. Because it provides a relevant forum for collective action, we predict that the hospital medical staff will be the surviving organizational model of aggregate activity.

Finally, the hospital medical staff of 1994 will retain the ethical basis for its existence. HMOs and IPAs and PPOs will come and go, part of a continuum of change in the dynamic restructuring of medical care in America. Entrepreneurs will surface, make their buck, and move on to greener pastures. What will remain is the professional ethic, the understanding that service to a suffering fellow man is the real touchstone of the whole effort. People will still experience sickness and injury and the fear of untimely death. They will still turn to a trusting relationship with a professional whose highest duty is their well-being. As Kaiser put it: "You can put together an entrepreneurial and compassionate ethic in one box. There is nothing wrong with providing a good service and making money. The bottom line now, however, is that every physician will become a manager, like it or not, because he or she will win or lose out depending on how well positioned the MD is in the changing market. Management of care becomes as important today as delivery of care."[6]

Let those who consider the predictions "far out" remember that the changes in the medical and hospital "industries" have been more profound in the past 10 years than in the previous 1,000 years. Let's bury the prediction in a time capsule to be dug up in 1994 and get about the task of shaping our future by our deeds, one day at a time.

Notes

1. Gallagher, T.M. The hospital: is it a place or a thing? *Health Care Mgmt. Rev.* Winter 1984.
2. Shortell, S.M. and Logerfo, J.D. Hospital medical staff organization and quality of care. *Med. Care.* 19:1041, Oct. 1981.
3. Relman, A. Money and medical ethics: will patients stop trusting doctors? *ACP Observer*, Aug. 1982.
4. Cunningham, R.M., Jr. *The healing mission and the business ethic.* Chicago. Pluribus Press, 1982.
5. Somers, A. And who shall be the gatekeeper? *Inquiry*, Winter 1983.
6. Kaiser, L.M. *Amer. Med. News*, Jan. 6, 1984.

Part II

Management Functions

Introduction

The environmental turbulence of the 1980s caused primarily by federal policy initiatives of deregulation, procompetition, and prospective pricing, significantly affected management functions in hospitals. Planning has matured from a simplistic long-range focus in a stable environment to a dynamic, aggressive process involving the governing body, senior management, and the medical staff. The outcomes of strategic planning, some of which were unthinkable 20 years ago, have led to implementation of logical and coherent, yet diverse, multidirectional strategies affecting internal resource allocation, utilization, and control as well as creating more complex inter- and intraorganizational arrangements. Increased accountability of hospitals to constituents, patients, governments, and third-party payors, including large corporate purchasers of health services, is part of the milieu—a given. Risk management and quality assurance are not only financially necessary for the hospital, but an ethical imperative. There is a new relationship between the hospital and its human resources, there is a new managerial attitude about them, and there are new methods for integrating them into new organizational structures.

The present environment with its new rules has caused one noticeable change between today's hospital and that of a decade ago, namely, a less sharp differentiation between hospitals and business corporations. Johnson insightfully distinguished between the two by describing a hospital as basically a social enterprise with economic overtones and a corporation as an economic enterprise with social overtones.[1] In some respects that distinction is now less precise. While retaining their social enterprise character, hospitals are tilting toward the economic overtones. A positive by-product is that hospital managers have become more adept and sophisticated in applying management functions. They pay more attention to strategic planning, the services provided by their hospitals, and resource consumption and control. As a result, methods to improve productivity through management engineering and operations auditing, information collection systems such as cost cen-

163

ter accounting and management information systems, and a product line management structure are now in place. They are the foundation for the hospital management of the 1990s.

As products, services, and structures have changed, so has the organizational climate. Once bastions of stability and predictability, hospitals have changed their character. No longer guaranteed the right of survival, and recognizing that fact, they are becoming economically lean and competitively mean. Aggressiveness and an eye on the economics, have resulted in hospitals positioning themselves to shape their destiny rather than merely reacting to events.

Strategic Planning

Hospital managers are now very adept at strategic planning that is overt, anticipatory, and long-term. Strategic planning deals with formulation (and reformulation) of organizational objectives and of overall organizational strategies to accomplish those objectives.[2] Strategic planning is externally and internally oriented and relies on assessment of the organization's environments. Integral to strategic planning is health services marketing, particularly the marketing audit that facilitates environmental linkage. Fig. II-1 illustrates the components of strategic planning: (a) objectives, (b) appraisal, and (c) choice of strategy; these are followed by the outcomes of strategic planning: (d) program implementation and (e) control.

Objectives

An organization's objectives constitute the goals, targets, or output desired. They are the ends toward which organizational effort, programs and activities are directed, and the reasons for obtaining, allocating, and using resources. Hospitals have primary and secondary objectives. Examples are delivery of quality health services to clients; financial solvency; growth in new patient and nonpatient areas; education and research; and social citizenship. For some hospitals in today's environment, survival has become the paramount objective.

The strategic planning process of formulating objectives and establishing their priority is influenced by external and internal stakeholders – individuals or groups who have a vested interest in what the organization does. External stakeholders typically include government, the community, unions, third-party payors including large corporations, and the medical community. Internal stakeholders include the governing body, managers, employees, patients, and medical staff. All affect what a hospital's objectives will be and their order of priority. The 1980s witnessed a changed relationship among stakeholders. Payors increasingly influenced hospital objectives. Most were concerned with costs, capacity, and productivity. Some argue that this increased influence has modified the role of internal stakeholders, who are becoming the defenders of quality of care.

The result of the formulation of objectives is a statement of the output the organization seeks to achieve. This statement corresponds to the solution criteria in the strategy choice process (Fig. II-1C); it is the focal point for gathering and allocating resources and the basis for deriving control standards against which organizational performance is compared.

Situation Appraisal

The situation appraisal or audit is critical to strategic planning because the identification, evaluation, and choice of strategy result from it (Fig. II-1B). The audit is a systematic, formal, in-depth collection of past and present information and expectations about the future pertaining to the hospital and its internal and external environments. This data base permits an identification of external threats and opportunities and internal weaknesses and strengths.

Analysis of the external environment focuses on the major macro forces presently affecting or likely to affect the hospital. This analysis requires evaluating and making assumptions about such areas as the economy, demographic changes, cultural and sociological trends, political stability and public policy toward health care, competition, and technological changes. Collecting and processing this information enables senior managers to identify environmental threats and opportunities. They are then able to choose strategies to lessen the impact of the former and take advantage of the latter.

Opportunities created by the external environment may include changing demographic and service patterns, an excess supply of physicians, abandonment of a service by another hospital, or development of a setting conducive to affiliating with a health maintenance organization (HMO) or forming a preferred provider organization (PPO). Threats are circumstances that can adversely affect the hospital. Intense competition from existing or new entrants into the service area, prospective pricing with an increasing fixed price patient mix, alternate delivery methods and locations, and fast-changing technology requiring major capital expenditures are examples.

Capability analysis evaluates the hospital's internal environment; from this analysis strengths and weaknesses are identified and inferences about comparative advantage are made. This can be done by examining the organization's functional areas. Included are the hospital's depth and breadth of services; its service area and market share; its efficiency in providing services, including work systems design and the qualities and capabilities of personnel; its financial strength, indebtedness, and patient-payor mix; and the skills, competencies, values, and experience of senior management, employees, and medical staff.

Information about weaknesses (W), opportunities (O), threats (T), and strengths (S) that can be identified in the situation audit (WOTS-UP analysis) becomes a critical ingredient in strategic planning and choice of strategy. Identifying opportunities and threats implies that strategies will be formu-

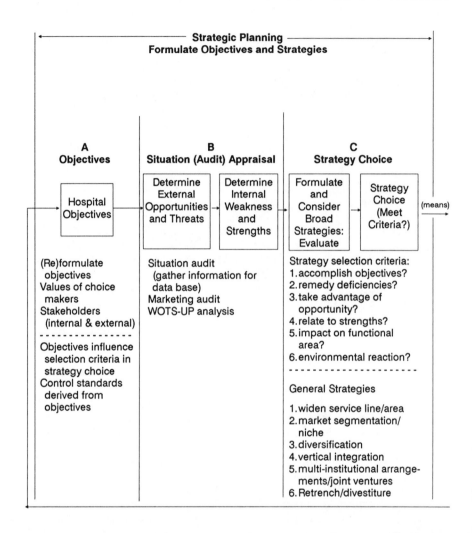

Figure II-1. Strategic and Operational Planning—Resource Allocation and Control Model. (See pages 166 and 167 for entire figure.)

lated to take advantage of the former and mitigate the latter. Strategies are evaluated using the criteria listed in Fig. II-1C. Will the strategy under consideration help accomplish the organization's objectives? Will it remedy a deficiency? Does it exploit an opportunity? Is it consistent with the organization's strengths? Does the organization have the capacity (physical resources, personnel, finances, technology) and capability to implement the

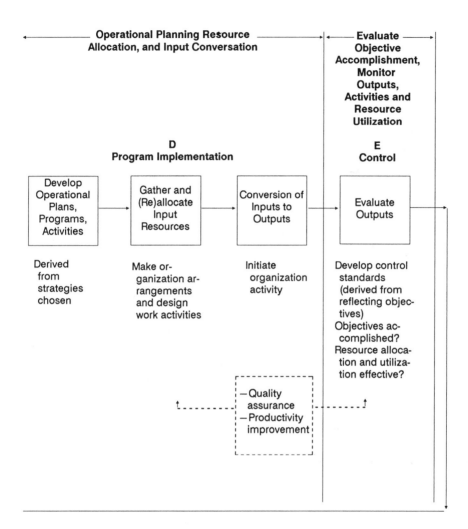

Figure II-1, continued.

strategy? What effect will the strategy have on functional areas such as administration, patient care, and financial resources? Finally, will the organization be able to cope with internal change and external competitive reaction if the strategy is implemented?

Choice of Strategy

Just as objectives are ends to be accomplished, strategies are means or ways to accomplish them. Strategies constitute the hospital's broad-based, comprehensive, integrative plans, which require a substantial commitment of resources. From them, detailed operational plans, programs, and activities are derived (including resource allocation among them) and implemented (Fig. II-1D).

Concurrent strategies can be formulated in broad areas such as influencing the external environment or targeting and supplying services to meet the needs of a specific clientele. One typology of hospital strategies described in the literature is downsizing, or becoming the low-cost provider and competing on the basis of price; increased market share; specialization; and diversification.[3] For clarity, a variant of this typology appears in Fig. II-1C. Included are (1) widening of the service line or area, (2) market segmentation (finding a niche), (3) diversification, (4) forward and backward vertical integration, (5) multi-institutional arrangements or joint ventures, and (6) retrenchment or divestiture.

Widening of the service line or area is a strategy hospitals choose to maintain or increase market share, to round out and complement and/or strengthen other existing services, and to adapt to changing environmental and client population trends. Examples are the addition of an attached hospital outpatient department, a satellite same-day surgery facility, a neonatal unit, an end-stage renal disease center, or a family practice center.

Market segmentation, or the decision to serve a particular market niche, is a strategy particularly suited to some hospitals. It involves identifying a target population by age, disease, class of people, or geographic area, and offering them a service such as prenatal care, oncology, psychiatric care, a birthing center, or an infertility unit.

Diversification, although similar to the first two strategies, involves offering programs and services that are not part of the acute care hospital's traditional core of inpatient care activities in order to enhance revenues. The services may be health care related (most often the case) or nonhealth care related; for example, a hospital may choose to provide construction consulting, data processing services, or productivity improvement programs to other organizations. Diversification into related health services not part of the core of inpatient services is increasing. Examples are rehabilitative services, wellness and health promotion programs, substance abuse programs, and home health care.[4]

Vertical integration involves establishing organizational arrangements whereby delivery of care (backward or forward) covers a range of "degrees of illness" rather than only one stage. The spectrum thus ranges from outpatient to chronic care. The most prevalent form of full vertical integration is exemplified by HMOs that provide outpatient care, acute inpatient hospital care, and long-term care often in an affiliated skilled nursing facility. A strategy adopted by many hospitals today is backward integration through establishing hospital-based or satellite same-day surgery facilities, and to a lesser degree forward integration by offering long-term, skilled nursing care and postdischarge home health care.

Multi-institutional affiliation as a strategy entails formalizing cooperative arrangements among independent provider organizations, or becoming a partner or subsidiary of a system that may offer management depth and access to capital advantages. ventures with physicians are another strategy. Common examples include radiology, emergency, and pathology services.

Finally, controlled retrenchment or divestiture is a strategy hospitals are increasingly adopting in order to survive, particularly when faced with conditions of excess capacity, weak cash flow, deteriorating breadth and depth of service, and technical obsolescence. The extreme case is facility closure. Less extreme is abandonment of selected services. A noteworthy example of a combination of strategies of controlled retrenchment and forward vertical integration for hospitals with excess beds is the closing of hospital wings and converting the beds to skilled nursing care.

Health Care Marketing and Strategic Planning

Health care marketing, particularly the marketing audit, is an integral part of strategic planning. Most authorities agree that marketing is a process by which one party receives something of value, such as a service, in exchange for something of value, such as paying a fee. Extending this notion of exchange results in the marketing concept, a process by which organizations seek to determine the wants and needs of prospective consumers and satisfy them with products or services.[5] If one accepts the basic marketing concept, marketing can be defined as "the analysis, planning, implementation and control of carefully formulated programs designed to bring about voluntary exchanges of values with target markets with the purpose of achieving organizational objectives."[6]

Ten years ago hospitals practiced inside-out marketing, in which the needs of the hospital were the primary focus. Today, hospitals practice outside-in marketing, in which consumer patient needs are identified and the hospital responds to them.[7] Traditionally, planning, implementing, and controlling programs to foster voluntary exchange focus on the four Ps: product, place, price, and promotion.

A hospital's product consists of the wide range of services hospitals provide, such as inpatient care, same-day surgery, emergency care, renal dialysis, and any additions to and deletions from the hospital's service mix over time. Nontraditional products are now offered, such as prescription services to other providers (nursing homes) and computer services to physicians.

Price has become increasingly important in the exchange relationship. It is no longer solely determined by the hospital. Some prices, particularly for Medicare beneficiaries, are mandated, whereas others are set by competitor and market forces. Price is also used for market penetration, or discounted as in the case of PPOs.[8]

Place is the physical location where services are provided. No longer are hospitals restricted to a single-site inpatient facility. Market outreach through freestanding primary care facilities and mobile health screening and service units are examples of extending place and altering the manner of distribution of service in order to attract and serve new customers.

Finally, promotion consists of those activities that inform consumers about the hospital's services, its place(s) of delivery, and, more recently, price. Compared to 20 years ago, advertising is now commonplace. No longer considered a characteristic of the snake-oil seller, promotion is seen as a legitimate way for the hospital to inform potential consumers about services.

The analysis and planning of marketing programs is predicated on the marketing audit. One author describes the marketing audit as incorporating three basic steps: identifying the information needed to evaluate the overall marketing effort (product, place, price, and promotion), collecting that information, and evaluating it.[9] As an information-gathering device, the marketing audit is a subcomponent of the strategic planning situation audit. Through activities such as marketing research (patient origin studies are an example), demographic analysis, and competitor analysis, the marketing audit provides information about internal strengths and weaknesses and external threats and opportunities as related to services provided, the manner in which they are provided, and their price and promotion. It assists hospitals in more clearly defining their potential patient population, assessing the population's health status and health care needs, and identifying ways to respond to those needs.

New Concepts and Consequences

The application of new concepts to strategic planning has increased hospitals' ability to cope with their environment. Three related, market-oriented concepts have altered the way managers view their hospitals and their outputs. They are strategic business units, portfolio analysis, and product line management.

Contemporary managers recognize that hospitals do more than provide patient care services. Diversification into nonrelated for-profit activities such as real estate is evidence of this. Strategic business unit (SBU) analysis provides an important conceptual framework for categorizing hospital activities and improving strategic planning by recognizing the distinctions among hospitals' services and among their markets. An SBU is an operating unit that provides distinct products or services to distinct customers. For example, a hospital may classify its SBUs into the following:

- Newborn and maternal care

- Child and adolescent care

- Adult medical care

- Mental health care

- Ambulatory/primary and outpatient care.[10]

The attributes of SBUs are that they can be allocated resources independently of others, they can be managed differently, and they can pursue separate and unique strategies chosen to respond to their external environment, yet they can contribute to accomplishing overall hospital objectives.

Portfolio analysis is simply strategic planning assessment, including a situation audit, applied to SBUs. It includes assessment of the SBUs' internal strengths and weaknesses and external threats and opportunities. Generally a market-driven two-axis matrix shows the SBUs' potential for growth (high or low) and market share (high or low). For an SBU with low market share and low potential for growth — for example, obstetrics — retrenchment or divestiture may be appropriate. One with high market share and high potential for growth, such as open heart surgery, warrants continued investment.

Another variant of portfolio analysis is the directional matrix presented in Fig. II-2. Its two axes show competitive strength (which could also include barriers to entry, market share, efficiency, quality of care, state of technology, and revenue produced) and future prospects (as affected by environment, competition, demographics, and other forces). Depending upon the strategic assessment and into which cell the SBU falls, different strategies are suggested.

The logical extension of SBUs is product line management. It is an organizational arrangement whereby one person is responsible for planning, resource use, control, and marketing of a service or product. This construct results in accountability and responsibility by the manager for volume, costs, and profits.

Prodded by DRGs, incorporation of SBU and product line management concepts into strategic planning is logical and results in many positive outcomes. First, hospitals now view themselves as a set of subunits providing different services to different clienteles. Second, strategic planning is now even more inextricably linked to marketing as hospitals consider the changing needs of existing and potential customers, as well as identify new opportunities and potential for market growth. Third, hospitals now pursue concurrent strategies for different SBUs. This is rational, but contradictory strategies (e.g., expanding same-day surgery while retrenching obstetrics) can lead to implementation of programs moving in diverse directions and having different effects on resource allocation and intraorganizational stability. Fourth, SBU and product line management allow enhanced control because they are predicated on sophisticated information and cost accounting systems. Finally, new organizational structures, often not functionally based (e.g., nursing service, surgery, housekeeping, administration), are required. The sheer dynamics and breathtaking speed with which new strategies and new structures have developed have created their own instability and altered the character of the hospital.[11]

FUTURE PROSPECTS OF HOSPITAL SBU OR PRODUCT LINE
(Including environment, competition, demographics, public policy, etc.)

COMPETITIVE
STRENGTH OF
HOSPITAL

(Including barriers
to entry for others,
market share, ef-
ficiency, quality,
state of technol-
ogy, revenue, etc.)

	Unattractive	*Average*	*Attractive*
Weak	Disinvest	Phased withdrawal Custodial	Double or quit
Average	Phased withdrawal	Custodial Growth	Try harder
Strong	Cash generation	Growth Leader	Leader

Figure II-2. Portfolio Analysis Model. Adapted from Lester A. Digman, *Strategic Management* (Plano, TX: Business Publications, Inc., 1986), p. 165, with permission.

Resource Utilization and Control

Once strategies have been chosen, derivative programs are designed or redesigned at the operational planning level, and resources are allocated or reallocated (Fig. II-1D). With proper organizational arrangements, including work processes and the appropriate mix of input resources, conversion occurs, outputs are generated, and hospital objectives accomplished.

Resource allocation and use in hospitals has always carried with it tag-along concepts of costs and quality. During the past decade they have become more than whispers; they have become a driving force for decision-making. It is imperative that managers, as stewards of resources, be able to function effectively in an environment where resources are limited and choices about use must be made. This necessarily implies prioritizing or even rationing. Cost control and productivity are much improved, yet managers and their constituents must be watchful to ensure that quality is not diminished.

Control

Planning and control cannot be separated. Planning determines the standards against which activity is compared; control is the process by which the comparison is made. Control ensures that results (outputs) of activity match expectations. Fig. II-1E shows how control standards—those criteria against which results are measured—are derived from and reflect objectives. Procedurally, controlling simply involves measuring results against standards (i.e., the expected results) and intervening should there be deviation.

Control is applied at two levels: outputs and activities. Output control standards are easily established since they tend to mirror objectives. Operationalizing standards means converting them into numerical measures such as length of stay, occupancy rate, number of outpatient visits, and cash flow and revenue-to-expense ratios. Control in hospitals also focuses on conversion activities (see Fig. II-1D) as they relate to design and implementation of programs, allocation of resources, or efficiency of resource utilization. Activity and resource utilization standards can be expressed in terms of staff turnover rates, supply consumption, equipment utilization, payroll expenses, and inventory levels.

Negative deviation from a standard is usually an indication that something is wrong. However, positive deviation may also suggest a problem. For example, activity control, such as monitoring of nursing service payroll expenditures, may reveal that those expenditures (actual results) are below budgeted levels (standards). Although initially this may appear to be beneficial, the cause should be examined. Is it because staffing is below authorized levels, perhaps resulting in deterioration in quality of care? Or is it due to high turnover of experienced personnel who are being replaced by less-experienced, lower-paid nurses? To take another example, it could be that maintenance and equipment expenditures are less than expected because staff are not practicing preventive maintenance or replacing obsolete equipment. This shifts expenditure burdens to future years.

Negative deviations are the clearer case for action. Even when feedback indicates that corrective action is warranted, there may be instances when the cause is beyond the manager's control. For example, supply expenditures might exceed budgeted levels (standards) because of increased prices or unavailability of less costly substitutes. Increased payroll expenditure may be due to a recently negotiated labor contract over which the departmental manager had no control.

The most familiar control technique is the budget. In health services organizations there are various kinds, including payroll, supply, equipment, revenue, capital expenditure, and maintenance budgets. Budgets are simply operational plans and expectations expressed in numerical terms, which are used as standards.

Quality Assurance

The financial constraints forced on hospitals have mandated improved control; in addition there has been greater demand for scrutiny of the content and quality of medical care. Third-party payors are very interested in minimizing cost through controls on utilization; they are less concerned with quality. The private sector, especially the Joint Commission on Accreditation of Healthcare Organizations (JCAHO), was an early leader in what was to become quality assurance. Federal government has shown interest in utilization proportionate to expenditures, especially hospital payments. Here, too, primary emphasis is on utilization. The change from professional standards review organizations (PSROs) to peer review organizations was a way to shake off the stigma of PSROs, which never met their initial promise, but at the same time to continue utilization review of federal beneficiaries.

Quality assurance is a vexatious problem for hospitals. It is required by organizations such as JCAHO, whose surveyors expect to find a quality assurance plan that includes specific efforts to improve quality. JCAHO is changing its focus from structure and process measures to much more emphasis on outcome. The importance of hospital programs to maintain quality is reinforced by legal actions for alleged malpractice. Ultimately, the chain of command leads to the governing body, which bears the brunt, both positive and negative.

After lurking in the background for several years, assertions that there is a medical malpractice crisis are once again making headlines. Rallies by physicians petitioning state legislatures for statutory relief are a highlight of the situation. In response to such pressures, most states have enacted tort reforms that limit noneconomic and punitive damages, modify the statute of limitations, and similarly reduce the patient's opportunity for redress.

The medical malpractice crisis of over a decade ago was largely precipitated by insurance carriers, who feared heavy losses unless they obtained large premium increases. This seems to be recurring. Insurance companies and physicians argue that there is a real problem, as evidenced by some specialties facing premium increases of 50 to 100 percent. However, there is ample evidence that hospitals' efforts to solve the problem of marginal or incompetent practitioners have not been very effective. Furthermore, legal claims filed represent but a small percentage of actual substandard care in hospitals. In this regard, all elements of the triad are at fault, and at risk. Lethargy with a dash of pusillanimity best describes the problem. Failing to act when substandard care or marginal practitioners are found is the most important element of the problem. The occasional unpatterned mistake that occurs in the best facility and to the best practitioner may not be forgivable, but it is certainly understandable and may not be legally actionable against the hospital. The outrageous cases are those where the pattern is clear, the problem certain, but there is inaction. Who would defend such behavior? More difficult to understand is that honest practitioners and governing body members would not want to be rid of the bad actors.

In 1986 Congress enacted the Health Care Quality Improvement Act, which when fully implemented will require that all hospitals report certain disciplinary actions against physicians and other practitioners to a national data base. Hospitals are expected to use that data base in credentialing decisions. One result will be that some hospitals will take fewer disciplinary actions against affected staff because of the significant results of doing so. On the whole, however, it is an important step toward improving the quality of clinical care.

Productivity Improvement

The single most significant external force in the past decade affecting the way managers allocate, use, and control resources has been the prospective pricing or fixed-price reimbursement systems adopted by increasing numbers of payors. These include mandated pricing by DRG as in the case of Medicare beneficiaries, market-imposed pricing as in the case of HMOs, or a discounting variant in the case of PPOs. Productivity improvement has become a prominent management responsibility as managers allocate and use resources.

Productivity is the relationship between organizational outputs and inputs. Traditionally productivity improvement has focused on this relationship to increase outputs relative to inputs consumed, or to maintain outputs with fewer inputs. One method for improving productivity is management engineering. It applies analytical and evaluative techniques to the resource allocation needs of new programs and determines whether present resource allocation and program design are both effective and efficient. Terms such as *methods improvement, operations analysis, management services,* and *health systems engineering* are used, but all refer to the same analytical and evaluative process. Examples of techniques are:

1. Designing and evaluating work systems, work centers, and work methods, including work simplification, standardization, and automation;

2. Establishing and evaluating work standards of job requirements, staffing needs, and human resource utilization;

3. Evaluating physical facility utilization, work layout and arrangement, floor space utilization, materials flow, traffic patterns, and scheduling;

4. Designing and evaluating production control, inventory control, quality control, materials handling, and information systems;

5. Performing value analyses of man-machine-material-technology relationships;

6. Evaluating paper flows and forms design;

7. Evaluating organizational structure and departmental interactions and interdependence;

8. Performing project analyses such as staff recruitment and retention, patient origin studies, ambulatory services patient flow, laundry, central supply, housekeeping, dietary, and equipment cost-benefit analyses.[12]

As internal consultants, management engineers use a multitude of evaluative techniques ranging from people and work process flow, process charts, and time study to sophisticated statistical analyses such as sampling, computer simulation, and modeling. Quantitative techniques and decision models both foster control at the activity level and are useful to managers in making resource allocation decisions. Techniques such as statistical sampling, forecasting, and regression analysis; cost-benefit analysis and capital budgeting (i.e., alternative equipment evaluations using payback, present value, and returns); decision theory; linear and goal programming; PERT and CPM; queueing theory; and simulation are examples.[13] They can be applied to all forms of scheduling (a major problem area for hospitals), staffing requirements, inventory levels, equipment requirements, and facility configuration. More than ever, today's hospital managers recognize the value of these evaluation approaches in achieving control and the power of quantitative techniques in making resource allocation decisions.

In an interesting and conceptually meaningful typology, Selbst extended productivity improvement beyond the program or work system level, which he termed "technical" productivity improvement, to a higher level labeled "organizational" productivity improvement.[14] At issue is not whether ancillary services scheduling is appropriate or whether the proper ratio of registered nurses to patients exists, but whether strategies and derived operational programs are appropriate given the hospital's strengths and weaknesses in specific markets and competitive environments. Efficiently doing the wrong things or pursuing wrong strategies does not lead to productivity improvement within the construct of using organizational resources.

Identifying proper SBUs and product lines through strategic planning has enabled managers to better understand and make decisions about where resources should be allocated and the results that can be expected from using those resources. Cost center accounting and operations audits are tools for evaluating the true cost of providing specific services and whether they should be continued, expanded, or discontinued. The evolution of management information systems (MIS) into integrated data base MIS provides the necessary information to fully understand present and alternate resource use and the consequences and opportunity costs of that use. Organizational productivity improvement will question whether those SBUs, product lines, or services appropriately use the organization's resources given the competitive environment and possible alternative uses.

Human Resources and Change

Hospital managers are focused on the hostile and competitive external environment and ways to respond to it. However, it cannot be their preoccupation. Given that the acute care hospital is both capital and labor intensive, the hospital manager's attention must include human resources, both their role in accomplishing organization objectives and how organizational change affects them.

Employees are the hospital's most important resource. They are the catalyst used in conversion of all other inputs (technology, material, capital, information) into outputs such as patient care. Success, efficiency, and effectiveness depend upon employees' skills, motivation, and commitment to the organization and its objectives. The innovative application of various strategies, new organizational structures around SBUs, and advanced technologies are only as good as the people who use them.

Human resource management activities include (1) those related to acquiring and maintaining the organization's human resources, and (2) those related to initiating organizational activity through people. The first, the staffing function, is centralized in the personnel department (increasingly called the human resources department). Staffing activities dealing with human resource acquisition are human resources planning, recruiting, employment testing, selection, and orientation. Maintaining human resources activities includes the formulation of administrative policies for promotion, training and development, performance appraisal, safety and health, and wage and salary administration including job design, description, and specification, and compensation. An additional responsibility of the director of human resources is collective bargaining.

Organizational Behavior

The hospital is an input-output system. It gathers resources (inputs) and through their utilization accomplishes objectives (outputs) (see Fig. i-4 in the Introduction to this book). The most important of these objectives is patient care. From a systems perspective, the hospital is a set of individual, social, and technical-structural subsystems — component parts that are interdependent and interact with, influence, and affect each other. This relationship is illustrated in Fig. II-3.

Organizational behavior is an expansion of the traditional management function of directing, or initiating organizational activity through people. It seeks to develop and determine a behavioral understanding of individuals, work groups, and their relationship to the technical-structural subsystem, which includes technology; structural elements such as organization design, work process, and job design; policies and procedures; authority relationships; and control systems.

The interaction of these three subsystems results in work being accomplished. The blend, or the degree to which they are in harmony or equi-

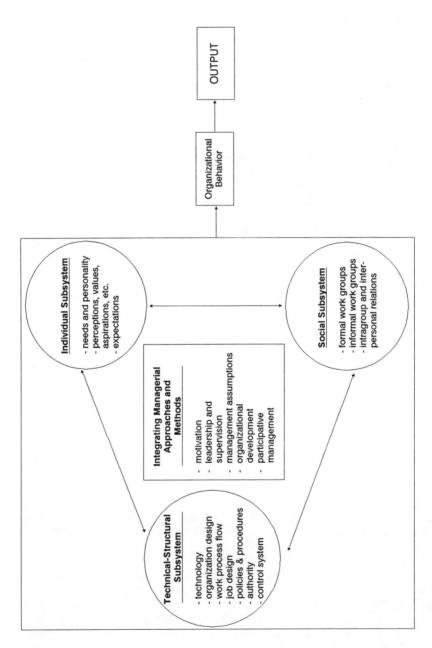

Figure II-3. Hospital subsystems.

librium, largely determines the effectiveness of task accomplishment and organizational activity—that is, whether objectives are accomplished. In today's environment changes to the technical-structural subsystem have had a measurable, and some would say adverse, impact on individual and social subsystems. Change and its impact are the focus of this section.

The Individual Subsystem

Initiating activity through people is what human resources management is all about. The motivation of individuals and externally or internally induced behavior is influenced by many factors. Among them are:

- Individual needs, shaped and affected by society, personal attitudes, expectations, aspirations, and previous experiences, including both positive and negative behavior reinforcement;

- Individual assumptions about behavior at work and the consequences of that behavior—behavior choice is largely based on the extent to which consequences correspond to behavior;

- The social environment, including formal and informal work group membership, and inter- and intragroup relationships, and the technical-structural environment including the formal organization;

- Managers' leadership and supervisory styles, along with the extent to which employees are involved and participate in work-related decision-making;

- The organizational culture, embodying the hospital's self-image and philosophy about the value and role of human resources.

The Social Subsystem

In hospitals, work is performed by formal and informal groups. The patient care team is the most prominent example of a formal group. The technical-structural subsystem establishes work relationships among people. Departmentalization into units, such as the nursing service, finance and accounting, the physical plant, and maintenance, or by SBU and product line, results in a formal grouping of people. Based on this design, methods for coordination and integration, authority-responsibility relationships, and work process flows result.

Informal groups coexist within the formal structure and formal work groups, and employees are members of both. Informal groups develop spontaneously and are not specifically designed by managers. Individual behavior is influenced by informal groups because they establish norms and standards of behavior for members and affect nonmembers. These standards may not be consistent with performance standards established by the organization's technical-structural subsystem. When they differ, peer pressure can cause individuals to conform to the informal group's norms.

Informal work groups have certain characteristics, including a structure of primary status, fringe status, and outstatus with an informal leader. Group members control the behavior of individuals through acceptance, nonacceptance (ostracism), or discipline. Informal groups develop because of physical proximity and sociological/psychological factors such as friendship, companionship, identification, and belonging affiliation. Outcomes of group activity typically include protecting the membership, role clarification, and limiting uncertainty.

The need for formal work groups in the hospital is obvious. They provide structure for task accomplishment through human resources. The need for effective informal groups is obvious, as well. Often, tasks can be accomplished through them more easily than through the formal organization. If informal group goals and norms are consistent with the formal organization, conflict is lessened and human resources are utilized more effectively.

Organizational Change

Change in organizations can be implemented by various methods. Among these are: (1) the decree approach, whereby managers simply announce changes; (2) the structure approach, whereby changes and alterations are made to the technical-structural subsystem with the individual and social subsystems reacting and adjusting; and (3) the individual and group participative approach, in which employees are included in decisions about change relating to their work.

Since the hospital's subsystems are interrelated and interdependent, changing one affects all. Further, conflict within organizations is not restricted to interpersonal clashes, but is often a function of organization design. Finally, organizational change, if systematically made and well thought out, can meet individual, group, and organizational needs concurrently.

Externally imposed and internally induced change is occurring in hospitals. Senior management responses through strategic planning have resulted in diverse multiple strategies and operational programs affecting structure, work systems, internal resource allocation, and utilization. The technical-structural subsystem is now measurably different and has affected the individual and social subsystems and their relationships. Finally, hospitals' perspective about the importance and use of human resources and how they fit within the scheme of strategic response is different. The culture has changed.

Traditionally, hospitals have been viewed as stable organizations with a well-defined self-image and philosophy that highly values human resources. It offered employment security and an atypical, yet smoothly functioning structure able to provide services on demand. Todays hospitals' self-image is blurred, and a new perspective toward human resources is emerging.

Decreased organizational stability and job security have changed employees' views about their employers and lessened motivation and commitment to the organization. With the tilt toward economic overtones, hospitals' previous attempts to improve productivity and contain costs through a rubric of behavioral-based approaches including participative management and quality circles are not pursued as aggressively. Two factors may account for this: First, the fast-changing external environment no longer affords the opportunity for resource-consuming innovation with limited immediate results; second, a shift has occurred in which management's focus is directed toward the technical-structural side of the organization to a greater degree than the human resources side. It is probable that the first factor has caused the second, because management has been preoccupied with the task of coping with the new requirements imposed by the environment.[15]

Some argue that this changed philosophy about human resources is undesirable. The literature supports this concern indirectly by citing the proxy measures of patient care and quality of care that are thought to be declining. The recent strategic changes have indeed been traumatic, yet are necessary for survival. As the immediate impact of change on the technical-structural subsystem and the consequences run their course, hospitals will redirect their attention and energy to their human resources. Equilibrium will be restored and hospitals will be much-improved organizations, producing outcomes substantially more positive than were present before the change.

Notes

1. Richard L. Johnson, "Revisiting 'The Wobbly Three Legged Stool,' " *Health Care Management Review* 4, No. 3 (Summer): 16, 1979.
2. For a good overview of strategic planning see: Farhad Simyon and Joseph Lloyd-Jones, *Strategic Management in the Health Care Sector: Towards the Year 2000* (Englewood Cliffs, NJ: Prentice-Hall, 1988). See also: Jonathon S. Rakich and Kurt Darr, "Outcomes of Hospital Strategic Planning," *Hospital Topics* 66, No. 4 (July/August):1988.
3. Dean C. Coddington, Lowell E. Palmquist, and William V. Trollinger, "Strategies for Survival in the Hospital Industry," *Harvard Business Review* 63, No. 3, (May-June): 129, 1985.
4. Frank G. Sabatino and Mary A. Grayson, "Diversification: More Black Ink than Red Ink," *Hospitals* 62, No. 1 (January 5): 36-42, 1988.
5. Pamela J. Bartlet, Charles D. Scheive, and Chris T. Allen, "Marketing Orientation: How Do Hospital Administrators Compare with Marketing Managers?" *Health Care Management Review* 9, No. 1 (Winter): 77, 1984.
6. Philip Kotler, *Marketing for Nonprofit Organizations* (Englewood Cliffs, NJ: Prentice-Hall, 1975), p. 5.
7. Paul McDevitt, "Learning By Doing: Strategic Marketing Management in Hospitals," *Health Care Management Review* 12, No. 2 (Winter): 24-25, 1987.
8. Dennis D. Pointer and Jack Zwanziger, "Pricing Strategy and Tactics in the New Hospital Marketplace," *Hospital & Health Services Administration* 31, No. 6 (November-December): 6-13, 1986.
9. Robert E. Sweeney, "The Marketing Audit—A Strategic Necessity: Marketing Management for the Mature Non-Profit," *Health Marketing Quarterly* 3, No. 2-3 (Winter): 94, 1986.
10. Gilbert D. Harrell and Matthew F. Fors, "Planning Evolution in Hospital Management," *Health Care Management Review* 12, No. 1 (Winter): 12, 1987.

11. Jonathon S. Rakich and Kurt Darr, "Outcomes of Hospital Strategic Planning," *Hospital Topics* 66, No. 4 (July/August):1988.
12. Jonathon S. Rakich, Beaufort B. Longest, Jr., and Kurt Darr, *Managing Health Services Organizations*. 2nd ed. (Philadelphia: W.B. Saunders, 1985), p. 264.
13. Keith A. Klafehn, Paul J. Kuzdrall, and Jonathon S. Rakich, "A Simulation Model for Hospital Bed Allocation

by Strategic Business Unit," *Proceedings of the Decision Sciences Institute*, November, 1989.
14. Paul Selbst, "A More Total Approach to Productivity Improvement," *Hospital & Health Services Administration* 30, No. 4 (July-August): 85, 1985.
15. Jonathon S. Rakich and Kurt Darr, "Outcomes of Hospital Strategic Planning," *Hospital Topics* 66, No. 4 (July/August):1988.

Bibliography

Adkins, Bobby and Stephen D. Smith. "An Information Revolution: The Transition to Expert Systems." *Computers in Healthcare* 8, No. 1 (January): 53, 1987.

Al-Fadel, Hashem O. "Clinical Engineering Productivity Improvement." *Journal of Clinical Engineering* 11, No. 5 (September-October): 355-359, 1986.

Alfirevic, Jay, Bruce Kroman, and Paul Ruflin. "Informational Needs for a Product Line Management System." *Healthcare Financial Management* 41, No. 3 (March): 60-65, 1987.

Baliga, B.R. and Brad Johnson. "Analysis of an Industry in Transition." *Health Care Strategic Management* 4, No. 12 (December): 5-14, 1986.

Barnes, James. "Good Marketing Takes a Lot of Strategic Planning." *Health Care* 28, No. 3 (April): 20-22, 1986.

Barrett, Diana and Susan R. Windham. "Hospital Boards and Adaptability to Competitive Environments." *Health Care Management Review* 9, No. 4 (Fall): 11-20, 1984.

Bartlett, Pamela J., Charles D. Schewe, and Chris T. Allen. "Marketing Orientation: How Do Hospital Administrators Compare with Marketing Managers?" *Health Care Management Review* 9, No. 1 (Winter): 77-86, 1984.

Bedard, Jean C. and Alton C. Johnson. "The Organizational Effectiveness Paradigm in Health Care Management." *Health Care Management Review* 9, No. 4 (Fall): 67-75, 1984.

Betz, Ronald P. and Howard B. Levy. "An Interdisciplinary Method of Classifying and Monitoring Medication Errors." *American Journal of Hospital Pharmacy* 42, No. 8 (August): 1724-1732, 1985.

Beyers, Marjorie. "Getting on Top of Organizational Change." *The Journal of Nursing Administration* 14, No. 11 (October): 32-39, 1984.

Bice, Michael O. "Corporate Cultures and Business Strategy: A Health Management Company Perspective." *Hospital & Health Services Administration* 29, No. 4 (July-August): 64-78, 1984.

Block, Lee F. and Christopher E. Press. "Product Line Development by DRG Builds Market Strength." *Healthcare Financial Management* 39, No. 12 (December): 50-52, 1985.

Boissoneau, Robert. "The Importance of Japanese Management to Health Care Supervisors: Quality and American Circles." *Health Care Supervisor* 5, No. 3 (April): 28-38, 1987.

Bolster, C.J. and Richard Binion. "Linkages Between Cost Management and Productivity." *Topics in Health Care Financing* 13, No. 4 (Summer): 67-75, 1987.

Boshard, Nick. "A Planning and Marketing Prototype for Changing Health Care Organizations." *Health Care Strategic Management* 4, No. 11 (November): 14-18, 1986.

Botz, Charles K. "Hospital-Wide Monitoring System Essential for Improving Productivity." *Dimensions* 63, No. 2 (March): 28-29, 1986.

Bradley, Donna. "Employee Credentialing." *QRB* 9, No. 11 (November): 345-346, 1983.

Brenner, Lawrence and William Jessee. "Delays in Diagnosis: A Problem for Quality Assurance." *QRB* 9, No. 11 (November): 337-344, 1983.

Buller, Paul F. and Ladd Timpson. "The Strategic Management of Hospitals: Toward an Integrative Approach." *Health Care Management Review* 11, No. 2 (Winter): 7-13, 1986.

Burik, David and David L. Marcellino. "Successfully Implementing a Multihospital Cost System." *Healthcare Financial Management* 41, No. 1 (January): 50-54, 1987.

Burton, Gene E. "Quality Circles in a Hospital Environment." *Hospital Topics* 64, No. 6 (November-December): 11-17, 1986.

Chaney, Harriett S. "Practical Approaches to Marketing." *Journal of Nursing Administration* 16, No. 9 (September): 33-39, 1986.

Chisholm, Rupert F. and James T. Ziegenfuss. "A Review of Applications of the Sociotechnical Systems Approach to Health Care Organizations." *The Journal of Applied Behavioral Science* 22, No. 3 (August): 315-327, 1986.

Clarke, Roberta N. and Linda Shyavitz. "Health Care Marketing: Lots of Talk, Any Action?" *Health Care Management Review* 12, No. 1 (Winter): 31-36, 1987.

Clemenhagen, Carol and Francois Champagne. "Medical Staff Involvement in Strategic Planning." *Hospital & Health Services Administration* 29, No. 4 (July-August): 79-94, 1984.

Cleverley, William O. "Financial Flexibility: A Measure of Financial Position for Hospital Managers." *Hospital & Health Services Administration* 29, No. 1 (January-February): 23-37, 1984.

————. "Financial Policy Formation: Principles for Hospitals." *Hospital & Health Services Administration* 30, No. 1 (January-February): 29-42, 1985.

————. "Promotion and Pricing in Competitive Markets." *Hospital & Health Services Administration* 32, No. 3 (August): 329-339, 1987.

————. "Strategic Financial Planning: A Balance Sheet Perspective." *Hospital & Health Services Administration* 32, No. 1 (February): 1-20, 1987.

Coddington, Dean C., Lowell E. Palmquist, and William V. Trollinger. "Strategies for Survival in the Hospital Industry." *Harvard Business Review* 63, No. 3 (May-June): 129-138, 1985.

Cooper, Robert B. "Market Strategies for Hospitals in a Competitive Environment." *Hospital & Health Services Administration* 28, No. 3 (May-June): 9-15, 1983.

Coulton, Claudia J. "Implementing Monitoring and Evaluation Systems in Social Work." *QRB* 12, No. 2 (February): 72-75, 1986.

Counte, Michael A., Diana Young Barhyte, and Luther P. Christman. "Participative Management Among Staff Nurses." *Hospital & Health Services Administration* 32, No. 1 (February): 97-108, 1987.

Covert, Richard P. "Management Engineering in the Hospital Environment." *Topics in Hospital Pharmacy Management* 3, No. 3 (November): 12-19, 1983.

Cowan, David Z. "Improving Productivity in the Health Care Industry." *Southern Hospitals* 52, No. 5 (September-October): 56-57, 1984.

Cushing, Maureen. "Informed Consent: An MD Responsibility." *American Journal of Nursing* 84, No. 4 (April): 437-440, 1984.

D'Aunno, Thomas A. and Howard S. Zuckerman. "A Life-Cycle Model of Organizational Federations: The Case of Hospitals." *Academy of Management Review* 12, No. 3 (July): 534-545, 1987.

Deane, Linda M. "Hospital Productivity Measurement in a Changing Environment." *Hospital Material Management Quarterly* 8, No. 3 (February): 59-65, 1987.

Deegan, Arthur X., II, and Thomas R. O'Donovan. "Budgeting and Management by Objectives." *Health Care Management Review* 9, No. 1 (Winter): 51-59, 1984.

del Bueno, Dorothy J. and Patricia M. Vincent. "Organizational Culture: How Important Is It?" *Journal of Nursing Administration* 16, No. 10 (October): 15-20, 1986.

Desai, Harsha B. and Charles R. Margenthaler. "A Framework for Developing Hospital Strategies." *Hospital & Health Services Administration* 32, No. 2 (May): 235-248, 1987.

Devolites, Milton and Myron Hatcher. "How to Evaluate the Effectiveness and Efficiency of Your Hospital's Operations." *Hospital Topics* 61, No. 5 (September-October): 10-15, 1983.

Donabedian, Avedis. "Criteria and Standards for Quality Assurance and Monitoring." *QRB* 12, No. 3 (March): 99-108, 1986.

_____. "Five Essential Questions Frame the Management of Quality in Health Care." *Health Management Quarterly* (First Quarter): 6-9, 1987.

_____. "Quality Assurance: Corporate Responsibility for Multihospital Systems." *QRB* (January): 3-7, 1986.

_____. "Quality, Cost, and Cost Containment." *Nursing Outlook* 32, No. 3 (May-June): 142-145, 1984.

_____. "The Quality of Medical Care." *Science* 200 (May 26): 856-864, 1978.

_____. "Twenty Years of Research on the Quality of Medical Care." *Evaluation & The Health Professions* 8, No. 3, (September): 243-265, 1985.

Eastaugh, Steven R. "Improving Hospital Productivity Under PPS: Managing Cost Reductions." *Hospital & Health Services Administration* 30, No. 4 (July-August): 97-111, 1985.

Eastaugh, Steven R. and Janet A. Eastaugh. "Prospective Payment Systems: Steps to Enhance Quality, Efficiency, and Regionalization." *Health Care Management Review* 11, No. 4 (Fall): 37-52, 1986.

Edey, Kim. "Productivity Improvement: Health Care Challenge of the 1980s." *Hospital Trustee* 7, No. 6 (November-December): 7, 23, 1983.

Ehrat, Karen S. "The Cost-Quality Balance: An Analysis of Quality, Effectiveness, Efficiency, and Cost." *Journal of Nursing Administration* 17, No. 5 (May): 6-13, 1987.

Fedorowicz, Jane. "Hospital Information Systems: Are We Ready for Case Mix Applications?" *Health Care Management Review* 8, No. 4 (Fall): 33-41, 1983.

Fera, Maureen and Gregory Finnegan. "Building a Productivity Improvement Team Through MIS Leadership." *Hospital & Health Services Administration* 31, No. 4 (July-August): 7-17, 1986.

Fetter, Robert B. and Jean L. Freeman. "Diagnosis Related Groups: Product Line Management Within Hospitals." *Academy of Management Review* 11, No. 1 (January): 41-54, 1986.

Fifer, William R. "Integrating Quality Assurance Mechanisms." In Roice D. Luke, et al., eds, *Organization and Change in Health Care Quality Assurance.* Rockville, MD: Aspen Systems, 217-230, 1983.

Files, Laurel A. "Strategy Formulation and Strategic Planning in Hospitals: Application of an Industrial Model." *Hospital & Health Services Administration* 28, No. 6 (November-December): 9-21, 1983.

Finkler, Steven A. "Ratio Analysis: Use With Caution." *Health Care Management Review* 7, No. 2 (Spring): 65-72, 1982.

Flexner, William A. and John W. Gunkler. "Confronting Organizational Culture." *Healthcare Forum* 29, No. 6 (November-December): 38-44, 1986.

Fottler, Myron D., Howard L. Smith, and Helen J. Muller. "Retrenchment in Health Care Organizations: Theory and Practice." *Hospital & Health Services Administration* 31, No. 5 (September-October): 29-43, 1986.

Gannon, John J., Dennis R. Roemer, and Randall J. Barbato. "Strategic Financial Planning Under DRG-Based Prospective Payment." *Topics in Health Care Financing* 11, No. 4 (Summer): 21-32, 1985.

Gilmore, Thomas N. and Mary Ann Peter. "Managing Complexity in Health Care Settings." *Journal of Nursing Administration* 17, No. 1 (January): 11-17, 1987.

Gluck, Frederick W. "A Fresh Look at Strategic Management." *Journal of Business Strategy* 6, No. 2 (Fall): 4-19, 1985.

Goodes, Melvin R. "Seizing the Competitive Initiative: Strategic Planning in the Healthcare Field." *Hospital & Health Services Administration* 29, No. 4 July-August): 30-39, 1984.

Hamilton, Robert D., III and Alan M. Zuckerman. "Strategic Planning: A Balanced View of a Balanced Portfolio." *Health Care Strategic Management* 4, No. 8 (August): 17-21, 1986.

Harrell, Gilbert D. and Matthew F. Fors. "Planning Evolution in Hospital Management." *Health Care Management Review* 12, No. 1 (Winter): 9-22, 1987.

Harrison, Fernande P. "Beyond Peer Review: The Medical Staff Role in the Price-Competitive Hospital." *QRB* 10, No. 9 (September): 262-268, 1984.

Heinzeller, Manfred. "Operational Auditing in Hospitals." *Topics in Health Care Financing* 10, No. 2 (Winter): 12-21, 1983.

Homer, Carl G. "Methods of Hospital Use Control in Health Maintenance Organizations." *Health Care Management Review* 11, No. 2 (Spring): 15-23, 1986.

Howell, Jon P. and Larry C. Wall. "Executive Leadership in an Organized Anarchy: The Case of HSOs." *Health Care Management Review* 8, No. 2 (Spring): 17-26, 1983.

Jaeger, B. Jon. "The Concept of Corporate Planning." *Heatlh Care Management Review* 7, No. 3 (Summer): 19-27, 1982.

Johnson, Brad. "Developing Strategic Planning Systems for Health Care Organizations." *Health Care Strategic Management* 4, No. 11 (November): 4-13, 1986.

Johnson, Everett A. "Thinking Conceptually About Hospital Efficiency." *Hospital & Health Services Administration* 26, No. 5 (Fall): 12-26, 1981.

Jones, Ronald H. "PERT/CPM Network Analysis: A Management Tool for Hospital Pharmacists Involved in Strategic Planning." *Hospital Pharmacy* 19, No. 2 (February): 89-90, 94-97, 1984.

Kaiser, Leland R. "Survival Strategies for Not-for-Profit Hospitals." *Hospital Progress* 64, No. 12 (December): 40-46, 1983.

Katz, Gerald, Leslie Zavodnick, and Elaine Markezin. "Strategic Planning in a Restrictive and Competitive Environment." *Health Care Management Review* 8, No. 4 (Fall): 7-12, 1983.

Kelley, Aaron C. and Mary Brady Brown. "Quality Circles in the Hospital Setting: Their Current Status and Potential for the Future." *Health Care Management Review* 12, No. 1 (Winter): 55-59, 1987.

Kellilher, Matthew E. "Managing Productivity, Performance, and the Cost of Services." *Healthcare Financial Management* 39, No. 9 (September): 23-28, 1985.

Kerschner, Morley I. and Jeffrey M. Rooney. "Utilizing Cost Accounting Information for Budgeting." *Topics in Health Care Financing* 13, No. 4 (Summer): 56-66, 1987.

Klinger, Charles A. "Information Systems Technology: Coming of Age." *Health Care Strategic Management* 3, No. 12 (December): 14-16, 1985.

Knoll, Robert J. and Thomas N. Howard. "What is Operational Auditing?" *Topics in Health Care Financing* 10, No. 2 (Winter): 1-11, 1983.

Kowalski, Jamie C. "Just-in-Time for Hospitals—So What's New?" *Hospital Materials Management* 11, No. 11 (November): 6-9, 1986.

Landsborough, Ron. "A Technique for Encouraging Employee Involvement in Improving Productivity." *Hospital & Health Services Administration* 30, No. 4 (July-August): 124-134, 1985.

Lehman, Malcolm E. "Quality Circles: Their Place in Health Care!" *Hospital Topics* 64, No. 5 (September-October): 15-19, 1986.

Longest, Beaufort B., Jr. "A Conceptual Framework for Understanding the Multi-hospital Arrangement Strategy." *Health Care Management Review* 5, No. 1 (Winter): 17-23, 1980.

Longo, Daniel R., et al. "Compliance with JCAH Standards: National Findings from 1982 Surveys." *QRB* 10, No. 3 (March): 81-86, 1984.

Lowe, Larry, "How to Avoid Chaos in the Transition to Product Line Management." *Health Care Strategic Management* 5, No. 4 (April): 9-13, 1987.

Luke, Roice D., and Robert E. Modrow. "Marketing and Accountability in Health Care." *Hospital & Health Services Administration* 26, No. 4 (Summer): 51-65, 1981.

MacStravic, Robin Scott. "Macro-Marketing in Health Care." *Hospital & Health Services Administration* 28, No. 3 (May-June): 54-61, 1983.

_____. "Product-Line Administration in Hospitals." *Health Care Management Review* 11, No. 2 (Spring): 35-43, 1986.

MacStravic, Robin E. Scott, Edward Mahn, and Deborah C. Reedal. "Portfolio Analysis for Hospitals." *Health Care Management Review* 8, No. 4 (Fall): 69-75, 1983.

Malhotra, Naresh K. "Hospital Marketing in the Changing Health Care Environment." *Journal of Health Care Marketing* 6, No. 3 (September): 37-48, 1986.

Manning, Martin F. "Product Line Management: Will It Work in Health Care?"*Healthcare Financial Management* 41, No. 1 (January): 23-32, 1987.

Margulies, Newton and John Duval. "Productivity Management: A Model for Participative Management in Health Care Organizations." *Healthcare Management Review* 9, No. 1 (Winter): 61-70, 1984.

May, John J. and Ed H. Bowman. "Information Systems for the Value Management Era."*Healthcare Financial Management* 40, No. 12 (December): 70-74, 1986.

McClure, Lynne. "Organization Development in the Healthcare Setting." *Hospital & Health Services Administration* 30, No. 4 (July-August): 55-64, 1985.

McColl, Cheryl M. "Managers and Staff." *Dimensions* 64, No. 1 (February): 37-39, 1987.

McDevitt, Paul. "Learning By Doing: Strategic Marketing Management in Hospitals." *Health Care Management Review* 12, No. 1 (Winter): 23-30, 1987.

McHugh, Mary L. "Information Access: A Basis for Strategic Planning and Control of Operations." *Nursing Administration Quarterly* 10, No. 2 (Winter): 10-20, 1986.

McLaughlin, Curtis P. "Strategic Planning Under Current Cutback Conditions." *Health Care Management Review* 7, No.3 (Summer): 7-17, 1982.

McManis, Gerald L. "Managing Competitively: The Human Factor." *Healthcare Executive* 2, No. 6 (November-December): 18-22, 1987.

McNash, Mark. "Management Engineering's Contribution to the Strategic Planning Process." *Health Care Strategic Management* 3, No. 4 (April): 4-7, 1985.

Mendenhall, Stanley, Robert Shepherd, and Edward Kobrinski. "Cost Accounting in Healthcare Organizations: Who Needs It?" *Healthcare Financial Management* 41, No. 1 (January): 34-39, 1987.

Minard, Bernie. "Managing the Hospital's Portfolio of Information Systems." *Health Care Strategic Management* 5, No. 1 (January): 16-22, 1987.

Morris, Dudley E. and Susan E. Rau. "Strategic Competition: The Application of Business Planning Techniques to the Hospital Marketplace." *Health Care Strategic Management* 3, No. 1 (January): 17-20, 1985.

Mullin, Robert L. "Diagnosis-Related Groups and Severity." *The Journal of the American Medical Association* 254, No. 9 (September): 1208-1210, 1985.

Nackel, John G. and Irvin W. Kues. "Product-Line Management: Systems and Strategies." *Hospital & Health Services Administration* 31, No. 2 (March-April): 109-123, 1986.

Nichols, Paul. "Market Oriented Strategic Planning, Revisited." *Health Management Forum* 7, No. 2 (Summer): 47-56, 1986.

Nowell, Antonia H., and Gadis Nowell. "Participation for Nurse Unit." *Hospital Topics* 64, No. 1 (January-February): 28-31, 42, 1986.

Orlikoff, James E. and Gary B. Lanham. "Why Risk Management and Quality Assurance Should Be Integrated." *Hospitals* 55, No. 11 (June): 54-55, 1981.

Pasmore, William, Jeffrey Petee, and Richard Bastian. "Sociotechnical Systems in Health Care: A Field Experiment." *The Journal of Applied Behavioral Science* 22, No.3 (August): 329-339, 1986.

Patterson, Dennis J. and Kent A. Thompson. "Product Line Management: Organization Makes the Difference." *Healthcare Financial Management* 41, No. 2 (February): 66-72, 1987.

Peters, Gregory G. "Reallocating Liability to Medical Staff Review Committee Members: A Response to the Hospital Corporate Liability Doctrine." *American Journal of Law and Medicine* 10, No. 1 (Spring): 115-138, 1984.

Pointer, Dennis D. and Jack Zwanziger. "Pricing Strategy and Tactics in the New Hospital Marketplace." *Hospital & Health Services Administration* 31, No. 6 (November-December): 5-18, 1986.

Polister, Pam. "Accreditation: Chance for Education as Well as Evaluation." *Trustee* 35, No. 9 (September): 30+, 1982.

Potter, Donald P. "Downsizing: It's Really Market Readjustment." *Health Care Strategic Management* 4, No. 4 (April): 19-23, 1986.

"PRO Rules Change Focus of Peer Review." *Hospitals* 55, No. 18 (September 16): 31, 1981.

"PROs." *Hospitals* 57, Nos.10 and 18 (May 16 and September 16): 59, 31, 1983.

Rakich, Jonathon S., Beaufort B. Longest, and Kurt Darr. *Managing Health Services Organizations.* 2nd ed. Philadelphia: W.B. Saunders, 1985.

Ready, R.K. and F.E. Ranelli. "Strategic and Nonstrategic Planning in Hospitals." *Health Care Management Review* 7, No. 4 (Fall): 27-38, 1982.

Reynolds, James X. "Using DRGs for Competitive Positioning and Practical Business Planning." *Health Care Management Review* 11, No. 3 (Summer): 37-55, 1986.

Rhee, Sang-O. "Organizational Determinants of Medical Care Quality: A Review of the Literature." In Roice, D. Luke, et al., eds. *Organization and Change in Health Care Quality Assurance.* Rockville, MD: Aspen Systems, 127-146, 1983.

Robertsen, John A. "Managing for Productivity Improvement." *Topics in Hospital Pharmacy Management* 2, No. 4 (February): 17-21, 1983.

Rosenberger, Herbert R. and Kate M. Kaiser. "Strategic Planning for Health Care Management Information Systems." *Health Care Management Review* 10, No. 1 (Winter): 7-17, 1985.

Ruppel, Ronald W. and Ted E. Grazman. "Operations Analysis Is the First Step in Planning." *Healthcare Financial Management* 36, No. 2 (February): 57-60, 1982.

Sabatino, Frank G. and Mary A. Grayson. "Diversification: More Black Ink Than Red Ink." *Hospitals* 62, No. 1 (January): 36-42, 1988.

Salter, Vera. "Product Line Management: Its Meaning and Future Promise." *Health Care Strategic Management* 4, No. 5 (May): 13-15, 1986.

Schlotman, Robert S. "Changing Industry Demands New Approach to Information Systems Planning." *Health Care Strategic Management* 4, No. 2 (February): 4-7, 1986.

Schneller, George O., Richard E. Kopelman, and John J. Silver. "A Combined Leave Benefit System for the Control of Absenteeism in Health Care Organizations." *Hospital & Health Services Administration* 27, No. 1 (January-February): 63-74, 1982.

Scotti, Dennis J. "Organizing for Strategic Planning in Smaller Not-for-Profit Community Hospitals." *Hospital & Health Services Administration* 29, No. 4 (July-August): 50-63, 1984.

Selbst, Paul L. "A More Total Approach to Productivity Improvement." *Hospital & Health Services Administration* 30, No. 4 (July-August): 85-96, 1985.

Shaffer, Ken, et al. "Successful QA Program Incorporates New JACH Standard." *Hospitals* 55, No. 16 (August 16): 117, 1981.

Shaffer, Michael J. "Integration of Clinical Engineering Into the Hospital Organization." *Hospital & Health Services Administration* 28, No. 5 (September-October): 72-81, 1983.

Shaffer, Michael, et al. "Clinical Engineering—An Enigma in Health Care Facilities." *Hospital & Health Services Administration* 24, No. 3 (Summer): 77-95, 1979.

Sheinfield Gorin, Sherri N. "Expect the Unexpected: Consequences of the Use of Productivity Indices." *Health Care Strategic Management* 3, No. 4 (April): 12-15, 1985.

Smith, C. Thomas. "Hospital Management Strategies for Fixed-Price Payment." *Health Care Management Review* 11, No. 1 (Winter): 21-26, 1986.

Smith, David P. "One More Time: What Do We Mean by Strategic Management?" *Hospital & Health Services Administration* 32, No. 2 (May): 219-233, 1987.

Smith, Robert J. "Integrating the Marketing Function: A Model for Strategic Management." *Health Marketing Quarterly* 3, No. 2-3 (Winter): 13-17, 1986.

Stearns, Gerry and Eric Joseph. "Passing JCAH Muster, Or Six Essential Ingredients for a Successful Quality Assurance Program." *Trustee* 38, No. 6 (June): 15-17, 1985.

Stevens, Barbara J. "The Role of the Nurse Executive." *The Journal of Nursing Administration* 11, No. 2 (February): 19-22, 1981.

Suver, James D. and Bruce R. Neumann. "Resource Measurement by Health Care Providers." *Hospital & Health Services Administration* 31, No. 5 (September-October): 44-52, 1986.

Sweeney, Robert E. "The Marketing Audit —A Strategic Necessity: Marketing Management for the Mature Non-Profit." *Health Marketing Quarterly* 3, No. 2-3 (Winter): 93-97, 1986.

"The QIP Form: the One-Page Quality Assurance Tool." *QRB* 12, No. 3 (March): 87-89, 1986.

Thompson, John S. "Diagnosis-Related Groups and Quality Assurance." *Topics in Health Care Financing* 8, No. 4 (Summer): 43-49, 1982.

Thompson, Richard E. "Guidelines for More Informative Quality Assurance Reports." *Trustee* 35, No. 12 (December): 33+, 1982.

Torrens, Paul. "What's Up Doc? Management. Technology. Systems." *Healthcare Executive* 1, No. 7 (November-December): 27-29, 1986.

Turban, Efraim. "Decision Support Systems in Hospitals." *Health Care Management Review* 7, No. 3 (Summer): 35-42, 1982.

Vraciu, Robert A. "Hospital Strategies for the Eighties: A Mid-Decade Look." *Health Care Management Review* 10, No. 4 (Fall): 9-19, 1985.

Wallace, Cynthia. "Hospital Turns to Staff for Cost-Cutting Help." *Modern Healthcare* 15, No. 4 (February): 108-110, 1985.

Weil, Peter A. and Leo Stam. "Transitions in the Hierarchy of Authority in Hospitals: Implications for the Role of the Chief Executive Officer." *Journal of Health and Social Behavior* 27, No. 2 (June): 179-192, 1986.

Weil, Thomas P. and A.T. Hollingsworth. "Strategies for Hospital Staff Reduction." *Health Care Strategic Management* 4, No. 4 (April): 14-18, 1986.

Weil, Thomas P. and R.W. Hoyer. "Determining Hospital Product Mix: An Exploratory Analysis." *Health Care Management Review* 12, No. 2 (Spring): 7-14, 1987.

Weinstein, Bernard M. "Situation Analysis and Strategic Development in a Public Hospital." *Hospital & Health Services Administration* 31, No. 6 (November-December): 62-73, 1986.

Wenke, Paul C. "13 Steps Toward Enhancing Productivity." *Hospitals* 57, No. 19 (October 1): 109-110, 111, 1983.

Williams, Kenneth J. and Paul R. Donnelly. "Straight Talk About Accountability." *Trustee* 35, No. 12 (August): 14-16, 1982.

Wood, Van R. and Jagdip Singh. "Strategic Planning for Health Care Markets: A Framework and Case Study in Analyzing Diagnosis Related Groups." *Journal of Health Care Marketing.* 6, No. 3 (September): 19-28, 1986.

Wyszewianski, Leon, John R.C. Wheeler, and Avedis Donabedian. "Market-Oriented Cost-Containment Strategies and Quality of Care." *Milbank Memorial Fund Quarterly/Health and Society* 60, No. 4: 518-550, 1982.

Zuckerman, Alan M. "The Impact of DRG Reimbursement on Strategic Planning." *Hospital & Health Services Administration* 29, No. 4 (July-August): 40-49, 1984.

Zuckerman, Stephen, et al. "Physician Practice Patterns Under Hospital Rate-Setting Programs." *JAMA* 252, No. 18 (November): 2589-2592, 1984.

Strategic Planning And Marketing

Selection 17, "What Does Strategic Planning Really Mean?" by Katy Ginn, offers a succinct presentation of the strategic planning process in health care institutions. This includes mission, objectives, analysis of internal and external environments, and choice of strategies. Selection 18, "Vertical Integration: Exploration of a Popular Strategic Concept" by Montague Brown and Barbara P. McCool, examines the implementation of this contemporary strategy in different settings, including investor-owned chains, multihospital systems, and managed care programs (i.e., HMOs, PPOs); under various market conditions, including those for tertiary and teaching hospitals; and the impact on physicians and competition.

Selection 19, "Marketing in the Academic Health Center" by Charles L. Breindel, offers an interesting marketing point of view for these organizations. The author's presentation of "demarketing" of services is meant to encourage lower cost alternatives, such as disease prevention, for low-revenue-producing clienteles. Myra Crawford and Myron Fottler in selection 20, "The Impact of Diagnosis Related Groups and Prospective Pricing Systems on Health Care Management," provides an extensive look at the impact of PPS on hospital management functions including planning, organizing, directing, and controlling. For each they present new constraints, conditions, and likely responses.

17

What Does "Strategic Planning" Really Mean?

Katy Ginn

Katy Ginn is a Consultant with Agnew, Peckham & Associates, hospital consultants, Toronto.

Discussions regarding the concept of strategic planning are becoming more frequent in today's health care institutions. What is really behind the name? Is it something which is appropriate in the hospital setting, or is it in fact there already, under some other name, or names? For instance, how does it relate to "role" or "mission"? Is it a "long-range plan"?

To answer these questions and even begin to assess the applicability of strategic planning to the health care industry, it is important to first understand what is meant by the term "strategic planning" and the assumptions and implications that lie behind it.

Strategic planning has evolved as a process which attempts to incorporate the various types of planning into a more encompassing business plan and a strategy for implementation. The objective of the process is to enable the organization to better adapt to the changes and pressures imposed by the environment. It provides the organization with the ability to direct its future, rather than forcing it to react to problems created by change.

Implicit in the process of strategic planning is a future orientation — "Who are we"?, "Where do we want to be in the future"? — and a view of the institution as a whole. It is a view which is concerned with the impact of external changes on the organization rather than with internal activities such as control of spending. It is an attempt to remove the constraints of current thinking in order to look at alternatives rationally.

The focus of the plan is on resource allocation decisions and priorities recognizing that few, if any, institutions can do everything they would like. It is a case of identifying the best value for the resources employed.

The strategic plan is intended as a tool which belongs to the organization as a whole, not merely the product of an exercise. In order to ensure that it remains dynamic and useful, the involvement and support of all levels of the organization in each step of the planning process is essential.

Much of the merit of the strategic plan lies in the process of its development. There are several distinct components which are worth examining.

The first step is the development of a mission or role statement. This is typically a broad directive establishing the thrust for the future. In strategic planning, the mission is an outcome of the assessment of the present purpose, an evaluation of internal strengths and weaknesses and an analysis of the threats and opportunities in the external environment.

The analysis of the external environment will project the most probable picture of the future as it affects the organization. It is not possible or worth monitoring all elements of the external environment. However, the most significant should be identified and are commonly grouped as social, economic, legal, political, competitive and cooperative factors. The weight or concern placed on each group will vary from institution to institution, depending on individual situations and the particular concerns of the community as a whole.

In conjunction with the environmental analysis, the organization must evaluate its capabilities to manage or compete in the external environment. This involves identifying major strengths and weaknesses within the organization. The headings under which these are generally grouped include financial viability, quantity and quality of programs, human resource skills at both management and provider levels, physical facilities and technical capabilities.

Considering the internal situation together with the assessment of the external environment enables the organization to define overall future direction and approach. For example, an organization may operate in an environment which is extremely unpredictable. The organization, therefore, has little potential power to exercise meaningful control and a reactive stance is likely the most appropriate philosophy. The situation which is more likely to face a hospital is an environment which is changing, but in broadly predictable terms. Assuming that the hospital is reasonably healthy in an overall sense, a preferred future may be defined and worked towards in an interactive manner.

Having identified key strategic issues through an assessment of internal capabilities and external threats and opportunities, the mission of the organization is then confirmed or redefined.

The next step in the planning process is the development of alternative strategies to deal with the key issues. Depending on the size of the institution and the issues, strategies are often considered at sub-unit levels such as departments, programs or projects. They are assessed for congruence with established goals and a perception of the internal and external environments. Strategies can be positioned based on merit and demand on resources. This allows the hospital to assess the contribution of various programs or departments to the overall effectiveness of the institution and ultimately allows it to make reasoned decisions and to establish priorities.

The remaining task in the planning process is the refinement of strategies to develop plans for implementation. For example, if the strategy is the development of a new program, the implementation plan will detail procedures, policies and workload projections, and will outline resource requirements such as manpower, financing, equipment and facilities.

In summary, the components of a strategic planning process include:

- an analysis of the internal and external environments;

- formulation of a mission statement;

- development of goals and objectives;

- identification of strategic alternatives;

- development of an implementation plan.

Involvement and support of all levels of the organization throughout the process is essential.

18

Vertical Integration: Exploration of a Popular Strategic Concept

Montague Brown and Barbara P. McCool

Montague Brown, M.B.A., Dr. P.H., J.D., in Chairman and CEO of Strategic Management Services, Inc., Shawnee Mission, Kansas.

Barbara P. McCool, R.N., M.H.A., Ph.D., is President of Strategic Management Services, Inc., Shawnee Mission, Kansas.

News headlines continue to proclaim the virtues of vertical integration, networking, regionalization, cluster markets, and other methods of organizing health care.[1] With insurers entering major joint ventures with providers (Aetna with Voluntary Hospitals of America [VHA]; Provident and Transamerica Occidental with American Healthcare Systems [AHS]; Equitable with Hospital Corporation of America [HCA]), it would seem that something fundamental is occurring that might presage a more vertically integrated health care delivery system.

The idea of vertical integration in health care easily stirs the imagination and holds the attention of policy makers, health administrators, and, increasingly, entrepreneurs. Those seeking to regulate expenditures want vertical integration to avoid duplication of services. Those seeking to ensure quality and efficiency attempt to own or control whatever resources a patient might need within an episode of illness or even a lifetime. More pragmatic people seek to bring downstream services and upstream services under their wings for many reasons: to stabilize markets, to use excess capacity, to secure profits from related services, and, from time to time, to capitalize on the prestige one hopes will enhance an entire line of services.

The concept of regionalization of health care services for a particular population, territory, or trade area has a long history: the Lord Dawson Report in England in 1920;[2] the Committee on the Cost of Medical Care in the United States in 1932;[3] the Commission on Hospital Care in 1956;[4] the

Reprinted with permission of Aspen Publishers, Inc., from *Health Care Management Review*, 1986.

Regional Medical Program in 1966;[5] and AHA's Ameriplan proposal,[6] which sought some form of integrated care for a geopolitical region.[7-10] Since these ideas seem to surface frequently, one can reasonably question whether the current enthusiasm will lead to major change or whether it merely represents another fad.

One should remember that earlier calls for regionalization and vertical integration came during times of physicians and hospital shortage. Access and comprehensiveness were big issues. Today, there is a surplus of hospitals, beds, and physicians, coupled with high cost and overuse. If these old ideas fit today, it will have to be for different reasons than those cited in earlier days.

The literature on the regionalization of health services discusses many, if not all, of the underlying reasons for vertical integration. However, the literature and rationale for regionalization go beyond the ideas of economy and medical efficiency to endorse political governance.

Many proponents of regionalization basically are seeking a way to govern. For those who prefer governance within the framework of the political system, regional health care systems can be directed by elected and appointed government officials and institutions. For others who prefer private, voluntary institutions, regional systems can work under a governmental charter or framework, but can be essentially self-directed by their own voluntary governing bodies. Those who sit at the supposed apex of a vertically integrated system seem to think it equally natural and desirable to have such a system governed and controlled by the medical elite at the academic health science center. In a pluralistic system such as the United States, regionalization represents a move toward greater vertical integration and centralization of control.

Whatever the motive, proponents of vertical integration generally share the arguments of economy, efficiency, quality, and access associated with the concept.

What is Vertical Integration?

Vertical integration is a term used in marketing and economics to describe complex systems that link resource development, manufacturing, distribution, and consumption. For example, food chains, when linked vertically, own and operate the farms, processing plans, and distribution systems, and provide food to their customer base in a variety of forms, including meal service. Their integration may also involve them in energy production for their farms, factories, and transportation systems.

In health care, vertical integration commonly refers to the ability of one provider system (i.e., owner or controlling entity) to provide all levels and intensities of service to patients and health care consumers from a geographically contiguous region when these clients present themselves to that system. Primary, secondary, tertiary, rehabilitative, custodial, and other care modalities are available within one system. In contrast, mere ownership of a variety of different service modalities in separate areas of the country should be analyzed as a form of diversification, perhaps, but not as vertical integration of service from a consumer's perspective.

In a system of vertically integrated services, a patient presents himself or herself for primary care and moves from one level to another as is medically appropriate, using the most economical and best service necessary and remaining within the ambit of the same provider. One can argue that the greater the extent that all problems are met by one provider, the greater is the vertical integration of that provider. A fully integrated system is capable of providing all services to all patients who present themselves for care.

In addition, since medical care has long been treated by consumers as a service for which one needs to purchase risk protection, a vertically integrated system will provide financial services, much as General Motors provides financial services such as loans to assist in buying a car so that consumers can use its products. Traditionally Blue Cross/Blue Shield provided such services independently of provider. Now providers are adding financial risk services to their portfolios to augment traditional financial risk services.

History of Vertical Integration

Hospitals and hospital chains were first attracted to vertical integration because of economies of scale and increase in market share. Economies of scale (quality, cost, production efficiency, profit potential, access to supply of inputs, and access and control of customer markets) relate to decisions about when to own, operate, control, or make an element or service versus contracting for, entering a joint venture, or buying it in the open market. These decisions are made with due consideration for quality of medical care, access for consumers, and competitive factors in the market.

Motivated by economy of scale issues and competitive concerns, the prudent strategist in previous times operated, merged, networked, or otherwise linked with as many elements of a vertically integrated system of hospitals and services as possible. This same strategist also sought to attract independent primary care physicians, who were often in short supply. The strategist sought to network with these physicians for referrals, education, and the economic opportunity brought about by their endorsement of the brand name (most prestigious, biggest, or best) of the system and its secondary and tertiary services.

Two-Stage Process

The strategist developed a two-stage process of vertical integration. In the first stage, he or she took advantage of the many economies of operation for hospitals and related services that were available, especially when there were units in contiguous geographic areas. For example, one top-notch management group with specialists could handle 10 or 20 hospitals rather well. Laundries, mobile diagnostic technology, educational systems, representation to government, access to capital, and the like provided attractive opportunities for systems of hospitals with a scale of approximately $300 million to $900 million in revenues.

The greatest opportunity to achieve economies of scale resided in a second stage of integration—control over medical referral patterns. This second stage depended more heavily on physician market competitive factors than on the known economies of scale in hospital operations. In other words, vertical integration had to overcome the resistance (i.e., the refusal to refer patients) of individual practitioners ready to attack any upstream competitor (hospital or specialist) that threatened their opportunities and their freedom to control their own patients.

Indeed, the experiences of voluntary multihospital systems in the late 1960s and 1970s show that integration of medical referrals is easier to attempt than to accomplish. These hospital systems set out to build regionally integrated cluster-type systems that would offer all levels of medical care: treatment in primary settings by independent practitioners; first-level hospital care; specialist care; and, ultimately, subspecialist care. What they found was that physicians insisted on vertical levels of care at one site, their primary site, and not someone else's primary base. Few, if any, voluntary systems achieved very good results in trying to influence referrals to the other geographically contiguous hospitals they owned. The system's ownership or management of additional hospitals simply did not overcome traditional physician referral patterns. Thus, voluntary hospital systems were able to achieve some degree of vertical integration of hotel-type support services (e.g., bed and board), management services, and capital economies, but not vertical integration of patient care.

Investor-Owned Chains

Investor-owned chains also have a history of showing supply-side gains but no real vertical integration. During the 1970s these chains, with their capital advantage, rushed into the most readily penetrable market areas that appeared to have been abandoned by privately owned hospitals: growth areas needing new capacity and overflow areas with breakaway physicians who, for their own competitive reasons, wanted another hospital.

As growth occurred in such investor-owned, horizontally integrated, single-site, and single-purpose hospitals, management specialization developed around organization building, reimbursement, and regulatory process. Shared purchasing, dedicated suppliers, and proprietary interest in manufacturing and distribution were always potential ways to gain additional revenue, but these options were not used much as long as no pressure existed on the pricing side, which controls utilization. Today, with more consumer sensitivity to the price of services, any savings in supply costs go directly to the bottom line, so the scramble for economies in hotel services makes much more sense. Any savings on cost in a price-oriented system benefit the provider's bottom line directly. Of course, the provider may lower prices, thus passing savings to buyers. Again, these economies of operation do not reflect real vertical integration.

Multihospital Systems

A number of multihospital systems have owned and operated prepaid plans, rehabilitation centers, nursing homes, and home care programs, and have offered many subspecialty medical services at one location or another. Such services offered in diverse locations represent a form of diversification but do not address the issues of integrated services for a defined population. Having such experiences and capabilities does, however, aid in positioning such firms for ultimately bringing their other resources into systems of vertically integrated services.

Current Interest in Vertical Integration

Since investor-owned systems historically have ignored the opportunities for integration upward into tertiary services and downward into risk services (e.g., ambulatory care, diagnostics), ventures such as Wesley Medical Center in Wichita, Kansas, Lovelace Clinic in Albuquerque, New Mexico, St. Joseph Hospital in Omaha, Nebraska, Humana's Louisville, Kentucky, operations, and similar deals came as a shock to the voluntary and university communities. Corporations thought to be interested only in the simple primary care hospitals in single-hospital or overflow-hospital markets were suddenly interested in hospitals with the potential for becoming the linch-pin in a vertically integrated system. The more skeptical observers, of course, seemed to think that such ventures were merely window dressing engaged in for prestige and for marketing purposes, not serious business ventures with their own merits. Less attention seemed to be given at the time to the inherent potential in aggressively seeking preferred provider status with multiple managed care systems or in building or buying such systems to complement the provider capacity in place.

Increasing Profitability

This new interest in vertical integration in markets where excess capacity exists is understandable as chains such as HCA, American Medical International (AMI), and others announce lower earnings from operations. Having maximized their economies of operations, these chains are now turning to vertical integration to increase their profitability from underutilized assets.

To achieve this goal, the chains must have a solid base of primary physicians, tertiary capacity, and as many ties as possible with insurance companies and managed care systems. Three tasks comprise the real competitive challenge to the chains and regional systems: (1) backward integration to risk services, (2) joint ventures with physicians, and (3) forward integration into referral services. Unless mastered, these tasks represent the Achilles' heel of the for-profit and not-for-profit regional systems.

Changing Competitors

Vertical integration may also play an increasing role among some hospitals in areas sparsely populated by chain operations. In fact, some observers have said that these hospitals may drop out of the national voluntary alliances, realizing that their biggest competitive threat stems from the potential vertical integration of other systems in their own regions, not from hospital chains.

Now, with the major move by investor-owned chains and voluntary alliances to join with insurance firms to vertically integrate backward into risk services, and with risk service firms striving to move subscribers into managed care systems in order to meet customer demand for more cost control, the entire range of assumptions about who is competing with whom is open for serious examination.

Management and Governance

In summary, the traditional development of voluntary regional systems, as well as national chains, is built on management, supply, and related economies, not true vertical integration of medical care. Until last year, the voluntary national alliances followed the pattern of the national chains by buttressing their potential advantages in operating costs and ignoring the development of an integrated system of medical referrals.

Even without full vertical integration, voluntary alliances and investor-owned chains can gain much from rebuilding horizontal, somewhat integrated, systems to take advantage of buying power, regional management system sharing, and intramarket program sharing. The biggest roadblock to this process is the notion of local prerogative and discretion. Hospital administrators, especially those who run the larger voluntary and investor-owned chains, have maintained and reinforced the notion that the local administrator has control and autonomy. But these concepts retard movement toward the greater efficiency that national buying and program (product) development afford.

Environmental Factors Supporting Vertical Integration

Four key factors tend to support vertical integration. First, the distribution of disease in populations dictates vertical integration. Most illnesses are common problems that can be treated by primary practitioners. Because of the relative frequency of these illnesses, primary practitioners can be supported by a relatively small population base. Secondary and tertiary practitioners deal with less frequent problems and thus need a population catchment area of much greater size. A population base in excess of a million may be required for some subspecialty practices, while a family physician can fill a practice in an area that has a few thousand families.

Secondary and tertiary practitioners must depend on the vigilance of the primary care physician to identify those problems requiring specialized care and then to refer the patient to a specialist when more complex diagnostic and therapeutic services are needed. Thus, it is the nature of complicated diseases and complex, expensive technology and specialized treatment to require some form of regionalization or, as has happened most often, a network of referral relationships that move patients to the specialist and then back to the primary practitioner.

Second, quality of care by secondary and tertiary practitioners can be ensured only when these physicians continue to develop their skills by serving large population groups. This is a quality of scale issue. It is also an economic value issue, since offering a service without maintaining quality will ultimately cost the practitioner business from sophisticated buyer groups.

Third, there is an efficiency issue involved. Volume helps decrease production cost (at least over some theoretical range of size), and in medical specialties it also increases quality (again, over some theoretical range of activity). Superior value can be produced if there exist the scale and market share to support those specialty services that work efficiently. A comprehensive system has the potential to attract a large volume of patients, thereby lowering the unit cost of services and specialized technology.

Fourth, there is an inherent appeal to the idea that wherever a person comes in contact with a system of care, there exists an incentive within that system that encourages quality performance and economic treatment, smooth and timely movement among services, and easy communication among caregivers. A good example of this is the perceived quality image of the Kaiser Permanente system.

Environmental Factors Inhibiting Vertical Integration

There are several key reasons the health care field has not moved toward the concepts of regional and vertical integration.

Physician Autonomy

First, physicians enjoy their independence as economic and medical practitioners. Physicians have always had a keen sense of the potential for hospitals to influence their practice patterns. This potential power and a potential counterweight to it are well known to any physician soon after he or she enters the profession. The question is how to control big, strong, financially well-heeled hospitals. Such hospitals can be controlled by keeping two hospitals viable and using both for patients and referrals. Patient referrals and hospital use patterns are potent tools of control, especially for the primary care physicians who are at the entry level of the medical system. Therefore, some physician groups would resist any movement by hospitals toward scale and increased leverage.

Of the many potential threats to physician autonomy, a hospital's dominance over specialty practices is the oldest and greatest. Physicians truly fear the potential of a dominant institution that fully controls their access to hospital and related services. Regional or vertically integrated systems greatly increase the potential for institutions to control physicians through their ability to shift referrals among competing physician specialists and among competing hospitals. If any geopolitical region had only one vertically integrated set of services, physician power to shift referrals and maintain power or leverage over hospitals would be lost or at least severely diminished. Whether the system is government owned, voluntary, or investor owned makes little difference.

Physicians appear to like the notion of vertical integration of their practices, within their practices, and for their practices where opportunities exist to achieve revenue, profit, quality, and efficiency. In theory, all the ideas that make vertical integration attractive to hospitals (and increasingly attractive to insurance companies) make vertical integration attractive to the practitioner, as long as it is under his or her control.

When there were not enough specialty physicians, there was no incentive for specialists to vertically integrate in order to pressure the primary care physicians for referrals. They did not need more patients. As long as this traditional referral pattern existed, specialists kept their autonomy and so did primary physicians. Perhaps even more important, any moves by secondary and tertiary physicians to invade the primary territory were, and still are, punished by the primary physicians whose referrals control the system of secondary and, especially, tertiary medicine. However, with the current surplus of specialists, increased vertical integration becomes an option.

Pluralistic System

The second, and supporting, set of reasons for the lack of any serious movement toward regionalization or vertical integration involves the history and underlying motives for societal support for a system of private and public hospitals. For many reasons, the United States has developed a pluralistic system (a variety of owners) of hospitals. This approach is supported by underlying beliefs about religion, ethnicity, and politics. It also suits the intensely competitive nature of medical practice. In the past, competing physicians could almost always find a religious group, a public body, or more recently an investor group to build a hospital for their use, as long as there was some assurance of getting a sufficient number of patients to fill the hospital, carry the debt burden, and secure profits for the equity investment required.

In the past, hospital owners took advantage of the cost-plus reimbursement system. When physicians wanted their own shop to free themselves from outside restrictions or the weight of colleagues more senior or more in control in existing institutions, hospitals made it easy for them to move. When growth occurred, all benefited. One could put a service in place and charge what one needed for a good return, so both physicians and hospitals profited.

Support of Status Quo

Another reason for the lack of vertical integration is the fact that the prepayment systems (basically Blue Cross and Blue Shield) were constructed to reinforce those existing arrangements, not undercut them. Insurance was cost, place, physician, and hospital neutral. More recently, with the advent of managed care programs, physicians and hospitals are under intense pressure to sign up with plans that force them to share economic risk for the care of patient groups.

Support of Multiple Delivery Sites

A fourth reason is that cost-based reimbursement, with its neutral stance toward organization and integration of services, basically supported the development of multiple delivery sites, various degrees of aggregation desired by the provider of service, and competition among all arrangements for the patronage of the individual patient. Under the cost-based system, professional desires regarding technology, place, and service configuration were paramount decision factors. There was no incentive to integrate services.

Now this approach faces rapid obsolescence because of buyer pressure, competitive prices for services, strict utilization review, increasingly fearful insurers who want to get ahead of the game in cost-effective managed care systems, and a real glut of hospitals, beds, services, and physicians. Faced with this obsolescence, many groups are now considering vertical integration.

Implementing Vertical Integration

What are the options for hospitals and multihospital systems to improve performance in multifacility markets, in areas with substantial concentration, and in thinly serviced markets? Before moving to find answers to this question, one should consider how justified the new-found and widely spread belief in vertically integrated systems really is. After all, vertical systems consistently have failed to materialize almost every time they have been attempted in this century.

Access to Physicians Who Control Referrals

The first factor in achieving a measured level of vertical integration is access to the full range of physicians who control referrals. This acknowledges that the vast majority of people are not in managed care programs. Thus, as utilization rates go down, physicians will seek to move their patients to the hospital most likely to offer the broadest service array for their patients. They will enter joint ventures for economic gain, but not if such ventures threaten to tie them up with organizations that lack services their patients may need, i.e., those systems that are not vertically integrated.

For example, in Houston, Texas, both HCA and AMI need access to the kinds of services available at tertiary hospitals like the Texas Medical Center, a large biomedical complex with multiple tertiary facilities. By contrast, in Wichita and in Denver, Colorado, those firms can provide internally almost all the care patients might require in a managed care system. Humana has a similar capacity in Louisville.

Availability of Managed Care Programs

The second factor in achieving a measured level of vertical integration is preferred access to and availability of health maintenance organizations (HMOs), preferred provider organizations (PPOs), traditional insurance, and other more directly managed care programs. The chains and voluntary alliances are moving to cover this area. Both have made attempts to enter the risk services business.

Any major move by VHA, HCA, or Humana into the full range of risk service products makes that organization's members major competitors with all other systems — hospitals, networks, and insurance. Up to this point, these organizations have been primarily competitors in the market for hospital services. By vertically integrating, they may become formidable in all levels of care and a real competitive threat to any providers that are not vertically integrated. As many of these systems form local alliances, they force others to form counterweight alliances to compete with them. Many older coalitions and status quo arrangements crumble under this pressure.

With alliances and chains bringing the kind of capital needed to capture managed care opportunities, all providers will begin to understand the ultimate power of a new strategy of vertical integration. Patients are the coin of the realm for physicians. Hospitals need them. Universities need them. Tertiary care systems need them. By vertically integrating, chains and alliances can have a stake in every market, and they will discover that having a stake in bringing patients to providers makes all other economic joint ventures with physicians seem insignificant by comparison.

Vertical Integration in Different Environments

Actually achieving economic advantages of scale in a horizontally integrated firm makes it possible to add all savings to the bottom line in a product priced or managed care environment. Thus shared and centralized services should be developed within cluster and concentrated markets, to the extent that they make economic sense. Even selective backward integration into supply areas, where the firm could benefit from any excess profits being generated by suppliers, can be lucrative in some areas.

Many economies of operation can be achieved by consolidating and centralizing business service functions of existing units. Ensuing economies of scale on purchasing, supplies, standardization of equipment, and the like can and should be done as soon as possible, after a thorough analysis of gain, line by line, area by area. Moves of this type are already under way by most alliances and firms. For each product, the unit of analysis may be as large as the company or as small as two units. For some lines of business, the proper unit for economies and competitive advantage may be larger than the parent firm itself. Risk service may well fall here. In essence, vertical integration takes on the persona of the environment in which it is developed. Several examples follow.

Concentrated Markets with Tertiary Capacity

In concentrated markets the major gain, beyond shared service economies, stems from the potential for moving patients among programs through physician referral. This is the key to vertical integration. Most approaches to influencing physician referral patterns have involved buying or entering joint ventures with primary care hospitals, or entering joint ventures for diagnostics, ambulatory care centers, managed care programs, PPOs, and other such risk products that can be used to direct patients. But for the near term (three to five years, and possibly longer), winning primary physician loyalty to referral physicians and referral hospitals is the key to achieving vertical integration of medical care capacity in markets where firms own or operate tertiary capacity. In such markets additional equity investments in all levels of services that can utilize existing assets (space and services) also may be attractive.

These concentrated markets should be organized around such concepts as medical care markets and major trade areas, areas within which the population normally seeks and receives 80 to 90 percent of its medical care. Management for the entire market should be under one manager. Such managers might report to a strategic business unit that has overall regional responsibilities for marketing, strategic analysis, investment, and general management of all company activity in the region.

Markets in Which Firms Have Several Primary Hospitals

In markets with limited tertiary capacity within the owned and managed system, it will be necessary for primary hospitals to create substantial joint ventures to link with tertiary programs. Only in this way can an organization gain the greatest returns from the care needed by patients who are initially attracted to primary care physicians and primary care treatment in dispersed hospital systems.

This is true for several reasons. First, any managed care, PPO, or HMO insurer wants to contract with the most complete network of providers. If significant types of referral care are not in one's own facilities, then the next best option is to enter a joint venture, network, or independently build and offer such services. In this way, hospitals can become attractive to managed care programs.

Second, under contracting market conditions that necessitate a choice of which hospital to save, physicians typically abandon the overflow or primary care facility in favor of the full-service facility or system. Physicians consider full-service facilities as the best alternative for serving their patients. Not coincidentally, these systems also help physicians maintain their own practice viability. Ironically, when one does not have major referrals for tertiary services, it is not as necessary to seek physician loyalty on referrals. Unlike the markets with tertiary care programs, in primary care markets there is less likelihood that physicians will want or need to move their patients from one hospital to another. However, as managed care continues to gain ground, those hospitals without the more complex tertiary abilities will lose business as physicians choose to save the more complex facilities needed for their patients. Thus, hospitals must band together with tertiary care systems in order to survive. Fortunately for those with primary care facilities, tertiary facilities are also in oversupply and need alliances for referrals, just as primary hospitals need their referral backup to make their linkage with managed care firms effective.

Third, the supplier with the greatest control over referrals will have the most capital available to offer the next level of technology for medical care and the most advanced systems will become more attractive to upscale consumers, a lucrative target market. For these three reasons, it is essential that primary hospitals link with one or more tertiary care facilities.

Independent Hospitals in Markets with Several Hospitals

The solo hospital in a market with several hospitals will need to pursue a niche strategy designed to hold what business it can while fending off competitors seeking additional patient days.

Several basic approaches can be developed to support a solo strategy. First, the hospital can link or network with a referral center and try to maintain utilization of primary care services. Second, it can seek to become a primary provider for all managed care plans as they develop. Under this scenario, the hospital must try to keep one plan from becoming dominant in the marketplace. Third, the hospital can try to become the primary provider for at least one managed care plan. When possible, securing an equity position in one or more managed care plans will aid in keeping the directed patient flow from becoming too narrow, or, if it does become narrow, this position will help the hospital to benefit from that flow.

Specialty hospitals will need to find ways to secure the specialty business from all managed care plans or link closely with the general provider most likely to deliver the largest part of the specialty referral market segment to them. Many specialty hospitals depend heavily on the routine work they receive to maintain their more esoteric services, so any strategy that cuts heavily into their overall business may threaten their ability to maintain these referral services.

Teaching Hospitals

Teaching hospitals basically fall into two categories: (1) the major university health science centers where much of the basic health science research is conducted. These centers have a teaching mission, with the hospitals devoted principally to research and education, and (2) the teaching hospitals that offer three or more major residency programs. These hospitals put more focus on patient service, with teaching and research being less primary activities.

Health Science Centers. The health science center is likely to have substantial financial support for both its research and its educational role, in addition to the support that is derived from providing patient services. To the extent that these outside support systems can be maintained and enhanced, the health science center will need and be able to compete in the marketplace for referrals from the sophisticated managed care programs. This assumes, however, that the health science centers can and do control their service cost and maintain relatively unique program offerings. Having a research base will continue to make such institutions attractive for the more difficult cases; managed care systems such as Kaiser Permanente, Health America, Maxicare, and others will always need help with their more complex cases. For such firms to try to keep their patients out of these centers of excellence will ultimately test their credibility as major suppliers. Barring a large market share for one firm, they will need to contract for such services for the foreseeable future. This represents a major opportunity for tertiary care suppliers. In fact, health science center and teaching hospitals might aggressively seek contracts to take on the management of the more complex cases before the insurance programs of such managed care companies decide to take responsibility for them.

Competitors for the more complex and specialized cases will come not from the managed care companies but from those tertiary and teaching centers that do not have major investment in and responsibility for research and teaching of medical students. Additional competition will come from those regional hospital systems and national hospital management companies that have strong regional networks and can offer tertiary services from within their systems.

At this time, it would appear that health science centers can compete effectively, provided they aggressively manage their costs (seek efficiencies) and are careful to seek the role of tertiary supplier for managed care systems early in their development. In other words, the game is just beginning. Many options remain open to those who see change coming, are open to meeting the challenge, and are aggressively examining their markets to determine when to join others, contract, or remain outside the competitive arena when appropriate.

Other Institutions. Those teaching institutions that depend heavily on patient revenues to support their teaching role are at greatest risk of losing some of their preeminence and their roles as centers of excellence. They are faced with the difficult situation of using price discounts to get volume, while simultaneously finding it increasingly difficult to support the residency programs that make it possible to maintain their center of excellence strategy. Ultimately, those who deal with this issue should survive. But they, unlike the academic health science center, will need to network with a large number of providers, managed care firms, and national alliances to secure aggregate volumes of patients necessary for their tertiary programs to maintain quality while performing efficiently.

Since state and federal supporters of academic health science centers are likely to aid their clients in maintaining their viability over the intermediate term of competitive developments, most teaching hospitals will not receive such support. For this reason, some will undoubtedly fail as major tertiary centers of excellence for some services. Maintaining costly specialized programs can be an unbearable burden in a price-sensitive market, especially when buyers seek lower cost.

It is likely that the teaching and tertiary care centers outside of health science complexes will have the greatest need to build regional networks, to link formally and informally with all possible referral sources, and to build as many managed care connections as possible. This expectation seems to be borne out by the large numbers of such institutions that have made up the initial membership of VHA, AHS, and Sun Alliance. Teaching hospitals also seem natural partners for investor-owned firms and managed care firms. The number of joint ventures between these hospitals and investor-owned firms indicates that teaching hospitals are aware that they have a stronger need for multiple alliances than do academic health science centers.

Alliances Between Health Science Centers and Management Chains. The alliance strategy is relatively new and none of the major linkages to date seems to preclude new initiatives to form alliances between the stronger academic health science centers and hospital management chains. Managed care companies also seem to want strong alliances with primary care providers and referral agreements with those tertiary care providers who wish to maintain their research and teaching capacity but who do not need to subsidize teaching and research programs. In other words, while teaching and tertiary hospitals would like to play a major role in primary care, both hospital chains and managed care companies want to retain this role for their own operations. Thus, it is likely that chains and managed care programs will be selective in seeking out tertiary referral lines with the major academic health science centers. They will reserve the primary and secondary care roles for themselves. In the process, they will bypass their close competitor, the teaching hospital, which has more limited tertiary capacity.

Managed Care Companies

Managed care companies are in the business of providing or negotiating for the provision of health care services purchased by employers or other groups. They are required to provide such services within the limits of a contract they make with these employers and groups. At one extreme is the owned and operated health service, such as Kaiser Permanente, which packages physician, hospital, and risk management services within its own family of companies. At the other end of the spectrum is the insurance firm, which contracts for risk and limits liability by specifying the range within which it will cover services or the amount of total payment. In other cases, employers may manage their own risk, specify eligible providers, contract for administration, and use excess insurance coverage to avoid large losses.

Increased Competition. Competition among managed care firms is increasing, putting pressure on premium price and thus pushing all suppliers in the direction of more tightly managed utilization and cost controls. As these firms compete for the buyers' attention, they will need to control utilization more and more and seek low prices from suppliers of services not offered directly by the managed care firm itself.

Probably the lowest-cost producers of primary care are family physicians. Some of the early HMO service suppliers sought out family physicians, general internists, and similar primary care providers as the core of their original network. Low-cost or low-price hospital providers and willing specialists have been secondary priorities. As patient volume has grown, specialists have been asked to take greater risks and hospitals have been asked to offer greater discounts in order to get the volume business offered by managed care firms that can select the provider for their clients.

Under conditions such as these, physician and hospital providers are under tremendous pressure to take the risk and start their own managed care firms. But in doing so, they must delicately balance their own risk management offerings so that they can gain market share while maintaining business and referrals from competing managed care firms.

Put another way, as providers develop their abilities to offer managed care services directly to employers and groups, they must do so in a fashion that does not simultaneously drive away business from other managed care firms (now competing firms) and from referring physicians whose practices are tied more directly to other managed care firms and hospitals.

If hospital and physician provider groups initiate their own risk services and managed care programs, they may lose referrals from these competing groups. On the other hand, if they have not positioned themselves to be the provider of choice in such groups, they run the risk of eventually being left out of more tightly managed groups.

Role of Insurance Companies. Managed care firms are, with a few exceptions, relatively new. Some have developed with little regard for utilization control and have depended heavily on the lack of tightly managed control for their profitability. As competition builds for the managed care premium dollar, the more loosely managed firms will lose out to more tightly managed groups. But as managed care firms succeed as a sector of the health care industry, it becomes more important than ever for any insurance firm wishing to compete for the full service benefit dollar to offer managed care. Therefore, health care managers now see, and can expect to see, many more insurance firms seeking managed care business, buying up established managed care firms, merging traditional benefit companies into managed care firms, and entering joint ventures between big benefits firms and provider networks and firms.

In short, the strategies of insurance and benefits firms are so new in their adoption and so tentative in their execution that it seems safe to conclude that the industry is only beginning to discover and answer many of the questions posed and implied here. Few of the strategies that have unfolded so far appear to be clear-cut winners. Few of the players seem secure in the belief that they have the answers. The only thing that seems certain is that change is here. For those who like the excitement of a game in its early stages, this is a great opportunity to participate in the definition of a new health care provider. For those who see only insurmountable problems, retiring to the sidelines of merging with someone more comfortable with the risk seems a more likely strategy.

For those who think that vertical integration is the right way to go, there is plenty of room to maneuver. They can mold the health care system into a more efficient and probably more vertically integrated mode of care. Who will do this is an open question. Where it can be done is similarly open. But since vertical integration runs counter to so many interests, it will remain a high-risk strategy, however it is implemented.

Assessment of Forces in the Health Care Field

Powerful forces are active in the health care field. Voluntary hospital alliances are flourishing as providers seek refuge in networks that will allow independent hospitals and independent physicians to retain control over their destinies in the face of impending radical changes in reimbursement that favor competitive pricing and full-service arrays.

Assumptions Underlying the Fears of Independent Hospitals and Physicians

Several assumptions are currently causing great anxiety among independent institutions and practitioners. One assumption is that the powerful hospital chains will use their ability to get market equity to buy up the good business opportunities to the exclusion of the voluntary hospitals. Just how such chains could come up with the new equity to perform this miracle is unclear. (It would probably require in the neighborhood of $50 billion in equity and a similar amount of debt to accomplish this feat.) Given the beating the chains have taken recently in the stock market, this scenario seems improbable. Therefore, the implication that the powerful companies will take over the field seems to be basically a fear tactic to encourage the forging of more horizontal and vertical voluntary alliances.

Another fear is that the powerful insurance and managed care systems will take over control of patients and usurp the role of providers in the system. This argument also assumes that only a few firms will dominate the industry. For this to happen, hundreds of benefits insurers would need to abandon the field; the full-service firms (HMOs) would have to become the sole, or at least dominant, model of delivery; and traditional providers would need to insist on high utilization under traditional methods of payment. Just the opposite seems to be occurring. Utilization is decreasing dramatically. Employers are managing their own care and benefits in a much more effective manner. Traditional providers are adjusting to this new approach, cost is coming down, and providers are accepting PPOs and other price-sensitive approaches fairly well. Also, more and more benefits companies are developing a wide range of approaches to ensure their survival in the marketplace. The world may be changing but it appears that many traditional owners (hospitals and physicians) are responding well to market forces. As a result, they are not losing their control over their hospitals and practices.

A third assumption is that businesses and personal consumers are ready and willing to make changes in how they consume health care services in order to secure a better price and value relationship. This assumption appears to be true. It is unlikely that the industry has fully explored consumers' willingness to change. However, this change is occurring incrementally. Many of the firms that moved first and fastest have experienced difficulty with their model approaches. As consumer groups move inexorably toward tighter controls of their own utilization, providers increasingly respond, albeit reluctantly.

Just how much of the market share will go to tightly managed care firms before traditional suppliers offer equally attractive utilization rates and prices, with greater freedom for consumers to choose physicians? Surely a 5 percent or 10 percent shift to HMOs is too little; but at 20 percent or 30 percent penetration, can traditional suppliers fail to respond? When the responses come, should there not be counter responses? The game has begun, but surely it is not yet decided.

Current Situation

As these fundamental changes occur, providers are indeed finding that circumstances can make for strange bedfellows. Disbelief that change will come has given way to fear that all is lost, only to be replaced by confidence in all-purpose alliances to fight the change. As the battle lines are drawn and readiness to do battle pervades, tenable options emerge with new lines of alliance, vertical and horizontal integration occur, and new partnerships begin to develop.

New Alliances. Vertical integration itself is beginning to emerge as an idea whose time has come. In the early stages many parties saw themselves at the core of such a system. They began the process hoping to solidify this coveted position. Some weaker, more timid players immediately threw in the towel and merged with the stronger partners. Others hedged and joined alliances to wait, see, and sample. A lot of money has been invested in these exercises but for the most part they were exercises, not the consummation of a vertical system.

Perhaps it is in these alliances that some of the potential for building vertical systems exists. Given the many different services offered for the total health care dollar, it may be that any given provider not only will be a strong part of one alliance, but will play an important role in many alliances. The United States is, after all, a pluralistic society. Many vendors, physicians, and hospitals are interdependent on the unique economies of specialized sectors of the health care economy.

Significance of New Delivery Systems. The HMO represents a particular subset of integration. The shared purchasing program represents another subset, and it is unlike the first, though important for its own merit. Maybe the health care industry is moving toward many different types of vertical integration. If new delivery systems do represent subsets of vertical integration, perhaps what is beginning will lead to a more vertically integrated system of services. But it is unlikely to lead to one or two or even a hundred or more super systems. It is more likely that the traditional mode of physician and medical care in general will evolve toward more efficient patterns. Pattern is the key term. In a pattern or set of relationships, more vertically related activities can evolve if and when they provide efficiency or provide a competitive or marketing opportunity for gains in terms of economy, medical care, or access.

Positive economic and medical care gains from joint ventures, networks, and diversification may occur without the parties involved giving up their control in these new negotiated relationships. Gains for consumers can occur without providers totally abandoning their traditional roles and missions. However, these roles will need to be redefined and renegotiated within the context of the larger societal goal of efficiency and access.

Total Integration Unlikely. It is unlikely, however, that health care will ever become fully integrated. It is possible, if not probable, that a totally owned and operated vertically integrated system would look and act much like a state owned and operated system, with all the barriers to innovation and change that this might represent. That is, the traditional notion of vertical integration may well be a bigger blunder in design than going along with the old cost-plus system despite that system's history of duplication and overuse.

If this is the case, total integration, vertical or horizontal, is undesirable. What is needed are the creativity and innovation that come from highly pluralistic approaches and the energy that comes from competitive behaviors within a pluralistic system that forces change, growth, or failure.

Rational Approach to Vertical Integration. As today's strategist explores vertical integration, he or she must look for an underlying rationale at each step. Is it for medical quality, efficiency, consumer acceptance, competitive advantage, or some related criterion? In analyzing the alternatives, issues of vertical integration and horizontal integration, corporate restructuring, diversification, merger, and alliance are great starting points, but as goals they fall short. They should be viewed as means or mechanisms for progress, not as goals or outcome measures. Indeed, there is a move toward greater vertical integration not because it represents an unalloyed virtue but because more general risk taking by larger groups of providers stimulates most cost-effective methods of care.

Totally owned and operated vertically integrated systems are not likely to occur as a result of market competitive forces unless all programs, resource requirements, and abilities can be brought to operate at the optimal level of utility simultaneously. This type of situation has never existed in any kind of organization. It certainly does not exist in medical care as it currently operates. Lumping everything into one organization would create a lump, not a set of orderly programs in harmony with one another and collectively meeting consumer needs.

Health care managers can and probably will network, enter joint ventures, and build and operate in a much more rational fashion — meaning more vertical and horizontal relationships. But these efforts will not result in a neat textbook example of what a vertical system might represent. The system will be pluralistic. It will meld together and it will break apart whenever the parts do not fit. It will have control and coordination between individuals, groups, and corporations with many voices being heard. The 1990s will not look like the 1970s, but many of the same owners and physicians will be doing many of the things they did in the 1970s with greater efficiency and sound value to consumers, and in competition with others seeking to serve similar markets.

In addition, they will be doing things with more and different partners than would have been envisioned in the last decade, or even today.

Notes

1. *Hospital Literature Index* 40 (1984): 207-8.
2. United Kingdom. Parliament. Consultative Council on Medical and Allied Services, Ministry of Health of Great Britain. *Interim Report on the Future Provision of Medical and Allied Services.* Cmd. 693. 1920.
3. Committee on the Cost of Medical Care. *Medical Care for the American People: The Final Report of the Committee.* Committee Pub. No. 28. Chicago: University of Chicago Press, November 1932.
4. Rosenfeld, L.S., and Makover, H.B. *The Rochester Regional Hospital Council.* Cambridge, MA: Harvard University Press, 1956.
5. Clark, H.T. "The Challenge of the Regional Medical Programs Legislation." *Journal of Medical Education* 41 (1966): 71-74.
6. American Hospital Association Special Committee on the Provision of Health Services. *Ameriplan: A Proposal for the Delivery and Financing of Health Services in the United States: Report of the Special Committee on Health Service.* Chicago: AHA, 1970.
7. Brown, M., and Money, W.H. "Promise of Multihospital Management." *Hospital Progress* 56, no. 8 (1975): 36-42.
8. Brown, M., et al. "Trends in Multihospital Systems: A Multiyear Comparison." *Health Care Management Review* 5, no. 4 (Fall 1980): 9-22.
9. Brown, M. "Multihospital Systems in the 80s — The New Shape of the Health Care Industry." *Hospitals* 56 (March 1, 1982): 344-61.
10. Brown, M. "Community Hospitals: Caring, Curing, Commerce. Systems Commerce and the Caring Tradition." Hospital Progress 64 (May 1983): 37-44, 62.

19

Marketing in the Academic Health Center

Charles L. Breindel

Charles L. Breindel is Associate Professor, Department of Health Administration, Medical College of Virginia, Virginia Commonwealth University, Richmond.

Most academic health centers share similar problems. They relate to the high cost of overhead for education and research and its effect on decreasing the attractiveness of high quality clinical health services. With payment systems favoring cost effective care producers, the plight of the academic health center (AHC) is further exacerbated in the competitive industry. For the AHC in an urban center, the final blow to effective competition is the realization that the market served by the center is dominated by indigent patients.

In reaction and response to these situations, marketing is coming into use in AHCs, just a few years after its discovery by and application to the remainder of the hospital industry. The temptation to invest heavily in advertising is great for AHCs in early stages of marketing, just as it was for hospitals in general when they first discovered marketing. AHCs, however, have the advantage of hindsight to realize that market research is necessary first to understand the market and its reception of health and medical services. However, while AHCs have learned from other hospitals about how and when to advertise, it appears that AHCs may soon follow their sister hospitals in a different direction which may prove to be costly and ineffective.

This article examines a new dimension, distinct from marketing thrusts of other hospitals, to the AHC marketing clinical services. By examining the markets of AHCs, noting their differences from other hospital markets and positing the scope of marketing for AHCs, a major new dimension for their marketing will be identified.

Reprinted with permission from *Health Care Strategic Management,* 5(1) January 1987, pages 8-10. Copyright 1987 by *Health Care Strategic Management.* All rights reserved.

Background

The dominant strategy of most hospital marketing for clinical services is to increase market share in general and by product line in particular. To this end, hospitals conduct market research to define potential and actual markets by product line and then define the markets into preferred segments often identified by their ability to purchase the hospital's products.

The goal of these marketing efforts is to increase the number of revenue generating transactions in an industry where payment per transaction is being cut by payers and insurers. The goal of these marketing strategies is to increase revenues through greater market share. It is not self-evident that market share increases equate to revenue increases. However, for many hospitals these two goals are nearly the same, so long as one is careful about payer mix in the implementation of market share increases.

There are two distinct segments in the AHC's primary clinical services market: users of tertiary care services and indigent patients. The former are characterized by possession of third party insurance, referral by a physician (often an alumnus of the medical school associated with the AHC), a broad geographic distribution and attractiveness to clinical researchers and educators of the center. On the other hand, indigent care patients are characteristically users of primary care, have no or insufficient resources to pay for care, are self-referring and come from a rather localized market area.

In developing the marketing for an AHC, two dimensions are generally used to define market strategies. Both are consistent with the dominant strategy of revenue enhancement. They are: expansion of the market for tertiary care and development of a new market for primary care. A third possibility, a combination of the two, will be addressed later.

Organizations focusing on expansion of the market for tertiary care utilize programs of networking such as development of an 800 number, hotlines, alumni contact programs, courtesy staff privileges for community physicians to admit patients and refer to esoteric consultants, mail distributions of AHC clinical staff and service directories, etc. All of these aim at increasing referrals and utilize the market exchange relationship of referral systems, rather than client self referrals.

The organization that focuses its marketing on the development of a new market for primary care is drawn to the middle and working class segments of insured individuals. For this focus, attractive marketing tactics are cultivation of HMO/PPO markets to attract large segments of insured individuals. Development of satellite delivery sites, establishment/expansion of cooperative programs with community hospitals, workplace programs of occupational health and occasionally recreational health and wellness programs are helpful. Campus amenities are also important for AHCs which have this focus in their marketing.

A New Focus

Negative marketing is one concept which has had some modest application in health care in the recent past but has not received much examination or analysis.

Negative marketing refers to the processes that decrease market exchanges between an organization and targeted segments of its market. It is also called demarketing. It has meaning for an organization in that it can define a substantial market segment with which to decrease exchanges. For most hospitals, such segments exist, but they are small. Hence, negative marketing tactics have not been implemented because of higher priorities for increasing market share in other areas. In addition, given the relatively small size of negative markets for most hospitals and the relatively larger size of potential positive markets, there is little impetus for negative marketing. Finally, there are social concerns about the appropriateness of a service organization trying to decrease services and/or utilization.

In actuality, hospitals have had some good experience with negative marketing. For example, attempts by hospitals to identify physicians who overutilize hospital ancillary services provide an example of determining negative markets. Also, the related identification of patients who approach limits on allowable lengths of stay in order to place them in nursing homes or at home is also a negative marketing tactic. However, these are usually the only instances of negative marketing.

For the AHC with two markets, tertiary care users and indigent care patients, there is yet another focus to marketing. It is negative marketing to the indigent care population in an ethical and practical manner. While this notion sparks immediate negative connotations of social irresponsibility, negative marketing does not necessarily mean ceasing to give care or giving less care to current indigent clients.

Negative marketing seems abhorrent because the goal of negative marketing is not often correctly conceptualized. The goal is not simply to decrease utilization by a segment but to improve the financial status of the AHC. In the short term, improving financial status generally equates to providing less care. But, in the long run it has another meaning, namely getting the indigent care segment to use services that are less costly or not to need to use services. In effect, negative marketing to the indigent care segment translates to long term goals of getting this market segment healthier and more informed about health promotion and illness prevention. From the AHC's point of view, this negative marketing is based on long term expectations of decreasing the cost of indigent care by lower utilization of services or through the use of less costly services.

Just how does this translate into tactical marketing for the AHC? First, the AHC must be able to define for its indigent care population product lines for which there is high uncompensated utilization. Targeted segments of actual and potential users must be identified, and strategies of primary prevention, education, and early detection developed to reach the targeted population segments.

In summary, negative marketing to indigent population groups implies investments in health promotion and prevention by AHCs. The challenge facing AHCs in implementing such negative marketing is the difficulty in demonstrating a cause-effect relationship between any primary prevention and health promotion and lower and less appropriate utilization of services in the future. Initial investments in negative marketing must be carefully selected, based upon products which offer a high potential for demonstrated improvements in appropriate utilization.

Examples of Negative Marketing

Negative marketing in the area of indigent care can be implemented principally in the areas of primary care. At least two areas are potential candidates for the AHC, pediatrics and obstetrics. In both these product lines there are high levels of uncompensated care for a center and both are high demand items for the indigent population.

For the obstetrics/neonatology line, an investment by an AHC in perinatal care for the indigent segment is one way to affect long term negative marketing. By offering a full range of screening for high risk, routine perinatal care and education, the possibility exists to decrease need for long maternity stays and neonatal inpatient care. In implementing such a program to cause negative market growth, the market plan needs to address where to deliver care, what to charge and how to communicate with the market segment.

In the area of pediatrics, provision of parental education relating to accidents and childhood disease management, in concert with primary prevention programs, may reduce the long term high utilization of inpatient services. Of course, by implementing such a negative marketing program, marketing issues such as place of delivery of care (mobile/stationery, hospital/home, etc.), pricing and promotion need to be addressed, just as in any other marketing plan.

Summary

In any market-oriented health care organization, a combination of marketing dimensions will determine strategies and tactics. Most hospitals identify market strategies to increase product-specific market shares. For the AHC, increasing product specific markets involves two dimensions, i.e., either increasing the referral and geographic market for tertiary care or finding new local markets for primary care.

However, since both dimensions are directed toward the overall financial goal of improving revenue flow, a third dimension to AHC marketing can be developed to focus on negative marketing to the indigent care segment. Such a dimension in marketing implies an investment by the academic health center in improving the health of the indigent population, decreasing disease and disability for the poor in the area and other prevention and promotion products.

If the AHC could define such negative marketing and demonstrate its success in reducing long term revenue losses, a whole new focus on the issue of indigent care emerges. The additional benefits in developing this third dimension of negative marketing include improved community relations and increased social responsibility. The AHC with a developed preventive medicine program already has the structure for planning and implementation of needed research and services.

20

The Impact of Diagnosis Related Groups and Prospective Pricing Systems on Health Care Management

Myra Crawford and Myron D. Fottler

Myra A. Crawford, Ph.D., is Research Assistant Professor, University of Alabama School of Medicine, University of Alabama, Birmingham.

Myron D. Fottler, Ph.D., is Professor of Management and Director of the Ph.D. Program in Administration - Health Services, University of Alabama, Birmingham.

The rapidly escalating cost of medical care, which has increased three times faster than the overall rate of inflation,[1] has brought about legislation designed to curtail the rate of inflation in expenditures by the Medicare hospital insurance trust. In March 1983, PL 98-21 (the Social Security Amendments of 1983) was passed and included a fixed-price prospective payment system (PPS) for hospitals, based on diagnosis related groups (DRGs). This PPS/DRG system is currently legislated for Medicare only, unless the state adopts a PPS that applies to all third party payers. This new law has set in motion significant changes in the way medical care is managed in America.

PPS and DRGs have been discussed and defined at length in the literature.[2,3] Although the potential for using DRGs as a management tool has been discussed,[4,5] the DRG system is not compatible with the traditional medical departments, staffing workloads, or case mix—especially severity of illness, length of stay, and intensity of nursing needs.[6,7] DRGs do not describe outputs in terms of traditional hospital services. The new system may discourage the acquisition of technological advancements. The concepts of profitability, "winners and losers," and competition have now been brought to the attention of an "industry" that has rarely considered the cost of the inputs, processes, or outputs.[8]

Reprinted with permission of Aspen Publishers, Inc., from *Health Care Management Review*, 1985.

Prospective payment involves determining hospital rates of payment for specific diseases in advance of treatment with predetermined reimbursement based on the DRG classification system. PPS replaces the retrospective cost reimbursement system in which payments for certain similar procedures varied by thousands of dollars in different hospitals. The current system has a phase-in period, as well as exclusions for certain types of hospitals and services in general facilities (long-term, children's, psychiatric, and rehabilitation). After it is completely phased in and as it is currently mandated, PPS/DRG will pay nearly 7,500 hospitals over the nation "the same rate for treating the same illness with only minor adjustments for local labor costs."[9]

Based on the International Classification of Diseases-9th Revision-Clinical Modification (ICD-9-CM), all cases are separated into 23 Major Diagnostic Categories (MDCs). The DRG coding system, which has been adopted for Medicare PPS, further classifies all medical diagnoses into 467 categories. Cases are further subdivided into medical and surgical categories and by other specific procedures, the patient's age, and the presence of complications or significant co-morbid disorders.

Although most hospitals are responding to the short-term management concerns of changes in record keeping and billing procedures, significant long-term issues remain to be addressed. Many of these issues have the potential for changing the manner in which hospitals are managed and the way in which hospital services are planned and administered. Although PPS/DRG is currently confined to those hospital patients who are reimbursed by Medicare, it is likely that this program, or a similar one, will be expanded to all third party insurance systems in the future. The predictors expressed here represent the most likely impacts of the new system on the majority of general care delivery hospitals. These impacts will vary, depending on the institutions, their location, teaching status, and size.

Management Implications

The potential impact of PPS/DRG will be on four basic management functions: planning, organizing, directing/motivating, and controlling. This issue is important because, while most early articles written about PPS/DRG express concern over the changes that will occur in hospital management, they predict only a few of the probable impacts.[10] None has assessed these possibilities systematically, yet such assessments need to be done in terms of the traditional management functions. Constraints, conditions, and strategies for managing under PPS/DRG are key considerations.

Because the evidence supports the likelihood that PPS will spread quickly to other third party insurers, these predicted impacts express changes that may be anticipated beyond those expected under the current circumstances in which PPS is limited to Medicare reimbursement. The empirical evidence for most of the hypothesized changes possible under PPS/DRG is scanty or nonexistent. These predictions, therefore, attempt to assess the likely outcomes of the new system, assuming that the DRG classification is maintained.

The Planning Function

Planning Constraints

Competition among hospitals will increase along with the regulations being imposed on them. (See Table 20-1.) Future legislation or regulation unknown at this time will continue to impose constraints on planning. The influence of government regulatory guidelines will increase substantially by virtue of the necessity of the hospital's adherence to the law. PPS/DRG is currently limited to Medicare, but the likelihood that such a system will be expanded to all third party payers is high.

An independent commission has been appointed to advise the secretary of the Department of Health and Human Services on changes in the current Medicare PPS. What additional regulations will be imposed on the system remains unclear until the newly established commission becomes fully functional.

Whether patients will have more influence on the medical care process under PPS/DRG is unclear. Their influence will have to evolve through the political process if they are to have an impact on regulations that will constrain current law (PL 98-21) and future legislation. How successful individuals can be in influencing medical care legislation or the regulatory process remains uncertain.

The influence of professionals from within the organization will necessarily increase as management attempts to gain their cooperation in implementing the program and in constraining costs. Although physicians formerly operated in most medical care facilities as outside contractors, they now have an increased stake in the fiscal viability and continuance of those facilities. The physician should become more actively involved in the facility's administrative planning process. Only physicians can define and refine treatment protocols and ensure that they work cost-effectively.

The influence of internal politics should decrease as the external constraints increase. The governing board, hospital administrators, physicians, and other health care professionals should work more closely together to meet the demands of PPS/DRG and to strengthen the position of their individual facility in its market. The need for consensus should reduce the influence of competitive internal politics. Failure to reduce internal conflict may result in an inability to make the difficult decisions required by the new system.

Market constraints will increase as competition increases. More facilities will attempt to increase their provision of profitable services, while reducing their exposure in less profitable areas. Hospitals will plan to reduce less profitable services and to support the profitable DRGs. This action could involve total institutional restructuring, resistance by internal and external individuals and groups, and alterations in the balance of hospital services in an entire community. Consequently, there will be more competition among

Table 20-1. Predicted Impact of DRGs on the Planning Function.

	Increase	Uncertain	Decrease
Planning constraints			
Influence of government regulatory guidelines	X		
Customer or client influence		X	
Influence of professionals within the organization	X		
Influence of internal politics			X
Market constraints	X		
Influence of third party payers	X		
Planning conditions			
Level of uncertainty and difficulty in forecasting future			X
Autonomy and flexibility in defining purposes	X		
Multiplicity of goals and goal conflict			X
Difficulty in establishing goal priorities			X
Importance of charismatic leadership in defining goals and objectives			X
Changes in goals, objectives, and programs	X		
Emphasis on planning resource inputs	X		
Emphasis on planning for results	X		
Emphasis on risk avoidance	X		
Marginal admissions		X	
Emphasis on inpatient services			X

facilities in providing profitable services. Those facilities unable to compete in terms of price and quality will risk failure.

The influence of third party payers on providers will increase when PPS is expanded beyond Medicare because of the necessity to verify performance and conformity to the guidelines and to refine the system further. These in-

Table 20-1, continued.

	Impact		
	Increase	Uncertain	Decrease
Planning conditions *continued*			
Emphasis on traditional services			X
Planning strategies			
Reexamine goals, priorities, strategies, and programs	X		
Target cuts and discontinue weak services	X		
Monitor environment	X		
Plan to diagnose outlook for specific-services/market segments in the long run	X		
Restrict domain (i.e., specialize) by emphasizing distinctive competencies	X		
Emphasize outpatient services	X		
Emphasize preventive services and health education	X		
Emphasize marketing services	X		
Emphasize referral arrangements	X		
Emphasize accurate departmental budgeting	X		
Emphasize discharge planning	X		
Plan to alter resources dependency	X		
Establish or strengthen a political unit	X		

surers already are voicing their concern about possible cost shifting by medical care facilities. The current law provides special consideration for states that will adopt all-payer PPSs. Maryland, Massachusetts, New Jersey, and New York have waivers from the system, and other states are planning to propose alternative systems.

Planning Conditions

Initial uncertainty about revenues will be resolved as base-year and case mix data are generated in each facility. Most facilities should then be able to forecast data that are sufficient and accurate for planning purposes. Relying solely on DRG data, however, without considering the impact of severity of illness and individual physician practice patterns may yield inaccurate information that could severely compromise the planning function.

As facilities respond to the market and begin to specialize services, autonomy and flexibility in defining purposes will increase. The multiplicity of goals and goal conflict will decrease because of increased specialization. This also will decrease the difficulty in establishing goal priorities. In the past, charismatic leadership often influenced the definition of goals and objectives. Under the new system, the increase of data will dictate more objectivity in planning and goal setting. The extent to which goals, objectives, and programs change will increase as institutions attempt to respond to changing markets.

The objectivity imposed on the facility by the constraints of PPS/DRG will increase the emphasis on planning resource inputs and results. The need for knowing all the significant variables in resource utilization will intensify. The desire to avoid risks will increase as accurate and timely data are available. The incidence of marginal admissions should decrease if facilities adhere to the law, which dictates a strong utilization process to monitor for abuses. As facilities learn how to manipulate the system, however, these admissions may initially or periodically increase.

Inclusion of a severity of illness index factor in the payment scheme could also diminish the profitability of marginal admissions and the transfer to public institutions of patients whose illnesses demand resources that exceed profitability. Consequently, the net effect is unknown at this time.

The likelihood that PPS/DRG will decrease the cost of medical care dictates that in the future more services will be given on an outpatient basis. The emphasis on inpatient services will decrease, as will the demand for traditional services that are not profitable and that can be provided in an ambulatory setting or in the home.

Planning Strategies

The result of PPS/DRG will be that hospitals will have to reexamine their goals, priorities, strategies, and programs. In particular, they will need to do a case mix portfolio analysis to position hospital services according to market attractiveness and the institution's relative advantage for each service.[11] As targeted cuts become clear and necessary, the ethical dilemma of discontinuing weak services or of entering a two-tiered system of care will create conflict and could result in indecision or a choice to continue a revenue-losing service to the financial detriment of the hospital. All services will need to be periodically reevaluated to determine short- and long-term viability.

The hospital will have to monitor its environment more closely and engage in long-term planning to diagnose the outlook for specific services or market segments. Many institutions will begin to restrict their domain by emphasizing their distinctive competencies. To lower the total cost of treating a particular category of patients that may be less profitable, they may also begin to substitute less expensive outpatient services for more expensive inpatient services. Moral and ethical issues concerning the type and extent of medical care delivered will surface.

The markets for preventive services and health education appear to be growth areas as hospitals seek methods to prepare patients to accept shorter lengths of stay and more appropriate use of services. The literature supports the use of health education programs to reduce hospitalization and shows psychological interventions to be cost-effective.[12]

These educational functions are currently supported outside third party payments. Such services are not included as part of payment by DRGs. As these and other markets grow and change, institutions will give greater emphasis to marketing profitable services and to developing referral arrangements with other institutions and individuals. Physician recruitment may be based on the particular services that an individual physician offers as compared with projections of patient demand for services by case mix.[13]

Financial resources will become increasingly scarce and more difficult to obtain. Department managers will need to develop the skills to forecast departmental needs accurately. They will also need the skills to develop a budget based on forecasted needs and to negotiate needed departmental resources. Because PPS rewards efficiency, efforts should be made to control the length of stay and to discharge patients as quickly as possible. Effective discharge planning will be an important tool for maintaining quality of care.

The insecurities stemming from PPS/DRG will cause hospitals to enhance their resource base by increasing the number of funding sources on which they depend. An example would be the development of management services contracts for helping other institutions manage under prospective pricing. These same insecurities should also cause institutions to establish or strengthen a political unit to provide advance warning of legislative or regulatory changes.

The Organizing Function

Organizing Constraints

As facilities are encouraged to restructure their departments and divisions, departmental autonomy in individual hospitals may increase. (See Table 20-2.) DRG classification, as currently constructed, does not adhere to the traditional medical care departmentalization; therefore, DRGs will probably stimulate changes in how medical care is organized. To be able to

Table 20-2. Predicted Impact of DRGs on the Organizing Function.

	Impact		
	Increase	Uncertain	Decrease
Organizing constraints			
Managerial autonomy in organizing	X		
External constraints on methods and spheres of operations		X	
Job enlargement	X		
Job enrichment		X	
Organizing conditions			
Top management concern with external relationships	X		
Linking pins for internal–external integration	X		
Importance of interorganizational cooperation for goal achievement	X		
Decentralization	X		
Span of control	X		
Degree of employee specialization	X		
Organizing strategies			
Participation in interorganizational networks for monitoring the external environment	X		
Centralization of decision making			X
Involvement of physicians in management functions	X		
Emphasis on vertical integration	X		
Participation in multihospital systems	X		
Emphasis on the role of medical records and finance departments	X		
Development of a new DRG coordinator role or DRG coordinating committee	X		
Development of management-related groups (MRGs)	X		
Reorganization of departments around MRGs	X		

relate costs and services accurately, the departmental structure and the DRG categories will need to be matched more closely.

Current regulatory guidelines do not dictate how a facility achieves the goal of cost reduction that is implicit in PPS/DRG. The methods and spheres of operations, therefore, may not be constrained from the outside, unless those regulations are changed.

As the economic constraints of PPS/DRG reduce the levels of staffing, the opportunity for job enlargement will increase. Efficient operations demand job enlargement by having employees trained in a greater number of operational functions. As fiscal constraints increase, however, the opportunity for job enrichment programs, i.e., adding more high-level functions, may diminish as facilities monitor every expenditure more carefully. In contrast, those employees who seek satisfaction through increased involvement in the planning and control functions of their jobs may see their jobs enriched as decentralization occurs. The net impact is uncertain.

Organizing Conditions

Top management concerns over external relationships will increase as a result of the close monitoring that the organization experiences. As a result, hospitals may increase the number of roles or positions linking internal and external environments. They may also feel the need to increase their interorganizational cooperation to achieve goals. For example, a director of management information systems may be promoted. In the new role, he or she may be more responsible for external linkages.

Internally, the organization will decentralize decision making to lower levels while requiring increasing accountability for results. As the number of middle-level mangers is reduced, fewer people will be responsible for greater numbers of employees. The span of control of supervisors will increase. The new decentralized structure will help department heads and middle-level managers to function as such by pushing decision-making authority to a lower organizational level.

Initially, hospital staffing will become more specialized as facilities' outputs become more specialized. Over time, however, staff functions may become less specialized as employees diversify to enhance their productivity. This will occur especially when positions go unfilled or are eliminated for economic reasons.

Organizing Strategies

The strategies of participation in interorganizational networks, decentralization of decision making, and increased involvement of physicians have already been established. More recently, hospitals have also been involved in horizontal integration, creating multi-institutional systems. Vertical integration should increase as facilities bring long-term care and outpatient facilities into their organizational structure. Access to extended care facilities will assist hospitals in shortening the length of stay in high-cost facilities. Preventive health care services should increase as hospitals attempt to educate the public in minimizing utilization of costly and unprofitable therapeutic procedures.

Nonprofit hospitals can improve both their access to capital and their potential for survival by joining together in multihospital systems. Although some hospitals have been reluctant to give up their autonomy by coalescing with others and pooling their assets, this restructuring does allow them to develop subsidiary for-profit enterprises and to exploit the equity market.

Some hospitals have pooled their excess revenues into joint revenue-generating activities; profits are then distributed to participating hospitals. These subsidiaries may provide hospital-related services, such as contract management, consulting, and purchasing systems, or they may operate other health-related businesses, such as home health care agencies, free-standing laboratories, rehabilitation units, health clubs, or surgicenters. Other hospitals may develop for-profit subsidiaries in areas less related to health care, such as real estate.

The necessity for increasing the quantity and quality of data will increase the emphasis on the hospital's medical records and finance departments. As economic concerns become the driving force in the system, the finance department will be responsible for providing timely, accurate, and more complicated data, as virtually any decision made by any department will come under increased scrutiny.

An increased need for an interface between these departments and for automation of the data collection process also demands an increase in the preparation of medical records personnel. The new medical record department's role has led some hospitals to bring medical records under direct control of the finance department in order to coordinate medical record and billing information.[14] This also provides the hospital with a data base for monitoring parameters that may have important effects on resource use, such as physician practice patterns and the severity of illnesses among patients. Although many members of the hospital management team will have to increase their efforts to achieve their hospital's goals, none will increase in influence as dramatically as those responsible for fiscal accountability.

The implementation process may also be enhanced if a new role of DRG coordinator is developed. Such a coordinator would serve as a liaison between hospital departments, would disseminate information, and would make recommendations based on analytical findings. This process may be enhanced if someone who has good working relationships with diverse groups of employees is appointed coordinator.[15] Another approach is to create a multidisciplinary DRG committee to develop organizational policies for working with DRGs.[16]

Some hospitals may choose to develop management-related groups (MRGs). These would be product-line teams who would use physician/management collaboration for cost containment and performance evaluation.[17] The administration would then use creative approaches to reward efficiency in product-line teams and to exert pressure on inefficient teams to reduce their utilization of resources. Because the usual department structure in hospitals is not currently compatible with either DRGs or MRGs, some institutions will probably make an effort to reorganize around MRGs. In this way, a group administrator could be held responsible for financial results within his or her group.

The Directing/Motivating Function

Directing/Motivating Constraints

The linkage between rewards and seniority or credentials is likely to be reduced in the new system. (See Table 20-3.) Because of financial constraints, management will, by necessity, have to emphasize performance rather than the traditional reasons for reward in a bureaucratic system. Under the new system, individual physicians and nursing services will be able to undertake detailed analyses of their respective cost performance and to evaluate their contribution to an institution's net revenue.

New legislation currently being considered by Congress would take effect in FY 1986 and would regulate professional fees as well as charges for services. In addition, the overall decline in spendable revenue will slow the rate of salary increases for employees in general. Employees who have come into hospitals primarily for financial remuneration will be likely to experience less satisfaction as the opportunities for rapidly expanding salaries decrease. Those who enjoy change and the necessity for living in a less stable environment may remain satisfied during the turbulent early years.

The long-term impacts on role conflict and role clarity are unclear. Role overload and associated stresses should increase and may have an adverse impact on satisfaction. Innovation will increase a facilities respond to their changing markets by developing new services and new ways of managing traditional services.

PPSs may cause conflict between administrators and medical staff. Administrators are responsible for the financial consequences of treatment plans employed by the medical staff. As a result, they will have a financial incentive to reduce unnecessary ancillary services and to expedite discharges. Physicians will tend to focus on meeting patient needs and to repudiate programs that depersonalize services and reduce quality. Administrators will try to develop ways to encourage physicians to adjust their medical practices.[18]

Directing/Motivating Conditions

As salary increases are constrained, noneconomic motivators for physicians and other employees should increase. A greater emphasis on charismatic leadership is expected in the motivation process. Although the importance of charismatic leadership in motivating employees appears to

Table 20-3. Predicted Impact of DRGs on the Directing/Motivating Function.

	Impact		
	Increase	Uncertain	Decrease
Directing constraints			
Linkage between rewards and performance and efficiency	X		
Employee job satisfaction		X	
Organizational incentives for conformity and avoidance of risk taking			X
Potential administrator conflict with physicians	X		
Directing conditions			
Importance of noneconomic motivators for physicians	X		
Importance of noneconomic motivators for nonphysician employees	X		
Importance of charismatic leadership in motivation	X		
Importance of administration's ability to manage change	X		
Management control of important employee incentives	X		
Importance of volunteer labor	X		
Directing strategies			
Willingness to make major, nonincremental and innovative changes	X		
Emphasis on internal communication needs	X		
Emphasis on employee training	X		
Emphasis on management of cutbacks and employee layoffs	X		
Emphasis on management of physician practice patterns	X		
Employee staffing levels			X
Substitution of less expensive for more expensive personnel	X		
Emphasis on participation of physicians in the implementation process	X		
Emphasis on labor–management cooperation	X		

contradict the earlier descriptions of the diminished influence of charismatic leaders in goal setting, these statements are not actually in conflict. Goal setting will now be primarily determined by economics, whereas implementation of those goals may still benefit from charismatic leadership.

One result of the changes required under the new system will be that the management of change will become increasingly important. Mangers will be selected on the basis of their ability to work with a variety of individuals and groups in managing change.

Management control of important employee incentives should increase, because a failure to differentiate rewards among high- and low-performing employees will be costly. PPS/DRG rewards efficiency, but DRG-based data alone are not sufficient to track efficient resource use. Performance levels will become apparent as the quantity and quality of data increase. Facilities will be able to determine precisely how much revenue is produced by service and by provider; rewards are more likely to be distributed equitably on the basis of performance.

The importance of volunteer labor will increase, and management will be encouraged to motivate volunteers to undertake activities currently being performed by paid employees. Although volunteerism has fallen with the increase of females in the job market, older persons who do not desire payment for services could assume many of these volunteer roles.

Directing/Motivating Strategies

To respond to the demands of PPS/DRG, such changes will often require major, nonincremental (i.e., fundamental), and innovative changes. These changes will require an increased emphasis on internal communication processes and employee training. This training must include DRG coding systems and decision-making processes, as well as methods for determining and minimizing costs of procedures and tests. Training will need to be undertaken for trustees, administrative staff, physicians, and other employees.[19] It is particularly important that department heads be trained to facilitate internal and external communications concerning PPS implementation and future changes.

Cutbacks and employee layoffs may be expected as fiscal constraints cause reductions in staffing levels. Management will need to learn to respond to these conditions using strategies that have rarely been exercised in the medical care environment. An example might be the development of an outplacement service.

Monitoring and controlling of physician practice patterns and employee staffing levels will increase. Staffing levels will become leaner and workloads heavier. Substitution of less expensive (less skilled, less senior) for more expensive personnel should also increase. Development of sophisticated severity measures and patient acuity systems, as well as other methods to determine appropriate staffing, will become more important.

The practice patterns of the medical provider may have to change if his or her present practice patterns are not compatible with the requirements of PPS/DRG (i.e., being too resource-intensive to be cost-effective). A hospital's ability to respond to the new system may depend on the ability of administrators to transmit PPS incentives to attending physicians.[20] Physicians will need to understand the way PPS incentives will affect them, the importance of timely and accurate documentation, and the impact of physician practices on other costs, resource use, and revenues. Physicians will need to participate in the DRG implementation process if the goals of PPS are to be attained.[21] Physicians must be made aware of the importance of and need for accurate and prompt entries in the medical record. They will also need to be kept informed of changes in certain services necessitated by data generated by the new system.

Organizations in which employees are represented by labor unions will begin to move toward more cooperative forms of collective bargaining.[22] This development of collaborative arrangements will take many forms, just as it has in heavy industry. Adversary relationships under the new system could be potentially fatal, because higher costs will no longer be automatically passed through to the payer as part of the overall cost.

The Controlling Function

Controlling Constraints

Hospitals will need extremely sophisticated computerized management information systems to deal with DRGs. (See Table 20-4.) As management information systems and data collection increase, the difficulty in establishing predictable and impersonal feedback mechanisms will decrease. Management will be able to identify problem areas with accuracy and speed. Difficulty in measuring results will decrease for the same reasons. The degree to which external authorities undermine internal managerial control will remain uncertain until the federal advisory commission acts and it becomes apparent if and how rapidly PPS proliferates. In any case, it is clear that institutions that are able to meet the external control standards will be rewarded in the new system.

Hospitals can expect additional internal paperwork, at least as measured by the computer printouts and attendant summaries generated. The amount of external paperwork may decrease, as in the example of simplified Medicare reports. The reporting requirements that will be demanded by future legislation or regulations are unclear.

Efficiency should be enhanced in PPS/DRG because it limits the amount that will be paid for specific services rendered to Medicare patients. This necessitates that less resources be invested by the hospital in the medical care of those patients. If the system proves to be inefficient, it will fail and another payment or controlling mechanism can be expected. If the system is success-

Table 20-4. Predicted Impact of DRGs on the Control Function.

	Impact		
	Increase	Uncertain	Decrease
Controlling constraints			
Necessity for sophisticated management information systems	X		
Difficulty in establishing predictable and impersonal feedback mechanism			X
Difficulty in measuring results			X
Degree to which external authorities undermine managerial control		X	
Rewards for meeting control standards	X		
Degree to which proliferation of controls undermines efficiency			X
Degree to which proliferation of controls undermines effectiveness		X	
Controlling conditions			
Standardization of service outputs	X		
Emphasis on control over inputs	X		
Emphasis on control over outputs	X		
Controlling conditions *continued*			
Success measured by larger budgets		X	
Patient length of stay			X
Evaluation by external agencies	X		
Control strategies			
Centralization of control function		X	
Control of physician practice patterns	X		
Development of information tied to individual performance	X		
Emphasis on inventory control	X		
Emphasis on internal utilization review and quality assurance	X		
Development and use of specific cost data by service	X		
Emphasis on cost containment	X		
Upgrading of reported case mix	X		

ful, this will tend to focus the attention of management on those services that respond positively to the demands of the system.

Effectiveness is rarely mentioned explicitly in discussion of PPS/DRG; its impact remains uncertain. Increased use of utilization review and the potential for malpractice litigation are expected to motivate effectiveness, i.e., quality of care. Departmental productivity monitoring coupled with performance standards and subsequent corrective action will provide a mechanism to improve efficiency. A periodic "sunset review" in which all services are systematically reviewed for adherence to hospital goals will be necessary. This review determines continuance or discontinuance. Based on this information, decisions concerning continuance and alteration of services will necessarily be made.

Controlling Conditions

The service outputs (i.e., patients) of the medical care system will increase as a result of the incentive to serve more patients for shorter lengths of stay. At the same time, this may decrease the diversity of treatment modes. The long-term outcome of PPS/DRG indicates that standardization of medical care procedures will increase. Management control over inputs and outputs will increase in order to elicit the type of data needed to operate in the new system.

Success may no longer be measured in terms of larger budgets but will be determined by the facility's ability to provide quality care within the constraints of PPS/DRG. Patient length of stay should decline, because the institution has a disincentive to keep the patient longer than necessary. Outlier cases will not only be carefully monitored, but may also be disallowed following review. An increase in evaluation by external agencies appears obvious as a result of increased utilization review and regulatory agency monitoring.

Controlling Strategies

The New Jersey experience with PPS/DRG has indicated that many functions will be decentralized and that the chief executive officer will be less affected than department heads. Who will retain, or gain, control of the organization, however, remains unclear. Control of physician practice patterns will increase as the chief of medical services increases monitoring of individual deviations from cost-effective procedures. Physicians are likely to exercise control over their own performance as peer pressure heightens.

Increased data management will result in an increased emphasis on inventory, internal utilization review, quality assurance, and cost per service. For example, departmental productivity and performance standards may be increased. The resulting integration of clinical and financial data can be useful in determining financial implications of alternative practice patterns.[23] This provides a natural communication link between administrators and physicians. The concern remains that facilities will upgrade the reported case mix in order to enhance their revenue. Although this may occur in the short run, the monitoring system should factor out such violations over time.

Management Emphasis

Although the current PPS for medical care based on DRGs is confined to Medicare patients, this approach will probably become the norm for the entire medical care industry. Proponents of this approach believe that it will enhance hospital and physician efficiency by providing incentives to decrease the average length of stay and the use of unnecessary ancillary services.[24] Whether this optimistic outcome is achieved will depend on how well medical care managers are able to incorporate the new approach into their management systems. Management is the crucial variable linking the initiation of the PPS to the attainment of the goals of that system.

Previous attempts by the federal government to regulate the health care system have fallen short of their goals. (PL 93-641 created health care systems agencies that had responsibilities, but no power.) That legislation also did not provide enough funding to achieve the stated goals. In effect, the opportunity for success was suppressed by inadequate funding.

The present legislation, however, is not likely to suffer the same fate. Under the new law, PL 98-21, the basis for reimbursement has been unalterably changed. The final impact of the new system will not be known for several years; however, what is apparent is that health care services delivery in the United States will be substantially different and not necessarily better.

The fundamental change that should occur as a result of PPS/DRG is the beginning of a medical care management focus on organizational outcomes. This approach will assist management in evaluating organizational activity by looking at the end product. DRGs will lead to product definition on the part of the medical care industry for the first time in history.[25] The performance of the organization can now be evaluated by examining resources consumed and outputs produced.[26]

The new system should also produce a better management information and control system, because it will require a unified data base rather than the separate ones that now exist.[27] Planning, budgeting, and controlling will be facilitated, if the data base is accurate and timely.

Changes in the administrator-physician relationship should also be expected. Failure to convince the physician to become a team member concerned with the financial health of the institution could lead to financial disaster. No PPS/DRG system can be implemented without the cooperation of the physician.

Finally, the future will see a growth in the team management approach, with an emphasis on employee communications and training. For a hospital to survive, it is imperative that interactions and communication among all personnel improve. This interaction will need to be goal oriented and not just window dressing. The new system will provide a commonality of interest among all those concerned with the provision of quality care delivered in the most efficient manner.

Notes

1. Schweiker, R. *Report to Congress: Hospital Prospective Payment for Medicare.* Washington, DC.: U.S. Department of Health and Human Services, December 1982.
2. Grimaldi, P., and Micheletti, J. *Diagnosis Related Groups: A Practitioner's Guide.* 2d ed. Chicago: Pluribus Press, 1983.
3. Grimaldi, P., and Micheletti, J. *Medicare's Prospective Payment Plan: DRG Update.* Chicago: Pluribus Press, 1983.
4. Bowman, R. "DRGs Help Trace Revenue Sources." *Modern Health Care* 10, no. 1 (1980): 92-94.
5. Barnard, C., and Esmond, T., Jr. "More Work Needed: DRGs—A Progress Report." *Hospital Financial Management* 36, no. 1 (1982): 48-52.
6. Horn, S., Sharkey, P., and Bertram, D. "Measuring Severity of Illness: Homogeneous Case Mix Groups." *Medical Care* 21, no. 1 (1983): 14-30.
7. Fox, R. "DRG's: A Management Control Tool in Hospitals and Multi-Institutional Systems." *Hospital Progress* 62, no. 1 (1981): 52-53.
8. American Public Health Association. "Social Security/Prospective Payment Bill Passes." *Washington News Letter* no. 4 (April 1983): 3-4.
9. Ibid., 3.
10. Crawford, M. "Implementing Medicare Prospective Pricing by Diagnosis Related Groups." *Alabama Journal of Medical Sciences* 21, no. 1 (1984): 96-100.
11. Hofer, C., and Schendel, D. *Strategy Formulation: Analytical Concepts.* St. Paul, MN: West Publishing, 1978.
12. Mumford, E., Schlesinger, H., and Glass, G. "The Effects of Psychological Interventions on Recovery from Surgery and Heart Attacks: An Analysis of the Literature." *American Journal of Public Health* 72 (1982): 141-51.

13. Grimaldi and Micheletti, *Diagnosis Related Groups.*
14. "Should Finance Be the Boss?" *Hospitals* 57, no. 4 (1983): 40.
15. Grimaldi and Micheletti, *Diagnosis Related Groups.*
16. Boerma, H. *DRG Evaluation: The Organizational Impact.* Princeton, NJ: Health Research and Educational Trust of New Jersey, 1983.
17. Lindner, J., and Wagner, D. "DRG's Spur Management-Related Groups." *Modern Healthcare* 13 (1983): 160-61.
18. Grimaldi and Micheletti, *Diagnosis Related Groups.*
19. Iglehart, J. "New Jersey's Experiment with DRG-Based Hospital Reimbursement." *New England Journal of Medicine* 307 (1982): 1655-60.
20. Schweiker, *Report to Congress.*
21. Lindner and Wagner, "DRG's Spur Management-Related Groups."
22. Fottler, M., and Maloney, W. "Guidelines to Productive Bargaining in the Health Care Industry." *Health Care Management Review* 4, no. 1 (1979): 59-70.
23. Averill, R., and Kalison, M. "Prospective Payment by DRG." *Healthcare Financial Management* 37, no. 2 (1983): 12-22.
24. Feldstein, P. *Health Care Economics.* 2d ed. New York: Wiley, 1983.
25. Marley, A. "Prospective Pricing Based on Diagnostic Related Groups: Managerial Implications." Master's thesis, University of Alabama at Birmingham, 1983.
26. Fox, "DRG's: A Management Control Tool."
27. Smith, H., and Fottler, M. *Prospective Payment: Managing for Operational Effectiveness.* Rockville, MD.: Aspen Systems, 1985.

Resource Utilization

In selection 21, "Fiscal Fitness: Ten Principles for Evaluating Financial Health," William O. Cleverley presents specific measures of hospital financial performance important to their survival. Steven R. Eastaugh in selection 22, "Organization, Scheduling Are Main Keys to Improving Productivity in Hospitals," emphasizes the importance of an output-driven staffing and scheduling system. Recommendations are made to enhance productivity. Selection 23, "Dispelling Productivity Myths" by Brian Channon, follows. The author of this article corrects some inappropriate assumptions about productivity improvement.

Selection 24, "Megatrends in Hospital Information Systems" by Ron Ladd, Tom Grudnowski, and Mike Dickoff, discusses the external forces, including PPS, affecting hospitals' information systems and contrasts present system attributes to those needed in the future. Michael J. Shaffer in selection 25, "Managing Hospital Biomedical Equipment," describes the impact of biomedical equipment in hospitals and the role of the manager in controlling it. Special attention is paid to the location of the biomedical equipment management function in the organization's hierarchy and the organizational relationships that are appropriate.

21

Fiscal Fitness: Ten Principles for Evaluating Financial Health

William O. Cleverley

William O. Cleverley, Ph.D. is Professor and Director, Center for Hospital Financial Analysis Service, Ohio State University, Columbus.

A critical question facing hospitals today is which of them will survive. More than 1,000 of them – 20 percent – may fail during the next 10 years.

What factors are likely to contribute to a hospital's failure? What can hospitals do to prevent failure? These are enormously complex questions, but not unanswerable. Insolvency is the primary cause of failure in many cases. Insolvency may relate to such problems as declining utilization, aging plant, or competition in primary markets, but the effects of these problems ultimately will show up in the hospital's financial statements.

This article has a twofold aim: (1) It will explain the fundamentals of managing for financial survival; specific measures of financial survivability will be discussed. Table 21-1 provides an assessment tool for measuring your own hospital's performance against these criteria. (2) It will examine Catholic hospitals' present financial health relative to other hospitals, and it will focus on specific areas that warrant close attention in the coming decade.

Following are the 10 basic principles for successful hospital operations:

1. Operating profits should cover replacement cost of assets.

2. Nonoperating sources of income are critical to product-line enhancement.

3. Growth of equity capital is the bottom line of survival.

4. A liquid operation is a must.

5. Additional debt capacity should be maintained to ensure future funding availability.

Reprinted with permission from *Health Progress,* 67(3) January/February 1986, pages 22-27. Copyright 1986 by the Catholic Health Association of the United States. All rights reserved.

Table 21-1. Hospital Financial Assessment.

Check your hospital's economic health by filling in the right-hand column.

Financial Health Measure	Formula	U.S. Norm	Your Hospital Value
1. Operating margin (price level-adjusted)	$\dfrac{\text{Total operating revenue} - \text{Operating expenses} + \text{Depreciation} - \text{Price level depreciation}}{\text{Total operating revenue}}$	-0.010	____
2. Nonoperating revenue	$\dfrac{\text{Nonoperating revenue}}{\text{Excess of revenues over expenses}}$	0.333	____
3. Return on equity	$\dfrac{\text{Excess of revenues over expenses}}{\text{Fund balance}}$	0.092	____
4. Liquidity ratio	$\dfrac{\text{Current assets}}{\text{Current liabilities}}$	1.84	____
5. Long-term debt to equity	$\dfrac{\text{Long-term liabilities}}{\text{Fund balance}}$	0.69	____
6. Average age of plant	$\dfrac{\text{Accumulated depreciation}}{\text{Depreciation expense}}$	6.94	____
7. Total asset turnover	$\dfrac{\text{Total operating revenue}}{\text{Total assets}}$	0.98	____
8. Replacement viability	$\dfrac{\text{Restricted plant fund balance} + \text{Unrestricted noncurrent investments}}{\text{Price level-adjusted accumulated depreciation} \times 0.50}$	0.37	____
9. Days in patient accounts receivable	$\dfrac{\text{Net patient accounts receivable}}{\dfrac{\text{Net patient service revenue}}{365}}$	61.5	____
10. Hard Times Index	$\left[\dfrac{\text{Liquidity ratio} - 1.84}{1.84}\right] + \left[0.69 - \dfrac{\text{Long-term debt-to-equity ratio}}{0.69}\right]$ $+ \left[\dfrac{\text{Replacement viability ratio} - 0.37}{0.37}\right] + \left[6.94 - \dfrac{\text{Average age of plant}}{6.94}\right]$ $+ \left[\dfrac{\text{Operating margin ratio} - 0.021}{0.021}\right]$	0	____

6. Older hospitals are often dying hospitals.

7. Getting the most from investment is critical during a capital shortage.

8. Setting aside funds for replacement and new product innovations is not a luxury; it is a necessity.

9. The hospital should collect revenue as quickly as possible.

10. Maintaining ability to withstand unexpected financial hard times is vital.

To examine these principles in detail, the actual experience of Catholic hospitals will be used as a benchmark. Financial indicator values from the Healthcare Financial Management Association's Financial Analysis Service (FAS) will be employed. FAS is a subscriber-based financial indicator service to which, at the time of this writing, 191 Catholic hospitals and approximately 1,400 hospitals nationally subscribed.

One caveat: Industry averages for financial ratios do not necessarily represent norms or standards. Values for specific indicators that are far different from industry averages may be both possible and desirable. For example, a hospital with a formalized policy of having no long-term debt would have leverage ratio values considerably different from hospital industry averages. Industry averages do, however, represent a good first effort at defining norms where no normative statements are possible.

Operating Profitability

Few people today contend that hospitals should be denied a profit. This is a giant step forward from prior public positions, but a question that often surfaces is how much profit a not-for-profit hospital should make from operations. To remain a viable concern during inflationary periods, an organization must cover the replacement cost of its fixed assets, and hospitals are no exception. Obviously, an x-ray machine that cost $100,000 five years ago and now costs $250,000 must be financed with an additional $150,000. Any business that fails to recover its replacement costs is financing itself toward bankruptcy.

How does one determine the amount of operating profit required to cover those replacement costs? A good indicator is the operating margin price level-adjusted ratio (OMPLA). This FAS ratio is an ordinary operating margin ratio, except that replacement cost depreciation rather than historical cost depreciation is used to measure capital cost. A hospital that fails to maintain a positive OMPLA is not earning enough from operations to replace its assets.

How is the average hospital faring with respect to this ratio? More to the point, how are Catholic hospitals doing? The following FAS data are illuminating.

	1980	1981	1982	1983
Catholic hospital median	-0.009	-0.011	-0.014	-0.005
U.S. hospital median	-0.015	-0.017	-0.015	-0.011

What do these data indicate? First, most hospitals, Catholic and non-Catholic, lose money. Simply stated, profits from operations are not sufficient to meet replacement needs. These needs will require funding from other sources. If grants, investment income, or expanded debt are not available, downsizing of the hospital is a virtual certainty.

Second, Catholic hospitals are better than the average U.S. hospital in this area, but not by much; improvement is still essential for long-term viability. Catholic hospitals should try to increase their OMPLAs to at least a breakeven level.

Nonoperating Income

Poor operating margins can be partially compensated by income from other sources. Most not-for-profit health care institutions, including hospitals, practice this form of subsidization. But how much is enough? What is a hospital norm?

FAS's nonoperating revenue ratio addresses this dimension of profitability directly. The ratio relates nonoperating income to total net income, or the excess of revenues over expenses. Following are data for this indicator:

	1980	1981	1982	1983
Catholic hospital median	0.290	0.222	0.330	0.268
U.S. hospital median	0.339	0.376	0.383	0.350

A slightly different picture from that of the first indicator emerges. First, Catholic hospitals do not earn as much from nonoperating sources as do non-Catholic hospitals. This offsets the favorable position that Catholic hospitals enjoy with respect to the OMPLA. Second, nonoperating income is crucial in any assessment of profitability. Though nonoperating revenue represents only 1 to 4 percent of total revenue in most hospitals, it accounts for about 30 percent of total net income.

Improvement in this area is critical to hospital viability. If future operating margins are constrained due to competition or price regulation, nonoperating revenue could provide an essential safety cushion.

Equity Growth

An unarguable rule of business is that viability requires increases in total asset investment. A comparison of most hospital balance sheets from five years ago with today's values will show that total assets have increased by about 80 percent. Much of this growth is not real; it represents inflated replacement costs and increases in working capital items such as accounts receivable. Nonetheless, the increase in investment must be financed with real dollars, and these real dollars must come from either equity or debt. Ultimately, equity is the key to sustained asset growth. No organization can long continue to finance its growth with debt. The return-on-equity ratio, then, is a key indicator of financial health:

	1980	1981	1982	1983
Catholic hospital median	0.085	0.098	0.093	0.105
U.S. hospital median	0.077	0.086	0.085	0.092

Catholic hospitals again appear to have a slight edge, having consistently earned a return on equity exceeding the national average. But a fundamental question remains: Is this rate adequate? The answer is probably not. If a hospital increases its assets at a rate greater than its return on equity, then it must increase its percentage of debt financing; and all hospitals, Catholic and non-Catholic, have in fact been increasing their assets in excess of their return on equity. Debt financing has risen dramatically as a result. Clearly, in light of the current reduction in the hospital industry's debt capacity, this trend must be slowed or stopped. Hospitals should attempt to set equity growth rates equal to expected asset growth rates.

Liquidity

Illiquid firms often fail, of course. But though liquidity is important, it must be considered in relation to profitability. An illiquid firm that is profitable will probably survive, but an unprofitable illiquid firm is dead. Why? Simply because profitable businesses can acquire short-term financing. Banks will loan money to good credit risks; they do not loan money to poor ones.

Nevertheless, it is important to maintain a reasonable degree of liquidity even if the institution is profitable. Data on liquidity ratios indicate that Catholic hospitals occupy a relatively poor position.

	1980	1981	1982	1983
Catholic hospital median	1.75	1.67	1.68	1.69
U.S. hospital median	1.92	1.87	1.82	1.84

The differences between Catholic hospitals and hospitals in general are significant and have been consistent over time. The values are not alarming, however, and managers should not overreact. Still, a poor liquidity position requires attention, and sufficient liquid resources should be maintained to meet future obligations.

Debt Capacity

Obviously, it is not good business to exhaust the hospital's debt capacity; the institution's financial flexibility will be impaired and it will be much less resilient in a time of fiscal stress. The ratio of long-term debt to equity is a good indicator of overall debt capacity:

	1980	1981	1982	1983
Catholic hospital median	0.73	0.68	0.81	0.78
U.S. hospital median	0.56	0.58	0.63	0.70

Not surprisingly, the data show a trend among U.S. hospitals toward less equity and therefore more debt. Among Catholic hospitals this trend is more erratic but still discernible. Moreover, Catholic hospitals appear to be more leveraged than the average hospital. Is this level of debt dangerous? Does it suggest that many hospitals have exceeded their debt capacity? These are difficult and complex questions. The hospital's ability to service the debt is clearly a factor. Businesses with good profitability can afford more debt; so can businesses with stable earnings. Do hospitals meet these criteria? Probably not, especially in the present payment climate.

In 1983 the average manufacturing firm's ratio of long-term debt to equity was 0.54. The hospital industry is highly leveraged by comparison. Hospital executives should define their corporate debt policy precisely. Few have done this yet.

Age of Facilities

Usually the failed hospital is an old hospital. It is one that has outlived its utility; it cannot provide the services needed by the community in an efficient or effective manner. Capital for renovation is urgently needed but unavailable. The hospital thus becomes a casualty of progress.

Renovations and equipment replacement give new life to old plant structures, and the average age of hospital plants is decreasing:

	1980	1981	1982	1983
Catholic hospital median (age in years)	7.56	7.49	7.14	7.10
U.S. hospital median (age in years)	7.30	7.18	6.99	6.94

Catholic hospitals are older than non-Catholic hospitals, and have been for some time. The gap is narrowing, but the difference still exists. Is the current difference significant? It probably is, since these values represent medians for a large number of hospitals. Variance in large samples becomes smaller and makes differences between median values more significant. If the average age of a plant exceeds 10 years, clearly it has a replacement need. In this case, unused debt capacity and a history of good earning power can be helpful. Without them, replacement may be difficult or impossible.

Revenue Generation

The more revenue that can be generated from a fixed plant investment, the more profitable the hospital will be. Total asset turnover is a measure widely used in business to indicate the efficiency of capital investment. The figures in this index for Catholic hospitals and for hospitals in general have converged:

	1980	1981	1982	1983
Catholic hospital median	1.00	1.04	1.05	0.98
U.S. hospital median	0.98	1.01	1.01	0.98

The 1983 values indicate that the typical hospital generates 98 cents of revenue for every dollar of total investment. Preliminary data for 1984 indicate a continuation of the downward trend, which may reflect declining utilization. Is this situation viable over the long term? Probably not. In an industry with low margins (such as the hospital field), turnover is the key. Grocery stores have low margins, but they turn their investment over rapidly. In short, they do not make a lot per unit sold, but they sell a lot of units. Hospitals do not make a lot per unit "sold," but neither do they sell a lot of units. Improvement in either turnover or margin is critical to long-term survival.

Replacement Funds

Most young couples anticipating home ownership know they must save money to make a respectable down payment and thus keep their debt service to a minimum. By the same token, a family with a stable income can afford a larger house if, and only if, it can save a greater percentage of the purchase price.

Unfortunately, many hospitals have ignored this simple principle and adopted the "new finance" which says, "Don't save anything; you can borrow it all when you need it." The result is a recent wave of construction programs financed with 90 percent or more of debt. Was this dangerous in the past? Yes, but perhaps not fatal. Today it is fatal. The "new finance" is dead and the old basics are back. Medicare may no longer enhance debt service ability. Replacement funds, funded depreciation, renewal funds—whatever they are called—are critical to survival.

How much should the hospital accumulate? The answer is simple. After the proportion of replacement needs that can be financed through debt is determined, that proportion is subtracted from one and the remainder is multiplied by the current replacement cost of the hospital's depreciated assets. FAS's replacement viability (RV) ratio measures the adequacy of available funds to meet replacement needs, assuming 50 percent debt financing. A value of one for the RV ratio indicates funds are sufficient on this basis. The following data indicate that hospitals are not setting aside enough funds to meet replacement needs:

	1980	1981	1982	1983
Catholic hospital median	0.28	0.27	0.26	0.33
U.S. hospital median	0.27	0.30	0.33	0.37

Ideally the values would be one. The 1983 values of 0.33 and 0.37 indicate that Catholic hospitals must debt-finance 83.5 percent of their replacement needs, and that hospitals in general must finance 81.5 percent of their replacement needs through debt. Can hospitals cope with such large proportions of debt? Not all of them, and none of them for very long. What is the solution? The board should formulate a policy for funding replacement needs. Only a few hospitals have yet done this. It may have been excusable before, but not any longer.

Minimizing Receivables

Prompt payment of accounts receivable is desirable in any business. Longer payment periods translate into greater investment of capital and therefore greater cost. This is not new information to hospital executives; rapid increases in accounts receivable have created cash flow problems for many hospitals in the past and will unquestionably be a factor in the future. FAS data for days in accounts receivable indicate that Catholic hospitals are in a favorable position compared with other hospitals:

	1980	1981	1982	1983
Catholic hospital median (days)	57.6	57.1	56.3	58.9
U.S. hospital median (days)	62.4	61.1	61.3	61.5

Is the present investment level excessive? Yes. Waiting 60 days to collect on a receivable is not good business, especially considering that many customers never pay off their accounts entirely.

Should the hospital cancel its Medicare contract? That may be rash, but clearly some action must be taken to minimize delays in payment. Closely monitoring the coding of physician diagnoses, requiring preadmission deposits, and using the services of collection agencies have been successful.

Maximizing Survivability

Is the hospital prepared for hard times? Does it have the financial flexibility to withstand a few years of reduced cash flow?

These are difficult questions, and the ability to survive hard times cannot be gauged by examining only one financial dimension. Yet many firms in other industries have grappled with the problem and concluded that the ability to withstand financial hard times is largely a function of the organization's ability to affect or manage its flow of funds. In a crisis, funds can be generated in five basic ways: borrow for the short term; borrow for the long term; use liquid reserves; sell assets; reduce operating expenses.

The author's "Hard Times Index" may be useful. It appeared in the newsletter *Hospital Bottom Line* (August 1984, pp. 1-2) and is a composite of FAS indicators that measure a hospital's ability to implement the five financial strategies just described. Positive values are favorable; negative values suggest a financial weakness. U.S. hospitals aggregately provide the norm in this instance:

	1980	1981	1982	1983
Catholic hospital median	0.104	-0.001	-0.390	-0.07
U.S. hospital median	0	0	0	0

Catholic hospitals appear to have less financial resiliency than the median U.S. hospital. The difference does not seem to be significant, but it does imply that in the future Catholic hospitals may fail at a slightly higher rate than the national average.

22

Organization, Scheduling are Main Keys to Improving Productivity in Hospitals

Steven R. Eastaugh

Steven R. Eastaugh, Sc.D., is Associate Professor of Health Services Administration, Department of Health Services Administration, The George Washington University, Washington, DC.

Productivity, in its simplest form, equals output divided by resource inputs.

Productivity can be improved either by expanding output or contracting inputs, or having the rate of change in output volume outperform the rate of change in input resources.

To paraphrase Peter Drucker, the noted management consultant, productivity is the first test of management's competence. You are a good manager to the degree that you can get the greatest output from your resource inputs, achieving the most value for the effort.

The productivity improvement issue has been around for two decades, but until now the will to act has been buried under the comfortable blanket of cost reimbursement. The economic shock to hospitals of prospective price payment may product a flurry of petty, short-sighted cost reductions.

Hiring freezes may prevent facilities from acquiring talented people who have the requisite management science skills to save the institution. Morale will decline if continuing education programs are sharply reduced, anticipated raises are chopped—and marketing and reorganization plans are cancelled. Fruitful cost reduction should not be so short run, superficial and spasmodic as to "cut a little fat," or so ruthless and indiscriminate as to impair the hospital's ability to survive in the long run. Any significant cost reduction effort must involve a significant reduction in the number of employees.

In 1984, the volume of inpatient days in the American Hospital Association (AHA) panel survey declined 9.1 percent, and admissions declined 4

Reprinted with permission from *Federation of American Hospitals Review,* 30(4) November/ December 1985, pp. 61-63. Copyright 1985 by the Federation of American Hospitals Review, Inc. All rights reserved.

247

percent — but personnel declined by only 2.3 percent. Consequently, the phrase "census-driven" flexible staffing became popular in 1984. However, staff per patient day increased by 7.3 percent. There is some truth in the argument that staff per patient day should increase somewhat as length of stay declined (5.1 percent), because the hospital is left with a larger proportion of acute (severe) bed days to serve.

As more staff are considered a variable cost, to be cut in line with declines in workload, the staffing ratio should level off in 1985. Based on 9 months of 1985 data, one would project a 3.6 percent decline in total staff, a 4.9 percent decline in inpatient days and an 8.2 percent increase in full-time employees (FTEs) per diem (see Table 22-1).

The critical point is that our objective should not become census-driven staffing. A staffing and scheduling system based on monitoring case mix complexity is a better alternative. To be output-driven (workload-based) in setting staff levels is superior to simply linking staffing to the census.

In the new world of the prospective payment system (PPS), the basic unit of productivity is the diagnosis related group (DRG) case treated, not the activity units accumulated. There has long been a need for a final product perspective in health care. Counting relative value units (RVUs) misses the target completely. It is largely irrelevant to measure "the product" with nurse relative intensity measure (RIM), or GRASP (Grace Reynolds Applications and Study of Peto, a nursing scoring system) points, and measure lab workloads with College of American Pathologists (CAP) points accumulated.

When talking in terms of RVUs, productivity experts lapse into a jargon that is an industrial engineer's version of the secret lodge handshake. Who cares if the RVU workload is improving because overreporting is on the increase? What matters to the chief executive officer (CEO) is that patient census has declined 10 percent, and cash flow declined 4 percent.

Keys to Improvement

The two greatest keys to productivity improvement are organization and scheduling. Much can be achieved by examining what is being done and how employees are being organized into work units (stage 1) and how labor and patients can be scheduled better (stage 2).

Stage 1

Initial Operational Assessment

Usually involving job and task redesign, this first step involves finding answers to two basic questions: (1) How many people should really be working here? (2) What is the best mix of staff and other resources?

Table 22-1. Aggregate Annual Changes in Utilization, Productivity, Staffing and Capacity, 1983-84, 1984-85 Estimate (AHA Panel Survey)

			1984	1985
A.	Utilization			
	— Inpatient Days		–9.1%	–8.2%
	— Admissions		–4.0%	–5.1%
	— Length of Stay		–5.1%	–3.0%
B.	Labor Input	1		
	$\dfrac{\text{}}{\text{Output}}$	= $\dfrac{\text{}}{\text{Labor Productivity}}$		
	— FTEs/Patient Days		7.3%	4.9%
	— FTEs/Admissions		1.8%	1.4%
C.	Staffing and Capacity			
	— Personnel (FTEs)		–2.3%	–3.6%
	— Part-Time Personnel		0.3%	–1.9%
	— Staffed Beds		–1.1%	–2.6%

Four basic actions make up the operational assessment: (1) review historical, current and budgeted staffing levels; (2) evaluate facility layout, equipment, intraunit functional relationships and interdepartmental coordination; (3) identify operational deficiencies and recommend improvements; and (4) analyze all forms and reports for appropriateness and timeliness of the information.

Operational assessment should focus on three principles: (1) don't organize for what is done only 5 percent of the time; (2) stream-line overlapping functions and excessive layers of supervision; and (3) reduce those departments that exhibit excess capacity.

The efficiency of standing orders and standard operating procedures (SOP), such as letting nurses restart IVs, need to be assessed. Nurse activities that need increased delegation to other staff should be evaluated — and anticipated changes coordinated. Nursing and ancillary departments should reorganize and retrain for improved productivity. Flexibility in staffing is the key to adjusting to the flux in demands during peak periods while keeping staffing levels down. Japanese hospitals, for example, use the "utility infielder" approach. They cross-train all staff in two areas.

Use an Adequate Reporting System

Functional procedural flow chart analysis and task evaluation are two key tools in operational assessment. Nursing productivity studies, in particular, are often hampered by poor information systems and support systems. Although some facilities allocate float nurses' work efforts back to the home department rather than to the understaffed units or subspecialty areas (like the operating room), other facilities draw all float pool personnel from an outside registry and define float time as a cost center, with no information concerning where the work effort actually should have been allocated.

In summary, operational assessment (a) yields better work assignments; (b) identifies "lost resources" and unnecessary activities, and (c) suggests ways to foster efficient interdepartmental coordination.

Stage 2

Who Can Be Scheduled Better

Three critical actors—the patient, the employee and the physician—must be scheduled better for improved productivity. Better scheduling of all three groups can reduce unnecessary activity flow, reduce costs and improve customer satisfaction by reducing waiting time for both providers and patients.

Preserve Employee Morale

A basic requirement of a scheduling system is that it preserves morale and meets the personal needs of employees for days off, vacations, birthdays and holidays. In addition, employees should "work smarter," but no individual experiences a perceptible shift toward working harder. Slack periods or "down time" simply decline in frequency and duration.

Use an Automated Scheduling System

Unfortunately, many hospitals use manual scheduling systems that are unresponsive to subtle shifts in workload and may be perceived as unfair. It is amazing that personnel are still manually scheduled in an industry that spends over $3 billion each week and that has such complex scheduling problems. If 12 nurses are scheduled over a month so that each nurse works 22 days (and disregarding all other constraints), there will be 1.5 million possible schedules. It is hard to imagine any human being who could find the best schedule. A computerized scheduling system, however, can select the best schedule without hours of paperwork, hassle and appeal. The computer can provide convincing documentation of fairness in demonstrating that weekend assignments and shift changes (mornings to afternoons and nights) have been equalized.

When caught understaffed, one can use float squads, float pools, further controlling of elective admissions, channelling of the more severe incoming cases to underworked units—and call-ups to incidental part-time staff.

Involve Your Physicians

Scheduling systems for physicians also can reduce costs through a reduction in the down time (wasted time). When an operating room mishandles the scheduling of cases, cost overruns result either from underuse or overtime wages. Changing utilization habits will improve productivity. Producing more services than are medically necessary—even if they are produced at a lower unit cost—has little to do with real increases in productivity per case.

When physicians order unnecessary RVUs of activity that provide no marginal information gain in diagnosis or treatment decisions, real productivity declines. If the hospital's product is now a DRG case treated and the total payment and clinical outcome are the same whether 3,000 or 7,000 RVUs of activity are ordered, the extra marginal resources drive up costs without any benefit to the patient or the hospital. Having employees work harder in ancillary departments will not be useful unless the extra information resulting from that work is valuable.

Stage 3

Provision of Incentives

It is a relatively easy task to reduce costs by cutting services or service quality. We have outlined a two-stage strategy that undertakes the hard task of managing cost reduction without service or quality reduction. Little attention has been paid to the use of motivational tools. The Henry Ford Hospital (of Detroit, Michigan) incentive compensation plan, initiated in 1983-84, is a prototype for using the bonus pay concept on an annualized basis to reward individual employees or departments (dividing up the bonus pool within the units or department). The provision of incentives will reinforce the changes made in Stages 1 and 2 of the productivity program.

Incentive pay offers substantial benefits beyond a reduction in the absenteeism. In the hospital industry, there are many jobs where individuals have considerable discretion over how they manage their work. Employees and medical staff have control over their personal commitment and their productivity. They can withhold it—or they can give it in exchange for something they value (cash, vacation time, nonmonetary rewards, etc.). Management needs to present carefully a philosophical and financial context for the announcement of incentive programs. Employee perception is critical. A system of perceived "bribes" will not change behavior, but incentive pay as a substitute for even more belt-tightening does improve productivity and morale.

Open Incentive Compensation Eligibility for All

Incentives help eliminate any danger of an organization becoming incapable of attracting good people—workers who can mobilize resources to maximize productivity. All such people do not come from the ranks of management. Therefore, incentives should not be offered exclusively to executives of the facility. As one IBM executive once summarized the issue: "If a $14,000 a year worker comes with an idea that saves $400,000, we don't quibble with rank. We pay them a bonus."

Employee entrepreneurs who push the standard operating procedure to the limits come from all classes of labor. Many such "change agents" will not bring forth their ideas unless (1) a friendly productivity-oriented environment has been established, and (2) they share directly in the benefits of "working smarter." If you foster a strong sense for performance and finding ways to do it better with your frontline people, productivity will improve.

Incentives can act as the glue that holds the entire three-stage productivity program together. If the people acting as entrepreneurs achieve improved productivity for the hospital, nonproductive workers and nonthinkers will be less willing (and able) to sabotage the process and throw a "monkey wrench" into the program. All employees will discover, over time, that the new program is not punitive. Entrepreneurs with the ideas and superior performers in daily activity should receive both incentive compensation (money, educational benefits, vacation, etc.) and professional recognition. But somebody at the top has to have the guts to initiate the process of starting a productivity program, acting as troubleshooter, targeting the problem areas and breaking a little crockery if needed.

What Must Be Done

The basic requirement of a successful productivity program is that the senior managers and trustees really must want cost reduction. The best productivity programs are rapid, large in scale, cost beneficial—and provide benchmarks for assessing future performance. Productivity improvement studies do not need to be multi-year and very costly. The first stage of operational assessment can be rapid (three to five months) and quite cost-beneficial. Substantial cost reductions can be obtained in the short run, while second and third stages of more refined improvements (scheduling systems, for example) and incentives are put in place for permanent, long-run cost containment. Timing depends on the size and scope of the facility and areas under study, but rapid plan development and implementation are essential both for financial and nonfinancial reasons. Allowing the assessment to go beyond a few months would create undue uncertainties among employees.

Start Big

The departments under study should be large if the gains are to be large. A 7 percent improvement in nurse production would dwarf a 37 percent improvement in labor productivity of central supply, pharmacy, housekeeping, laundry, plant and maintenance, for example. The frequent management complaint—"We have the best laundry costs and the worst hospital cost increases"—only illustrates a major point. Significant cuts in the big cost area of a hospital cannot be avoided in the vain hope that cost containment either can be easy or confined to cosmetic reductions in staff. Merely conducting an overhead variance analysis and cutting the number of housekeepers, administrative residents and interns will not get to the heart of a hospital's productivity problems.

Ask the Right Questions

Trustee and senior management should ask critical questions: What staffing ratio do we really need? How did other hospitals get expanded output with much lower growth in staff? What new equipment and organizational changes can be used to reduce staff and make the work force more effective? Examples from other institutions can convince management that new methods of organizing and scheduling can be made to work. Normative comparison of "best actors" among peer hospitals (those exhibiting the best levels of productivity) also can be useful in making ballpark "guesstimates" of the potential for staff reductions.

Things to Avoid

If a hospital has to undergo staff reduction, there are a number of inefficient ways to do it. An old favorite—and one that doesn't require much analysis—is to reduce every department's budget across the board. A variation of this approach is to exempt direct patient care areas of the facility and cut only nonpatient care staff across the board.

However, patient care departments often provide the greatest opportunities for achieving efficiencies that will allow reductions in cost without reductions in quality or access.

Another staff reduction strategy involves imposing a hiring freeze on all departments and forcing staff reduction through attrition. One hears of policies that say—"Departing employees will not be replaced unless their jobs are essential." If the job is not "essential" in the first place, why should it continue to be filled just because the incumbent does not elect to resign or retire?

The emphasis has been on labor productivity—which is natural in our labor intensive organizations. But we should not overlook capital and materials management productivity. Badly managed hospitals often experience many years of reduced available equipment life when their maintenance programs are poorly planned and executed.

It is quite possible to determine the optimal number of staff in each area of the hospital with a case mix-driven, workload-based staffing system. Having more than that number of staff simply wastes money. It does not provide better quality care. A tight ship is usually a quality ship, and when departments are more productive, achievement of an increasingly higher quality service is much more likely.

Hospitals with more employees and supplies than they actually need do not produce a higher quality service. The observation that a lean hospital also can be a quality hospital will be confirmed during 1986-87 as professional review organization (PRO) data on quality of care is made public by hospitals. Productivity programs do not cut muscle and bone. They cut fat and fluff. Quality does not improve merely by increasing the number of staff available. Poor response time to a patient's call bell, slow transport time and slow lab turnaround almost never are resolved by adding more staff.

One should avoid the textbook, timid, normative productivity program that usually involves the creation of a nonthreatening productivity task force. That approach features the creation of systems to measure "output activity units." One misguided manager summarized his charge as "not cost control, but rather tabulating units of activity that help justify current staff allocations. We know the ruler of measuring productivity is correct if changes to be suggested are minimal." It often takes years before any serious analysis can be accomplished — and the staffing target norms are outdated. Management can be lulled into believing that productivity need only be sufficient to reside in the "happy middle" of MONITREND staffing norms. However, the norms are declining rapidly as hospital payment rates tighten. Hospitals may find that the happy middle norms of 1986 will not assure a good future.

Adam Smith (the noted economist) wrote extensively on the relationship between progress and the "law of comparative advantage": If each good or service is supplied by the most productive producer, all in society will be richer.

To be against productivity is to be against medical progress. Productivity gains will help underwrite our future improvements in service delivery and technology. These programs will provide the linchpin to insure that we continue to deliver a quality service at an affordable cost for all concerned.

23

Dispelling Productivity Myths

Brian Channon

Brian Channon is Director, Center for Performance Enhancement, Chatsworth, California.

In today's changing and uncertain marketplace, intense competitive pressures, coupled with severe cutbacks in state and federal monies, pose stiff challenges to hospitals and governing boards. Price competition, provider contracting, insurance company audits of patient bills, business coalitions, and new low-cost producers are forcing the traditional hospital to retool into a competitive health delivery system or risk significant financial losses.

Now as never before, productivity can be the survival strategy. It can help a hospital recover costs, increase profits, improve the quality of care, and ultimately establish a more secure position in the marketplace.

While implementing productivity management programs at several hospitals, I have encountered much misunderstanding of productivity as a concept. For maximum effect, the concept must become a way of life for every manager. Disposing of some myths that surround productivity may assist in reaching that goal.

An increase in productivity can be defined as the reduction of the ratio of input to output, where input is hours worked and output is "units" of service rendered. The ratio is lowered when any of the following occurs:

1. Hours worked decrease while units of service stay the same.
2. Hours worked decrease at a rate faster than the rate of decrease in units of service.
3. Units of service increase while hours worked stay the same.
4. Units of service increase at a rate faster than the rate of increase in hours worked.

The following are some of the more widely held myths about productivity.

Reprinted by permission from *Hospitals,* Vol. 57, No. 19, October 1, 1983. Copyright 1983, American Hospital Publishing, Inc.

Productivity = Volume

Not necessarily true. Volume, or number of units is only one element of the productivity equation. Hours worked must also be considered.

	1981	1982
Hours worked	4000	5500
Number of x-rays	4000	5000
Hours/x-ray	1	1.1

Productivity = Efficiency

Efficiency improvement refers to working faster in the performance of an activity.

	1981	1982
Time per x-ray	10 min.	8 min.

In the example above, the efficiency with which an x-ray was performed in 1982 improved by 20 percent. But efficiency improvement and productivity improvement are not synonymous.

	1981	1982
Time per x-ray	10 min.	8 min.
Hours worked	4000	4000
Number of x-rays	4000	4000
Hours/x-ray	1	1

In the example above, the efficiency of the x-ray procedure improved without a corresponding change in department productivity, as reflected by the ratio of hours worked per x-ray. The improved efficiency led to an increase in department idle time, not an increase in productivity. Productivity would improve only if action were taken to increase units or reduce hours worked.

Understanding the distinction between efficiency and productivity is especially critical when evaluating the effect of automated laboratory equipment on productivity. For example, the hypothetical figures in the table below show an apparent increase in productivity after automating a lab test procedure. This apparent increase in productivity, however, is in fact only an increase in efficiency. Productivity will be improved—and dollar savings created—only if management acts to ensure that more lab tests are completed in the 3,333 hours, or that fewer hours than that are spent completing the same number of tests.

	Pre-automation (1981)	Post-automation (1982)	Savings
Time per test	7 min.	5 min.	2 min.
Number of tests	100,000	100,000	
Hours spent	11,666	8,333	3,333
Wage per hour	$12	$12	
Total wages	$139,992	$99,996	$39,996

Productivity = Revenue

Managers often equate productivity with revenue. There is a strong correlation between productivity and revenue, but they are not synonymous. Although revenue per FTE (full-time equivalent employee) is a traditional yardstick of performance, it does not provide a reliable measure of productivity. In the example below, revenue increased, because of an increase in charges, but productivity did not increase.

	1981	1982
a. Revenue	$900,000	$1,000,000
b. FTEs	100	100
c. Revenue per FTE (a/b)	9,000	10,000
d. Average charge per x-ray	$90	$100
e. Number of x-rays (a/d)	10,000	10,000
f. FTEs/x-ray	.01	.01

Productivity = Time and Motion Studies

One of the more common productivity myths equates the time and motion study with productivity measurement. In fact, the time and motion study is only a method of developing time standards, which identifies staff requirements.

The time and motion study is frequently advocated by those who find that the standards it establishes are statistically precise. It suffers, however, from three major deficiencies: 1) it is time-consuming, 2) the methodology it employs frequently bypasses manager involvement, and 3) it promotes over-emphasis on the importance of standards development.

Managers should question whether there are more efficient ways to develop standards than time and motion study—that is, whether the incremental increase in precision measurement it offers over other, less time-consuming methods justifies its use.

Managers should also note that numerous studies have illustrated the importance of manager involvement in standard setting. The widespread use of management by objectives (MBO) underscores the importance of such involvement. Most administrators would probably agree that standards set by outside consultants — as many standards developed through time and motion studies are — have contributed to the failure of many efforts to improve productivity. The imposition of external standards may cause managers to resent the standards and attack them as unrealistic. Standards "owned" by the manager, on the other hand, tend to lead to improved department productivity.

Finally, management should recognize that the time and motion study exaggerates the importance of standards. A standard establishes the optimum time required to complete a certain activity — again, for example, an x-ray. The problem in hospital productivity is not so much that, according to the standard, the x-ray technician should be taking an x-ray in eight minutes rather than ten minutes. Rather, the problem is that the radiology department is not doing enough of what it is supposed to do — take x-rays.

Standards development merely sets the stage for productivity improvement. It is a vital piece of the productivity concept, but by itself, it does not make productivity improve. Productivity improves only when management acts to increase units of service or reduce hours worked.

For all these reasons, the Center on Performance Enhancement (COPE), the consulting subsidiary of Health West Foundation, Chatsworth, California, recommends a negotiative approach in establishing time standards. The negotiative approach, which involves both the manager and a time and motion consultant, is significantly less time-consuming and intimidating than the time and motion study, and promotes acceptance by the manager. Under this approach, the manager and consultant work together to:

- Outline department activities. The manager and consultant analyze department activities which facilitates the development of standards specific to the department.

- Assign time values, or standards, to each of the activities. Involvement of the manager in this step ensures that the standards reflect the department's physical layout and the mix of employee skills in the department. It also ensures that productivity improvement does not compromise service or quality and strengthens the commitment to attaining the standards.

- Negotiate goals. Once the standards have been assigned, the administrator, manager, and consultant meet to discuss and agree to details regarding the standards. This meeting provides an opportunity for the administrator to show his concern and commitment to the productivity effort. Frequently, intermediate productivity improvement targets are set at this time.

Productivity = Effectiveness

"Effectiveness" refers to the accomplishment of results without serious regard for the resources consumed in the process. For example, the table below shows a hospital's attempt to increase patient days by 25 percent in 1982.

	1981	1982	% increase
Patient days	10,000	12,500	25
Hours worked	60,000	87,500	38
Hours/Patient day	6	7	17

The hospital was effective in meeting its objective, but because the number of hours worked in meeting the objective increased more than the number of patient days, productivity actually declined.

Productivity = Appropriate Utilization of Skills

Even a productive radiology department may not be using its staff appropriately. A work distribution chart, which lists department tasks and the percentage of time spent on them by each classification of employee, may disclose, for instance, that highly paid medical technologists are performing tasks better suited to a lab assistant. The chart may also be used to determine which tasks take the most time, that tasks are spread too thinly, and that the work load is spread unevenly.

Productivity = Being Busy

In conversations with managers, I sometimes hear the following: "I know my department is productive because the staff is working a lot of overtime and is always busy. Sometimes the employees work through their afternoon break." Administrators often state the corollary: "I observed an employee in the lab reading a novel, so the department must be overstaffed." Although observation of employees at work can provide valuable insight, there is no substitute for monitoring productivity, the ratio of hours worked to units of service. The unit of service selected should answer the question, "What is our department 'in business' to do?" For example, in the following table, which department is the busier, and which is the more productive?

Department	Units of service	Units per day	Hours of other activities	Idle time
Physical therapy	Hours of therapy	2	6	0
Speech therapy	Hours of therapy	4	2	2

Physical therapy, with no idle time, is the busier, but only because it is spending many hours on activities it is not in business to do. Speech therapy is more productive, because it is doing more of what it is in business to do, even though it has idle time. Although idle time does indicate a potential for improved activity, lack of idle time does not mean that there is no potential for improved productivity.

A misdirected focus on being busy results in an "activity trap," in which activities take place that may not increase a department's output.

Productivity = Staff Reduction

Unfortunately, many managers equate productivity improvement with staff reduction. In fact, however, productivity improvement may require adding to staff. Planners of a program to increase productivity should consider the evils of both overstaffing and understaffing. Although overstaffing may lead to employee boredom and under-utilization of skills, understaffing may result in employee stress and turnover.

Productivity is the Only Game in Town

Productivity does not and cannot measure the extent to which a department is satisfying the needs of the patient, medical staff, employee, or community. Nor does productivity measure quality, although there may be a strong correlation. Management must be aware of the limitations of monitoring productivity and must also monitor other, equally important indicators.

In the 1980s, the public is resisting ever-increasing health care costs, and health care financing is changing rapidly. Both these facts make it imperative for hospitals to implement management controls that will help them identify where the greatest potential for improved performance exists.

Although productivity is only one aspect of performance, it is an important one. Commitment to the concept of productivity will be highest and most beneficial when the concept is integrated with budgeting systems, goal setting, reward and recognition, and the hospital's performance appraisal system.

24

Megatrends in Hospital Information Systems

Ron Ladd, Tom Grudnowski, and Mike Dickoff

Ron Ladd is Corporate Director, Management Engineering, Western Reserve Care System, Youngstown, Ohio.

Tom Grudnowski is a Consulting Partner, Arthur Andersen & Co., Minneapolis.

Mike Dickoff is a Consulting Manager, Arthur Andersen & Co., Minneapolis.

This article describes how hospital information systems are evolving to meet the new information needs of hospital administrators. Hospital personnel responsible for planning and implementing information systems can use the ideas presented here to develop information systems which will keep their organizations competitive through the 80s and beyond.

Healthcare Industry Forces Change

Much has been written about the "revolution" in healthcare which has been spawned by Medicare's movement to a prospective payment system (PPS) for hospital payment. While Medicare's influence on the healthcare industry is great, it is important to understand that *all* aspects of a hospital's business environment have changed drastically over the past few years. A useful model for analyzing an industry is the Five Forces Model pictured in Fig. 24-1. This model depicts the "environment" of an industry as the ongoing interaction among existing competitors, buyers, suppliers, substitutes and new entrants. Fig. 24-1 illustrates the characteristics of the healthcare industry of five years ago, while Fig. 24-2 illustrates current industry characteristics. Recently, all of the "five forces" impacting a hospital's environment have changed significantly.

Reprinted with permission from *HIMSS Journal*, Healthcare Computing & Communications Magazine, 4(2) February 1987, pp. 37-41. Copyright 1987 by Health Data Analysis, Inc. All rights reserved.

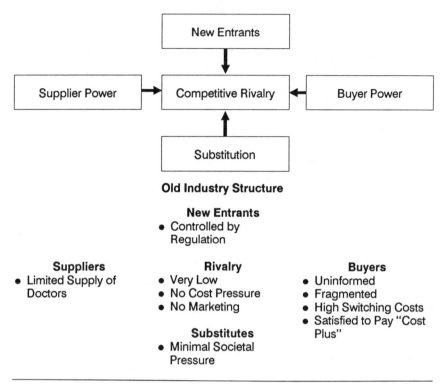

Figure 24-1. The Five Forces Model: Old Industry Structure.

Impact on Information Systems

The healthcare industry changes reviewed in this article appear to be permanent and irreversible. The result of these changes is an increased competition for patients and profits. Hospital chief executive officers are increasingly turning to their hospital's information systems to support decisions regarding strategic hospital direction, and to improve the cost-effectiveness of their operations. They are finding that traditional hospital information systems are inadequate for supporting these needs. In order to more effectively support chief executive officers and other executives in formulating and meeting long-term strategic objectives and operating goals, hospital information systems are undergoing a metamorphosis from:

- Charge based

- Department based

- Recordkeeping functions

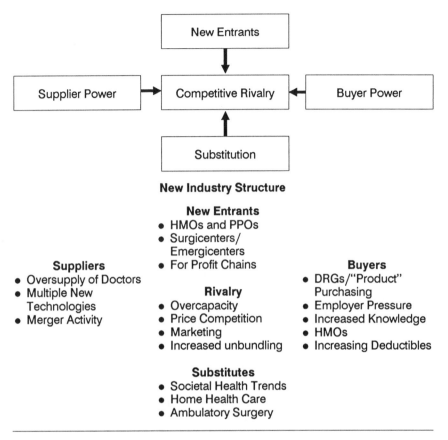

Figure 24-2. The Five Forces Model: New Industry Structure.

- Hospital inpatient
- Transaction systems
- Stand-alone
- Turnkey

to:

- Cost based
- Product based
- Productivity functions

- Multi-provider, multi-patient type
- Strategic systems
- Integrated
- Customized

These seven "megatrends" in hospital information systems are described in the remainder of this article. For each megatrend we have outlined:

- The business need(s) driving the trend.
- Strategies for implementing hospital information systems required by these trends.

We should note that, in developing this list of megatrends, we have deliberately omitted "technical" trends relating to computer hardware and software (e.g., shared systems to in-house systems). The "delivery system" used to effectively implement the trends described in this article could vary significantly depending on hospital size, organizational structure, new technological innovations, and other variables. The trends outlined in this article are independent of these variables and must be considered by all hospital information systems decision makers.

Charge-Based Systems to Cost-Based Systems

Although systems must continue to record and monitor the hospital "charges" (i.e., gross revenues) associated with patient services, it has become much more important to be able to monitor the costs of specific services rendered to hospital patients. Increasingly, hospital survival is based on the number and type of patients or other cost-related outputs, rather than on hospital charges. In order to analyze profitability of patient groups and to negotiate new contracts with its buyers, hospitals must have better cost information.

Strategies

1. Develop "foundation" systems which concentrate on costs rather than revenue as the basic information required to perform services. Comprehensive cost accounting/cost management systems illustrate this strategy.

2. Establish a firm commitment to the accurate generation of information for decision-making, i.e., the engineered standards approach as contrasted with the "ratio of costs to charges" method.

3. Communicate to all levels of management that cost management requires a re-orientation and structuring of practice for measuring performance. Prospective payment requires a new style of management.

Department-Based Systems to Product-Based Systems

Financial reporting profitability analysis, which in the past has been presented by department, now focuses on "product lines" (i.e., groupings of treated patients such as DRGs). The trend toward product line analysis was generated primarily by the introduction of Medicare's PPS reimbursement system. However, product line information can be extremely helpful in analyzing the competitive position of the services the hospital offers to buyers and physicians.

This trend solidifies the transition toward cost-based systems, in that the product line profitability analysis described above requires product line cost information.

Other uses of product line information include the analysis of physician treatment profiles (used by physicians to study variations in utilization of services across clinical services or by specific physicians), and in carrying out planning and marketing (i.e., "product management") activities.

There are many examples of hospitals which generate and use product line reporting for reimbursement analysis. This "case mix" reporting has become a standard feature of most hospitals' periodic reporting procedures. It is more unusual, however, to find hospitals which are actually using product line reporting for detailed physician utilization analysis and/or for sophisticated planning and marketing analysis. The trend toward this type of analysis is moving slowly, partly because systems which support this type of analysis are not in place. More importantly, there is an extreme shortage of hospital personnel trained to do this work. Over the next several years, the role of the hospital "product manager" (i.e., an administrative person responsible for all aspects of a group related hospital service such as open heart surgery) will evolve and drastically increase the demand for product line information.

Strategies

1. Identify levels of management and operational variables which are: (1) department-based; and (2) product-based. Develop reports taking these characteristics of information into account.

2. Establish levels of management accountability consistent with levels of reporting required.

3. Develop and incorporate product-line information into institutional planning to achieve objectives.

4. Provide systems support for "product-line managers" who coordinate information related to the provision of major hospital products.

Recordkeeping Functions to Productivity Systems

While information systems have primarily been used in the past to record financial and clinical information, systems are increasingly being used to increase the productivity and effectiveness of hospital personnel. Given the cost reduction pressures placed on all hospitals, the implementation of systems which can be justified through tangible savings or which can improve the quality of patient care at existing staffing levels are often favored over the implementation of systems offering primarily intangible benefits.

Systems designed to enhance productivity can do so in one of two ways:

- Productivity improvement—some systems actually improve the productivity of large numbers of hospital personnel by automating functions which had previously been manual, providing much more timely access to information, reducing communications time between two points, reducing error rates and consequently error correction time, and/or eliminating redundant tasks. Patient care systems such as order communications/results reporting tend to provide these types of benefits.

- Productivity monitoring—some systems effect productivity improvements by providing hospital managers with enough timely and detailed information to effectively manage departmental productivity and to adjust staffing to meet demand. Productivity reporting which is based on productivity standards can offer these benefits.

Strategies

1. Document and implement cost/benefits criteria for justifying information systems.

2. Develop and implement productivity monitoring systems by department, in order to properly update and maintain product-line labor costs.

3. Utilize productivity information by department as a major method to support the management style required by the prospective payment system.

Hospital In-Patient Systems to Multi-Provider, Multi-Patient Type Systems

With many hospitals expanding outpatient services, offering new services such as home healthcare, merging with a physician group and/or becoming part of a chain, systems must increasingly be able to support much more than pure hospital inpatient situations. Often, the requirements of the non-in-patient processing are significantly different than those for in-patient processing. Systems support for new ventures is often required on very short notice, as hospitals react quickly to opportunities for providing innovative or competitive services in the marketplace.

Beyond the absolute business need of being able to bill and collect for all services rendered by the hospital, other benefits of being able to combine in-patient, out-patient, physician and other services in the same system include:

- Business office productivity tends to increase when personnel are only required to work with a single system for all types of accounts.

- Systems which combine hospital and physician charge information will be extremely valuable in the future for developing "joint bids" for contractual opportunities (i.e., hospital and physician costs) of services purchased for their employees or subscribers.

Strategies

1. Define and implement information systems requirements relative to market share objectives by type of service provided, data elements required by service provided, and information delivery systems available to fulfill multi-patient needs.

2. Establish common resource networks for hardware and software utilization to comply with multi-provider, multi-patient-type needs.

Transaction Systems to Strategic Systems

Traditional hospital information systems primarily serve as "transaction processors." Hospital functions served as a repository of detailed transactions such as patient charges vendor invoices, purchase orders, payroll checks and related activities. These systems automate many of the clerical tasks within the hospital, and provide some level of management reporting regarding transaction volumes and patient services. However, they provide hospital executive management with little useful information for strategic and tactical decision making relating to functions such as:

- Pricing

- Addition/deletion of services

- Physician relations

- Marketing analysis

- Departmental productivity

Transaction system data tends not to be organized in a manner which easily supports these functions. The data coming from transaction systems must be summarized, analyzed and generally revised before it can be made useful for anything other than a cursory management analysis.

The term "decision support system" is often used to describe a system which will support an executive's strategic planning needs. Unfortunately, the decision support system term has been so abused that it has many diverse connotations. We do not believe that the concept of an infinitely flexible decision support system which will answer any "what if " question which a hospital CEO can imagine can realistically be developed in the foreseeable future.

We do, however, project a definite trend toward the development of specific strategic support systems which support these functions. These systems are difficult to develop because they require a very specific understanding of goals between hospital executives and hospital information systems personnel. Executives must outline the types of "questions" they would like the system to answer, and information systems personnel must understand the reasoning behind these questions. The tasks for each group are difficult at best, in that hospital executives are faced with the need to do analyses regarding pricing and product profitability which are much different than they have been required to do in the past. At the same time, information systems personnel are often very unfamiliar with the "business environment" in which the hospital operates.

We believe that the successful strategic support systems of the future will exhibit the following characteristics:

- Transaction data will be drawn directly into strategic support systems and used as the basis for strategic reporting. This will ensure a consistent basis of data for all reporting within the hospital, thus minimizing confusion and ensuring that strategic decisions are based on accurate, "actual" information.

- External data will be compared to internal data where appropriate. Strategic and tactical analysis often requires the comparison of internal hospital results with those of local competitors or of similar hospitals from other markets.

- Data will be presented to executives in an exception-oriented, easy to digest manner. Lengthy reports will be the exception, not the rule. Rather, strategic support systems will allow executives to extract, from large databases of data, only the small subset of data relevant to the analysis currently being done.

Strategies

1. Develop and implement a strategic business systems plan with structured direction for information systems development.

2. Establish and monitor return-on-investment ratios for information systems projects as related to institutional performance objectives.

Stand-Alone Systems to Integrated Systems

Stand-alone systems for different areas of the hospital are rapidly being replaced by integrated systems which share a common source of data. These systems reduce confusion over conflicting information generated by systems which do not communicate with each other.

True integration across all applications is difficult to achieve because no software vendor offers a complete set of hospital application systems which share a common database and provide adequate functionality and systems performance. Clearly, this is not a trivial task, as several major software vendors have attempted for several years, without success, to build such an integrated set of applications.

Hospitals striving for integration are dealing with this void in the marketplace by purchasing large "blocks" of application systems from individual vendors and then building interfaces and "bridges" from one block of applications to another. Another alternative which is becoming more popular is the creation of an "integrated database of information which can be used for generating administrative reporting. These databases are often created by extracting data from multiple "nonintegrated" systems and loading these data into a flexible database management system format. Using this approach, data can be extracted and reported in many different ways.

Strategies

1. Develop management criteria for identifying "stand-alone versus integrated" information systems applications.

2. Establish management approved information systems architecture for developing applications.

3. Define and implement communications criteria for software/ hardware interfaces.

4. Document current and long-term information systems integration objectives for strategic planning and systems development direction.

Turnkey Systems to Customized Systems

Turnkey systems which "pre-define" all processing functions are being replaced by customized systems which can be modified to suit the individual needs of a hospital. These systems provide a degree of flexibility that allows hospital management to analyze data in relatively unstructured ways rather than being bound by a fixed set of reports generated on a periodic basis.

These customized systems are needed not only by large, complex hospital organizations, but also by small community hospitals faced with increasingly complex contractual arrangements and competitive pressures.

While the use of software packages by hospitals will continue to be prevalent, hospital information systems directors are increasingly being faced with the need to hire and retain personnel qualified to modify software packages to meet unique needs. Project management and systems analysis skills are becoming increasingly important as systems, hence systems implementation projects, become larger and more complex. The management of system "integration" requires personnel who understand not only the technical aspects of systems, but also the business functions which the systems support.

The human resources problem in the information systems area is similar to that experienced in the marketing, planning, cost accounting and product management functions within hospitals. These functions are either new to hospitals and/or have increased dramatically in importance during the recent past. Therefore, people possessing these skills are in very high demand, with special strategies required to recruit, develop and/or retain these personnel.

Strategies

1. Establish and maintain applications "Steering Committees" directed by managers who will use information systems in order to define all functional requirements.

2. Document criteria for evaluating functions of external software to assess integration potential with internal hospital information systems.

3. Define and implement "functional knowledge" criteria for internal information systems personnel.

Summary

The "megatrends" identified for hospital information systems in this article require an innovative shift in hospital management perspective. Hospital chief executive officers and decision-makers must adopt a new model for planning and utilizing hospital information systems resources. Because of changes in the healthcare environment, prospective payment strategies for using information are very different from former retrospective reimbursement methods.

The purpose of this article has been to identify emerging "megatrends" for structuring future hospital information systems. The primary cause of these significantly different demands is the prospective payment system.

Medicare DRGs will probably expand into an all-encompassing payment plan which will alter the essence of hospital information systems. This article has reviewed the challenges of these "megatrends," and provided some preliminary management strategies for addressing these new demands on healthcare professionals.

25

Managing Hospital Biomedical Equipment

Michael J. Shaffer

Michael J. Shaffer, Sc.D., is Professor of Anesthesiology, and Director of the Bioelectronics Laboratory, The George Washington University Medical Center, Washington, DC.

Hospital chief executives are responsible for complex organizations that integrate biomedical equipment into medical services delivery. Concomitantly, the hospital is buffeted by external forces such as high cost of technology and malpractice risk exposure. As diagnostic and therapeutic advances continue at breathtaking speeds, hospital managers must be aware of the impact of biomedical equipment and become more competent in controlling it.

Biomedical equipment is the complex equipment with a patient connection that is used for diagnosis, therapy, and monitoring. As Table 25-1 shows, it also may include housekeeping equipment such as testing, data processing, and recordkeeping devices that may not have a direct patient connection but are complicated enough to warrant special consideration.

Before the 1970s biomedical equipment was relatively simple and could be bought, used, and maintained with minor on-the-job training. Between 1970 and 1975, largely because of the introduction of integrated circuits, sales of patient monitoring equipment tripled,[1] its complexity increased, and patient safety became a matter of concern. The medical device industry of the 1970s grew from $3 billion to $12 billion in total shipments in 1980.[2] Simultaneously, product liability litigation and awards increased. In 1976, the Food, Drug and Cosmetic Act was amended to establish the Food and Drug Administration's Bureau of Medical Devices to regulate medical device manufacturers.[3] Also during this period many new professional and institutional standards were generated by groups such as the Joint Commission on Accreditation of Healthcare Organizations (JCAHO), the National Fire Protection Association (NFPA), and the Association for the Advancement of Medical Instrumentation (AAMI) to govern hospitals' arrangement and use of equipment.

Table 25-1. Types of Biomedical Equipment.

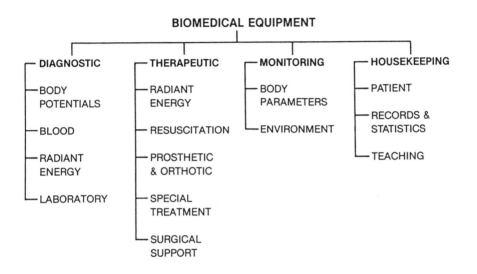

Hospitals reacted by establishing three levels of effort for handling biomedical equipment.[4]

Level 1: Corrective maintenance to repair broken equipment

Level 2: Preventive maintenance to ensure reliability

Level 3: Management to assure cost effectiveness

Corrective Maintenance

The corrective maintenance technique adopted for each piece of equipment is based on the information provided by manufacturers and on the skills of the staff. One of four modes applies:

1. Manufacturers provide adequate information and diagnostic facilities for hospital staff to identify and repair circuit board failures.

2. Manufacturers' documentation and diagnostic facilities are limited; in this case:

   a. failed circuit boards are identified by substitution and returned for repair or exchange;

    b. the hospital employs sophisticated test equipment such as a logic analyzer to identify the failure; or

    c. hospitals rely on manufacturers or maintenance contractors for support.

For the hospital the first option is the most cost effective; option 2 (a) requires the availability of a substantial number of replacement circuit boards; option 2 (b) demands higher skills of staff and, perhaps, additional training; option 2 (c) can be expensive. Costs of annual maintenance contracts are often as much as 30 percent of capital equipment cost.[5]

Preventive Maintenance

Preventive maintenance must be done under a formal protocol to ensure equipment operability. The JCAHO requires that it be done at least semiannually. This frequency may be decreased after actual failure rates are taken into account, and if the safety committee agrees.[6]

Preventive maintenance protocols developed by manufacturers are likely to include excessively complex and time-consuming tests as protection against product liability. In this event, maintenance staff who have multiple priorities and economic restrictions may find they are unable to allocate the resources necessary to comply with these procedures.[7] Hospitals may tend toward substituting simplified protocols that enable them to meet the only standard actively imposed on them: that of passing JCAHO surveys and/or state inspections. Hospitals' attitude is typified by such claims as, "Our maintenance program is fine; it got us through our survey without a contingency."[8]

Of late, preventive maintenance has been further complicated by the proliferation of microprocessors in the equipment and the flexibility they afford. A switch may no longer have a single function but rather multiple functions that are selected by software programs. For example, from 1970 to 1985, the number of controls and displays on the typical anesthesia machine grew by a factor of five, and alarm indications by a factor of 20.[9]

Management

Effective equipment management is essential to avoid equipment abuse and ensure proper operation and maintenance. This management has five objectives:

1. Select good equipment

2. Comply with standards

3. Assure proper use

4. Monitor performance

5. Support improvements.

These five objectives are examined in depth below.

Select Good Equipment

As applied to new equipment, this objective demands that the shortcomings of old equipment be known, hospital needs and constraints defined, and new equipment selected to meet those needs and constraints.

Shortcomings of old equipment can be indicated by the presence of idle equipment, excessive repair costs, incidence reports and malpractice actions, and queues waiting to use the equipment. These shortcomings may result from equipment limitations such as excessive gadgetry and early obsolescence; however, they may also be caused by personal dislikes, inadequate inventory or status control, or inadequate maintenance or instruction.

Selection of equipment should be based on logical analysis, not emotion. Features such as portability, maintainability, operability, reliability, adaptability, and safety and suitability for the environment, as listed in Table 25-2, should be considered. The effects of equipment on facility services such as furniture, water, space, cooling, heating, lighting, power, and drainage have to be considered in calculating implementation and operating costs. A balance sheet showing the equipment's costs versus its benefits is a useful management technique. On one side are the capital amortization and operating costs; on the other are income generated and intangible features such as quality, frequency of use, potential for risk, and potential for better procedures, accuracy, communications, availability, and skills mix.

The selection process should include seeking the opinions of others. Manufacturer demonstrations of the most suitable equipment should be arranged at the hospital or by site visits to determine the opinions of technical and clinical users. The FDA's Center for Devices and Radiological Health has a voluntary reporting system for hospital-detected anomalies, and a mandatory reporting system for manufacturer-detected anomalies. The center processes 2,400 voluntary and 14,000 mandatory reports annually, which are available to the public. The Emergency Care Research Institute, a private organization, publishes a consumer guide called *Health Devices,* hazard bulletins, and results of literature searches. These reports are available to subscribers.

Comply With Standards

Failure to demonstrate compliance with regulations and professional standards places in question a hospital's concern for patient care. The hospital must be aware of others' mistakes and of the standard of care created by product liability case law.

Table 25-2. Important Features and Considerations in Choosing Biomedical Equipment.

FEATURES	CONSIDERATIONS	
PORTABILITY	STRENGTH WEIGHT	SIZE
MAINTAINABILITY	IN-PLACE/BENCH DOCUMENTATION	MEAN TIME TO REPAIR SPARES
OPERABILITY	DATA INPUT ACCURACY	CONTROLS DISPLAYS
RELIABILITY	CALCULATED	MEAN TIME BETWEEN FAILURES
ADAPTABILITY	STANDARDS MODULARITY	LEVELS CODES
SAFETY	LEAKAGE EXPLOSION	GROUNDING TOXICITY
ENVIRONMENT	VIBRATION CORROSION INTERFERENCE	NOISE STORAGE CLEANLINESS

The FDA categorizes biomedical devices into two classes. In class 1 are those devices for which general controls are adequate to ensure safety and effectiveness. More hazardous devices are placed in class 2, for which general controls and performance specifications are required. Performance specifications include maintenance procedures that may have to be adopted by the hospital. Also, hospital licensure authorities will demand that biomedical equipment be type-approved by an acceptable standards testing laboratory, and they will specify acceptable laboratories. Those usually acceptable include Underwriters Laboratories, ITT Research Institute, the Canadian Standards Association, Underwriters Laboratory of Canada, and the City of Los Angeles Electrical Testing Laboratory.[10] Manufacturers will get their type approvals from one of these laboratories. Equipment untested by acceptable laboratories may require additional evaluation to convince the licensure authority of its safety and efficacy.

From the hospital construction and equipment aspect, the NFPA has issued its standard NFPA-99 for health care facilities. This document includes relevant standards, recommended practices, and manuals developed by the association.[11] These are professional consensus standards, which as such are not mandatory, but some parts of which are adopted as mandatory by hospital licensure and accreditation authorities. AAMI also develops standards for biomedical devices based on a consensus of its clinician, engineer, and manufacturer membership.

From the hospital operations aspect, the JCAHO *Accreditation Manual for Hospitals* includes management of biomedical equipment in its section on "Plant, Technology, and Safety Management." This chapter covers the need for an inventory, for testing at less than 6-month intervals unless exempted, for test records, and for a corrective maintenance procedure, user/operator instructions, and operator training.[6] Regular supervision is required to ensure that these guidelines and standards and any changes are followed.

Ensure Proper Use

In ensuring proper use it is important that purchased equipment be inspected on delivery to see that it meets the manufacturer's specifications and does the job for which it was ordered. Studies show that, in some cases, 40 percent of some high technology equipment failed to meet manufacturer specifications when delivered.[12] When needed, acceptance demonstrations should be demanded of the manufacturer.

Much biomedical equipment is part of a system. Fig. 25-1 shows that equipment hardware may be controlled by software programs, which, in turn, may follow the direction of mathematical algorithms. These programs and algorithms are essential to the hardware's performance, yet may be treated as proprietary information by the manufacturer. The hardware may have to rely on adequate facilities and operating and maintenance staffs, who may need equipment-specific organization, procedures, and training. Finally, both hardware and staff may have to be configured to function under contingency conditions in which some form of partial operation is continued.

Implementation of the system should be in accordance with good documentation and practices, including:

- Facility and equipment interface specifications
- Layout diagrams
- Contractor specifications and liaison
- On-site installation and checkout support
- As-built drawings
- Operating and maintenance manuals

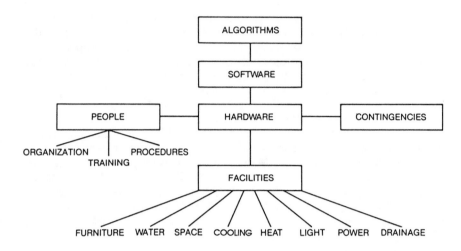

Figure 25-1. Internal and External Interfaces of Biomedical Equipment.

- Acceptance test specifications and demonstrations
- In-service training
- Recommended spare parts lists
- Warranty, loaner, and corrective maintenance support agreements.

The JCAHO lists many of the regulations, policies, and procedures that should be produced by hospital departments. These range from testing of anesthesia equipment before to special care unit actions in the event essential equipment breaks down.[6] It also requires:

1. Identification, development, implementation, and review of departmental safety policies
2. A hazard surveillance program
3. An incident reporting system including a recall system
4. Provision of safety-related information for operation and in-service education
5. Safety program monitoring
6. A reference library of patient safety documents.

As mentioned previously, instruction manuals have grown in size and complexity, and because of frequent software changes they quickly become obsolete. Consequently, manufacturers tend to limit the number of copies of manuals they supply to one or two per machine, regardless of the number of users. Because they do not have manuals readily available or time to study the mass of information, users tend to rely on repetitive practical experience. Accordingly, greater emphasis is being placed on equipment-oriented seminars and mandatory in-service education. It should be recognized that, in general, physicians support the use of equipment, nurses are reluctant, and administrators must be satisfied it will be worthwhile.

Monitor Performance

The performance of biomedical equipment should be constantly monitored to ensure proper performance. Part of operator training is learning to observe and detect unacceptable results.

Training should be performed with legal obligations in mind. In the event of equipment failure, the hospital may be liable if the defect was patent, or it the hospital was negligent in selecting a repairperson. If the equipment was operational, the hospital may be liable if the patient sustained injury from application of the device or through misplaced reliance on it. The hospital may also be liable if it failed to:

- Employ equipment routinely used elsewhere

- Keep abreast of technological advances

- Keep equipment standards up to date

- Advise patients when proper equipment is unavailable

- Apprise the patient of where such equipment is available, or

- Inspect and test the equipment for defects before use.

Frequent technical inspections should be performed to obtain operator comments and observe performance firsthand. Manufacturers should be encouraged to provide adequate simulation and test mean values in their systems to confirm proper operation with minimum perturbation.

In the early 1970s emphasis was placed on procedures to protect personnel from electrical shock. This was later broadened by a need for risk management whereby corrective action was assessed according to propensity for patient harm. The current emphasis is on cost-effectiveness, which reflects monetarily on the results of risk management, among other things. Accordingly, widespread use is made of microcomputers at the departmental level to measure performance of hospital services, schedule staff and patients, process medical data, and provide statistical records. Departmental use of microcomputers has the advantage of allowing easier and faster modification to meet special requirements than can be furnished by a central management information system.

Support Improvements

During system implementation and performance evaluations it may be necessary to make equipment modifications or use special units, adaptors, and cables to integrate the system or improve its operation. Improvements may be made to hardware or software. It is important that the changes be properly checked out, documented, and approved for quality. Procedures, drawings, manuals, and warranties may require amendment, and in-service education may be required to communicate them.

With respect to hospital-fabricated devices, the FDA recognizes two categories: [3]

    a. Devices custom-built for a physician or a patient

    b. Devices covered by an investigational device exemption.

The latter are controlled by the hospital's institutional review board alone or in conjunction with the FDA, depending on whether they constitute a nonsignificant or a significant risk, respectively. Although it is not clearly stated by FDA, hospital-originated devices should receive the same treatment as described above for improvements, if they are to be used by staff or on patients.

Implementation

Biomedical engineering has three subspecialties:

1. Bioengineering for research medical devices

2. Medical engineering to develop and design devices for industry

3. Clinical engineering to maintain and manage devices in hospitals.[13]

To implement the five management objectives, larger hospitals will establish a clinical engineering department comprising several clinical engineers for the management function and one or more biomedical equipment technicians for maintenance. The engineers support the technicians as needed.

Since the biomedical equipment used in hospitals embraces many engineering specialties, including mechanical, electrical, electronic, control, computer, and environmental engineering, it is appropriate that the clinical engineering staff be broad based. Preferably, the engineers will have engineering degrees and be licensed professionals and/or board certified by the International Certification for Clinical Engineering and Biomedical Technology. Currently, only about 400 clinical engineers are certified in the United States.

As to effectiveness, it must be recognized that many physicians, nurses, and hospital managers perceive an engineer to be someone who maintains the heating, lighting, and general hospital facilities, not someone from whom they should regularly seek advice.[14] The problem can be reduced by adjusting the position of the clinical engineering department in the organizational hierarchy and the distance across which it communicates. A clinical engineering department that reports directly to hospital administration may be too far away organizationally from users to develop close mutual ties with them and thus influence their knowledge of the equipment.[4] Administrative departments tend to arrange core service units in vertical reporting structures with relatively few crosslinks in the communication flow. Thus, a clinical engineering staff that identifies with and reports to one of the medical departments or to the medical director, rather than to an administrative department, not only occupies a higher niche in the hospital's hierarchy but benefits from an improved communication structure. The medical department selected should be one headed by a physician willing to represent and encourage the effectiveness of the clinical engineering service. Otherwise, experience has shown that engineers will be exposed to interdepartmental pressures and politics they cannot control.[15] Clearly, there is no single preferred organization for all situations; the personalities of the participants are still a predominating factor.

To manage the increasing amount and complexity of biomedical equipment used in critical care areas, some hospitals have encouraged standardizing and pooling equipment for common use. In the organizational structure in Fig. 25-2, critical care technicians have been added as a separate entity reporting to a medical department to store, set up, calibrate, and manage pooled equipment. These technicians should be trained to assume initial responsibility for identifying, perhaps by substitution, equipment needing repair. By virtue of their supportive operational relationship with medical departments, they will be able to identify educational needs and coordinate engineering in-service training. By doing so, the critical care technicians act as a valuable integrating medium for the clinical engineering department and its diverse clients.[16] Fig. 25-3 depicts a typical hospital hierarchy involved in equipment operations. It shows plant operations and central supply as departments that manage, inspect, and repair the facility and centrally controlled equipment. Critical care technicians and clinical engineers report through the medical structure. Critical care technicians set up and check out their equipment; clinical engineers manage, inspect, and repair it and the medical department's biomedical equipment.

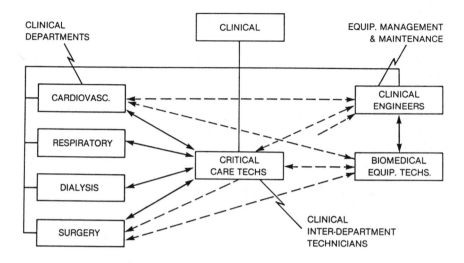

Figure 25-2. Engineer-Technician-User Interactions.

The Future of Biomedical Equipment Management

The United States hospital system is undergoing a reorientation that may also affect the acquisition of new technology. Multihospital chains manage over 30 percent of American hospitals, and investor-owned systems operate 1,000 acute care hospitals in addition to home care services, long-term care facilities, and health spas. Moreover, not-for-profit hospitals are establishing for-profit subsidiaries; individual entrepreneurs are developing freestanding surgical and emergency centers, "doc-in-a-box" offices, and a variety of clinics. These changes may require that clinical engineers provide shared services on a multihospital basis, either as a systemwide centralized service, or independently for the fragmented configuration. It is expected that centralization will create other management burdens, and fragmentation may cause smaller facilities to be undersupported for economic or geographic reasons. Either way, care must be taken to ensure that changes do not affect the standard of care.

Diagnosis-related groups (DRGs) are being used to reduce hospital costs, and reimbursement for care provided by Medicare is based on the diagnosis, not the amount of treatment given. Other third-party payors are expected to adopt similar approaches. Hospitals in which costs exceed DRG reimbursement will have to restrict services to those they can perform most cost effectively and/or reduce their equipment acquisitions or overhead ser-

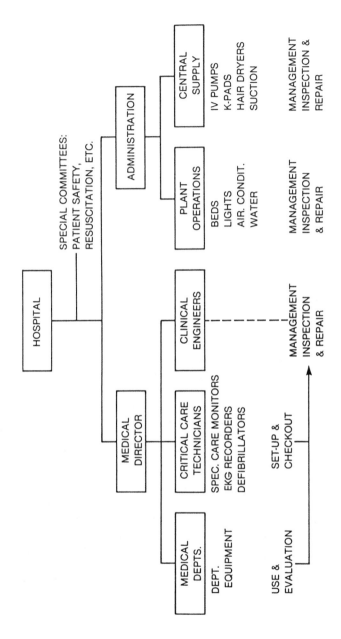

Figure 25-3. Organization of Biomedical Equipment.

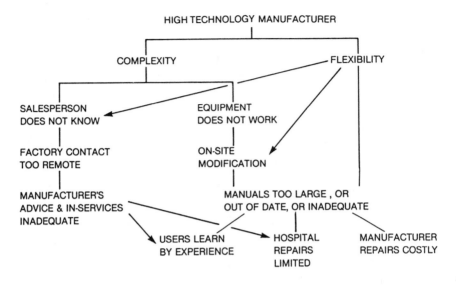

Figure 25-4. Complications of High Technology Patient-Supporting Equipment.

vices. Additional data processing services probably will be required to monitor performance statistics and to reassign priorities.

New high technology equipment controlled by microprocessors typically falls into one of two categories: The first enables medical departments to better support patients; the second enables them to better manage their affairs with more appropriate recordkeeping, billing, and statistics. The first category, although ideal in purpose, is a mixed blessing and can cause the hospital to lose control of its equipment. As shown in Fig. 25-4, high technology equipment is complex and flexible. Salespersons may no longer understand its details and may attempt to have the hospital deal directly with the manufacturer's engineers early in the transaction. When this happens, benevolent local representation is lost, and channels become too long for effective communication. Complexity causes the operator's and service manuals to become too large for ready consumption. Flexibility enables equipment changes to be made more easily—so much so that the manuals cannot be kept up-to-date. Both factors lead to increased reliance on expensive manufacturer maintenance.

Accordingly, it is anticipated that in the next decade clinical engineering will be involved more deeply in three areas:

1. Technology assessment to expand the equipment selection function by assessing such factors as:

a. whether new equipment is an extension of an existing service or a new service requiring new staff resources

b. capability for optimum level of quality, affordability, financial and liability risks, joint venture, or freestanding environment

c. life expectancy.[17]

2. Training with respect to human-machine relationships, developing the clinical engineers' receptivity to communicate on equipment matters, and enhanced use of interactive training aids.

3. Computer applications in performance evaluation by means of on-line recordkeeping and data base management.

It has been said that biomedical equipment takes some of the guesswork out of patient care decisions. It betters patient care when it is properly selected and maintained and when it is used by people who understand it and know what to do if the expected does not happen. Absent any of these components, the patient's well-being may be in jeopardy.[18]

Notes

1. Stetler, C.J. "The Medical Device Amendments of 1976—Prediction for the Future." *Medical Instrumentation* 11(190) May-June 1977.
2. Schoellhorn, R.A. "Industry's Achievements and the Task Ahead." *Medical Device & Diagnostic Industry* 4(3) March 1982.
3. Food, Drug and Cosmetic Act (Public Law 94-295), as amended, 1976.
4. Shaffer, M.J. "Integration of Clinical Engineering into the Hospital Organization." *Hospital & Health Services Administration* 28(5) 72-81, September-October 1983.
5. Shaffer, M.J. "Medical Equipment Maintenance." *Clinical Engineering News* March 1974.
6. Joint Commission on Accreditation of Healthcare Organizations. "Plant, Technology, and Safety Management." In *Accreditation Manual for Hospitals,* 1988.
7. Ben-Zvi, S. "An Urgent Plea for Realistic Preventive Maintenance Procedures." *Medical Instrumentation* 16:2, 115-116, 1982.

8. American Society for Hospital Engineering. *Medical Equipment Management in Hospitals.* 2nd ed. Chicago: American Society for Hospital Engineering, 1982.
9. Schreiber, P. *Safety Guidelines for Anesthesia Machines.* North American Drager, B86-001 MP10M, 1984.
10. Shaffer, M.J. and Gordon, M.R. "Clinical Engineering Standards, Obligations, and Accountability." *Medical Instrumentation* 13:4, 209-215, 1979.
11. National Fire Protection Association. Standard for Health Care Facilities, NFPA 99-1984.
12. Ben-Zvi, S. "The Selection and Evaluation of Medical Instrumentation." *Medical Instrumentation* 5:428, January-February 1971.
13. Institute of Electrical and Electronics Engineers. "Medical Engineering Program Expectations." *IEEE Engineering in Medical & Biology Group Newsletter* 61:7-10, 1977.
14. MyIrea, K.S. and Silvertson, S.E. "Biomedical Engineering in Health Care—Potential Versus Reality." *IEEE Transactions* BME-22, 116, 1975.

15. Ben-Zvi, S. and Gottlieb, W. "The Hospital Instrumentation Department: Delivering Clinical Engineering Services to the Hospital Community." *Journal of Clinical Engineering News* 4:5, 1, 1976.

16. Shaffer, M.J., Kuhn, J., and Coakley, C.S. "Clinical Engineering Education in the High Technology Hospital." *Medical Instrumentation* 18:5, 280-282, 1984.

17. Millenson, L.J. and Slizewski, E. "How Do Hospital Executives Spell Technology Assessment? Planning." *Health Maintenance Quarterly*, First Quarter, 4-8, 1986.

18. Hargest, T.S. "A Clinical Engineer's Viewpoint of Medical Instrumentation." *Medical Instrumentation* 14:4, 215-217, July-August 1980.

Quality Assurance
and Risk Management

Selection 26, "The Epidemiology of Quality" by Avedis Donabedian, looks at two groups: providers and clients. In his literature review, the author finds relationships between quality of care and provider attributes: in the case of physicians, their training, experience, specialization, age, and hospital affiliation. He finds little consistent correlation between quality and client attributes such as age, sex, or occupation, but he notes indications of a relationship for the socioeconomically disadvantaged. In selection 27, "Relating Quality Assurance to Credentials and Privileges," Benjamin Gilbert emphasizes that the hospital's governing body is responsible for assuring medical staff competency. This includes scrutiny of physicians at initial application as well as continued review of privileges. Court cases are presented along with a checklist for review of medical staff privileges.

In selection 28, "An Integrated Approach to Liability," Edie Siler urges the integration of quality assurance, infection control, and risk management activities in hospitals. Incentives for and benefits from this integration are discussed. Risk management is examined more closely in Selection 29, "Developing Patient Risk Profiles," written by Walter J. Jones, Buddy Nichols, and Astrid Smith. The authors present a patient risk profit, including age and diagnostic status, that can assist managers to monitor high-risk situations more closely. Other steps for reducing risk are also presented. Finally, Paul L. Grimaldi and Julie A. Micheletti discuss in selection 30, "PRO Objectives and Quality Criteria," the importance of establishing PRO admission, procedure, and quality objectives. They stress the importance of cooperation and involvement of physicians and hospital personnel.

26

The Epidemiology of Quality

Avedis Donabedian

Avedis Donabedian, M.D., M.P.H., is Nathan Sinai Distinguished Professor of Public Health, Department of Medical Care Organization, School of Public Health, University of Michigan, Ann Arbor.

The epidemiology of quality is the study of the distribution of quality at any given time and of changes in its distribution through time. Time, place, and person, the traditional triad of descriptive epidemiology, apply to the study of the quality of medical care as well. But the epidemiology of quality seems to be distinctive in having, simultaneously, two sets of populations to which it pertains: one of providers and another of clients. This duality, if nothing else, should invest the epidemiology of quality with a peculiar appeal.

Knowledge of the distribution of quality among the providers of health care services (whether these providers are individual practitioners, teams, organizational units, or entire institutions) is the product of the more usual studies of quality that throw light on the relation between structure, on the one hand, and either process or outcome on the other.[1] Often, the more immediate purpose of these studies is to demonstrate that certain attributes of providers can be used to indicate a greater or lesser likelihood that good quality will be delivered. In this way, structural attributes become indirect measures of the quality of care as well as indicators of where the quality of care is likely to be deficient and, therefore, worthy of more assiduous supervision. But more fundamentally, elucidation of the relation between structure and performance is central to the science of health care organization, insofar as such a science can be said to exist. We must understand the determinants of performance, for example, if we are to design a more effective system of health care.

The distribution of specified levels of quality among various groupings of the consumers of care is, of course, the ultimate measure of success or failure in achieving the social objectives of a health care system. It is necessary, therefore, to know who receives better care and who worse, and what the reasons for the inequality are.

We see that the epidemiology of quality has functions analogous to those of the more familiar epidemiology of health states: It is both a method of scientific inquiry and a tool for action. To the extent that health states are used in studies of quality as a measure of outcome, the two epidemiologies do, in fact, overlap, except that in order to serve the epidemiology of quality, observed disparities in health states must be attributable to corresponding differences in antecedent care.

It is not the purpose of this paper to deal with the epidemiology of quality as a method of scientific inquiry. The paper will merely offer a review of what we know about the relation between attributes of providers and clients and the quality of care that they, respectively, provide and receive. The reader can look elsewhere for a general discussion of the definition and measurement of quality[2] and for a detailed assessment of the methods used in the studies from which most of the information in this paper is culled.[3]

Even as a vehicle for the empirical findings, this paper, though reasonably detailed, is incomplete. First, studies that do not offer, or lead to, reasonably direct judgments on the quantitative or qualitative adequacy of care have been omitted. The vast literature on patterns of differential utilization was, therefore, excluded. Quality was then defined quite narrowly so that attention focused on the technical care provided mainly by physicians. The consequent omission of client satisfaction is a particularly limiting exclusion. Finally, even within the narrower field delineated above, the information gathered in this paper is meant only to be illustrative rather than exhaustive.

It is also important to realize that there are no national studies of quality from which we could obtain an undistorted picture of the level and distribution of quality, either here or abroad. For that purpose, and also to obtain a picture of temporal trends in quality, we must depend on reports of mortality, morbidity, longevity, and use of service — reports that are, insofar as their implications for the quality of care are concerned, extremely difficult to interpret. What we do have is a rather large assemblage of studies, using methods that vary in accuracy and stringency, to assess diverse aspects of the quality of care provided by selected practitioners to circumscribed populations at different periods. As a result, there is little we can say about the levels of quality in the United States as a whole, besides noting that almost invariably performance seems to fall far short of the criteria and standards used to judge the quality of care. And because one expects that as medical science progresses these criteria and standards will become correspondingly more stringent, there is little to be learned about secular trends from comparisons of current studies with those in the past, even if on other grounds the comparison might seem appropriate. For the same reasons, what is said concerning the factors that influence quality should also be treated with caution, even though in this case we can be somewhat more assured of the general applicability of the observed associations, particularly when they are repeatedly encountered and seem to be reasonable in the light of what we know about the health care system in general.

Variability and Localization

The distribution of behaviors that directly or indirectly connote quality reveals an astounding degree of variability among geographic areas, practitioners, and institutions. Particular attention has been paid in recent years to the poorly understood variations in the incidence of surgical procedures among small areas within the United States,[4] within other countries,[5] and among countries.[6] There is also considerable variation among practitioners and institutions in any given, rather circumscribed geographic area, and even among practitioners within a given institution. Adherence to the implicit or explicit criteria of good care has been observed to vary among general practitioners[7] and internists[8] practicing in an area. The same is true for physicians in a set of associated group practices.[9] There are wide variations in the cost of care provided by physicians in a group practice[10] and by physicians and other practitioners in a university-affiliated clinic.[11] The number and cost of diagnostic procedures vary considerably among physicians who practice in a geographic locale,[12] a hospital,[13] or a group practice.[14] The propensity to remove normal tissue in primary appendectomies is astoundingly variable among physicians in a hospital and also among the staffs of different hospitals, each taken as a whole.[15]

Hospitals and ambulatory care institutions are known to vary with regard to other aspects of quality as well. For example, hospitals have been observed to differ greatly in the proportion of unjustified hysterectomies performed in them,[16] in the incidence of postoperative fatality and complications,[17] in the occurrence of preventable maternal mortality,[18] and in the adherence of their staffs to the implicit or explicit criteria of appropriate use and quality.[19] The quality of care provided by organized ambulatory care settings has been observed to be similarly variable.[20]

Greatly variable though the practice of health care may be, the variability is far from random. Questionable practices, on the contrary, are known to be highly concentrated or localized. It has been observed, for example, that relatively small proportions of physicians account for a relatively large share of questionable drugs[21] and injections.[22] The concentration of tonsillectomies[23] and of other surgery[24] in relatively few hands raises the suspicion that those who are responsible for most of the operations may be doing too many, whereas those who are doing too few are not able to maintain their surgical skills.

Variability and localization are the twin necessities of epidemiology. What remains is to identify the attributes with which appropriate use and quality are associated.

Training, Experience, Specialization and Age of Practitioners

The key attributes that influence physician performance (beyond the possible influence of personality traits, a subject concerning which I have no information) are apparently training, experience, and specialization.

The effect of training is illustrated repeatedly in the literature. General practice has been observed to be of higher quality among physicians who were better students,[25] who were educated in certain categories of medical schools,[26] and who had longer periods of certain kinds of training,[27] there being a mutually reinforcing effect when two or more of these attributes coexist.[28] Generalists taken as a group, however, are usually found to maintain a lower standard of practice compared with their more highly specialized colleagues, at least when judged by criteria that usually correspond more closely to the opinions of specialists.

Specialists appear to perform better than generalists in many aspects of ambulatory and inpatient care. Specialists use x-ray examinations more appropriately,[29] give fewer questionable injections,[30] use the hospital more appropriately,[31] more often comply with the implicit or explicit criteria of hospital care[32] and of ambulatory care,[33] and are responsible for fewer "preventable" perinatal deaths.[34] There is evidence, moreover, that the effect of specialization is contingent on a specialist's restricting his or her domain of practice to the cases that fall strictly within the corresponding area of specialization.[35] Furthermore, organizations that as a whole are more specialized in their functions appear to provide better care.[36]

Training and specialization are, of course, intimately related to experience. There are two additional components to experience: 1) years in practice and 2) volume of similar cases treated or of nearly identical procedures performed each year. As concerns the second of these two (the volume of care), there is evidence that larger hospitals provide better technical care,[37] though not necessarily care with which patients are satisfied.[38] But institutional size is an attribute with several connotations; experience with larger volumes of similar cases, either by individual practitioners or by the hospital's staff as a whole, is only one of these. It is interesting to find, therefore, that fatality following certain surgical procedures is lower in hospitals where more of these procedures are performed[39] and that preventable maternal deaths are judged to occur less often in hospitals where a large number of deliveries take place.[40] A contrary observation, perhaps attributable to adverse factors associated with hospital size, is a positive association of the annual number of births with neonatal and maternal mortality in a national sample of hospitals.[41]

The effect of the experience that accrues with longer duration of practice seems to be obscured by the obsolescence of medical knowledge that apparently occurs at the same time. As a result, advanced age seems almost always to be associated with lower levels of performance. Although if is not clear whether it is good or bad to do so, older physicians use fewer laboratory tests and x-rays.[42] Other observations, more clearly indicative of quality, have shown that older physicians with more years in practice use x-ray procedures less appropriately;[43] more often use questionable injections;[44] perform less appropriately as general practitioners in a community,[45] as family physicians in group practice,[46] and as physicians in a variety of ambulatory care settings;[47] and provide hospital care that is less likely to conform to preformulated explicit criteria than that provided by physicians in their intermediate years of practice.[48] In a study that found a bimodal pattern that is the opposite of this last one, the best pediatricians in one community were found to have been in practice for either less than 12 years or more than 40; but on the whole, the longer general practitioners were in practice, the lower their adherence to the criteria of ambulatory care.[49]

Because these studies of the relation between age and performance are all cross-sectional in design, having observed only contemporaneous differences among physicians, we cannot tell how much of the difference between the young and the old is due to a failure of the latter to acquire new knowledge of skill and how much is the result of a loss of knowledge or skill originally possessed. It is also likely, as the foregoing comparisons between pediatricians and general practitioners imply, that under certain circumstances that now can only be surmised, the balance of these two tendencies (the acquisition and loss of competence) will remain favorable, at least until extreme old age inevitably takes its toll.

Conditions of Office Practice

The performance of physicians is also influenced by the conditions in their own practices and in the organizations or institutions where they work. For example, general practitioners in rural North Carolina in the early 1950s seemed to do better work when they had a larger variety of certain kinds of equipment (a microscope, a clinical centrifuge, an electrocardiograph, an apparatus for determining basal metabolic rate, and a photoelectric calorimeter) in their offices.[50] Seeing patients by appointment was found to be correlated with higher levels of performance by general practitioners in rural North Carolina,[51] by general practitioners in the Canadian provinces of Ontario and Nova Scotia,[52] and by family physicians in an association of group practices in New York City and vicinity.[53] Family physicians in this last setting were also observed to provide better care if they had a full-time office assistant or if they used a medical record with a larger format.[54]

Physicians who are very busy may begin to provide less complete care (as judged by the records they keep) when the number of patients seen each hour becomes too large.[55] As physicians become busier, their office records have been found to show evidence of less compliance with criteria for history taking and physical examination while there is greater compliance with criteria for laboratory tests.[56] This suggests that the latter could be a substitute for the former.

Financing and Organization of Care

There is also evidence, not always fully convincing, that financial incentives may influence practice. It appears that physicians who own x-ray equipment are more likely to use it, and to do so less appropriately;[57] that more surgery is performed when surgeons are less able or willing to make charges beyond those approved by an insurer;[58] that appendectomies are probably less often justified when the hospital stay is financed by a Blue Cross Plan;[59] and that patients who have help in paying for their hospital stays experience overstays more often and understays less often than do patients who pay the entire bill themselves.[60] These observations can be supplemented by a wealth of evidence showing that when prepayment is combined with group practice, there is a more parsimonious, and perhaps more appropriate, use of services.[61]

Participation in an organized group, clinic, or similar institution can be expected to alter radically the terms and conditions of practice, bringing about corresponding changes in the quality of technical care. It has been observed, for example, that the quality of ambulatory care for children is better in hospital outpatient departments than in office practice, at least as judged by entries in the medical record.[62] In rural North Carolina, general practitioners who worked in associations of two or more were observed to provide better care, perhaps because they were on the average better qualified by education and training, were younger, and had organized and equipped their practices in a manner more favorable to good performance.[63] No such relationship between quality and working in an association of two or more was observed for general practitioners in the Canadian provinces of Ontario and Nova Scotia.[64]

In the same vein, a more recent study in Hawaii suggests that physicians in multispecialty groups did not provide ambulatory care that was indisputably better than that provided by solo practitioners.[65] The physicians in such groups did, however, clearly use the hospital more appropriately, and provided better hospital care, than did physicians in solo practice.[66] But this association between belonging to a group practice and the nature of hospital care was explained by the fact that the groups employed specialists who restricted their practice to the domains of their respective specialties.[67]

It would be interesting and important to know whether group practice exerts an effect on quality through mechanisms in addition to the mere selection of the physicians who participate in the group, important though that is. Evidence for more subtle forms of influence may be inferred from observations that the quality of care provided by family physicians in a set of associated group practices was better when the physicians had a longer affiliation with the group, gave more of their time to the group, and spent more time in the facility owned by the group.[68] The importance of an active hospital affiliation is confirmed by the observation that the quality of ambulatory care was better when the physicians had such an appointment, when the appointment was at a higher rank, and when more hospital visits were made.[69] But, as if to highlight the complexity of the physician-hospital relationships there was no association in rural North Carolina between the quality of office care and the degree to which the physician was "active" in the use of the hospital, though the better doctors were more selective and skillful in their use of hospital services.[70]

There is some evidence about the association between access by patients to an organized practice and the outcome of care. The incidence of first at-

tacks of rheumatic fever has been observed to be lower after the establishment of a comprehensive care center in a low-income area.[71] Enrollees in
one prepaid group practice plan received more prenatal care and experienced a lower rate of neonatal mortality than a sample of the general
population, the advantage being greater for blacks than whites.[72] But a more
recent study in another community shows that the enrollees of a prepaid
group practice received less prenatal care but had an equal level of neonatal
mortality, leading the investigators to suggest a higher degree of efficiency in
the attainment of a given outcome.[73]

Hospital Characteristics

Of all the organizations that provide health care, hospitals are perhaps
the most likely to control the quality of care provided in them. The attributes
of hospitals, alone or in association with the characteristics of the physicians
who work in them therefore, can be expected to have a large influence on the
quality of care. I have already alluded to the possible effects of hospital size.
More important by far appears to be the teaching function of the hospital,
particularly when that function is reinforced by a close affiliation with a medical school.

Teaching hospitals are more often appropriately used.[74] Appendectomies in teaching hospitals more often appear to be justified.[75] The care
provided in teaching hospitals more often conforms to implicit and explicit
criteria of quality, at least as shown by the medical record.[76] Case fatality was
found to be lower in teaching hospitals in England and Wales,[77] and preventable perinatal deaths were lower in teaching hospitals in New York City compared with their voluntary or municipal counterparts that had no teaching
functions.[78]

There are some disquieting exceptions to this general harmony of praise.
In one national study of obstetrical care, maternal mortality, neonatal mortality, and the stillbirth ratio were all higher in hospitals affiliated with medical schools, conceivably because differences in case mix were not adjusted
for.[79] The same possible explanation does not hold for some other studies
that, having made extensive corrections for differences among patients, still
found that adverse postoperative events and teaching status — when the latter
was indicated by measures such as medical school affiliation, the presence of
residency training, or the number of house staff per hospital bed — were either
unrelated[80] or were perhaps positively related.[81]

Information about the quality of care in proprietary hospitals is fragmentary; it is also difficult to interpret, since these hospitals differ so much from
one another and are so influenced by the circumstances of time and place.
After an adjustment for differences in length of stay was made, the case
fatality for patients hospitalized in proprietary hospitals was reported to be
higher than that for patients in voluntary hospitals in Los Angeles County in
1964,[82] but not unequivocally so in New York City in 1971.[83] By contrast,
during 1950-1951, preventable perinatal deaths occurred less frequently in the

proprietary hospitals of New York City that in any other category of institutions except voluntary teaching hospitals.[84] But again in New York City, care in proprietary hospitals, at least for a certain segment of the population during 1961 or 1962, was much more often inappropriate and of "less than optimal" quality, particularly in the hands of physicians to whom only the proprietary hospitals would grant privileges.[85]

Seeing how much importance is given to hospital accreditation, it is remarkable how little is known about its relationship to the demonstrated quality of care. This may be because all the better hospitals are already accredited, so that the contribution that might be specifically attributed to accreditation is difficult to tease out. In one study of national scope, no significant association was found between accreditation status and postoperative fatality for three conditions after differences in case mix had been corrected for.[86] Among other fragments of information on the subject, hospital case fatality adjusted for length of stay is lower in accredited hospitals[87] and accreditation seems to be associated with somewhat higher quality when otherwise similar voluntary hospitals are compared but not when similar accredited and unaccredited proprietary hospitals are compared.[88] A study of 30 hospitals in the Chicago area, all accredited, showed that the more detailed ratings of medical departments by the surveyors of the Joint Commission on Accreditation of Hospitals were associated, when favorable, with lower case fatality rates, after adjustment for differences in length of stay, and with better reputations for the hospitals among knowledgeable informants.[89]

Hospitals no doubt influence quality partly through the facilities and equipment they provide and partly through selecting the physicians and other personnel who are permitted to work in them. There appears to be, however, yet another effect, one mediated through organizational controls. In any event, there is an interaction between the characteristics of hospitals and the attributes of the physicians who practice in them. The formal qualifications of individual physicians seem less important indictators of quality in a hospital affiliated with a university than in one that is not. By contrast, the less able the hospital and its medical staff are to control the practice of medicine in the hospital, the more likely is the care received by patients to depend on the qualifications of individual physicians.[90] Irrespective of university affiliation, the quality of technical care seems to be best in the hands of highly trained physicians in tightly organized hospitals and worst in the hands of less highly trained physicians in hospitals with looser forms of organization.[91]

A growing number of studies draw on the theory of organizations to explore the relation between quality and the details of organizational structure and behavior. These studies offer possible explanations for some of the more obvious correlations we have known about, but they also reveal new associations we had not suspected and occasionally find difficult to understand or believe.[92] We find, for example, that although hospital size, teaching status, or a higher proportion of more qualified personnel is sometimes not associated with better outcomes (either surgical or both medical and surgical), such outcomes seem to be better when there are higher levels of coordination in the hospital as a whole, in patient care wards, or in operating rooms,[93] and when there is greater control over the privileges and activities of the surgical staff.[94] By contrast, one study unexpectedly revealed that when nursing administrators had a greater degree of power in their own "domain," postoperative mortality was worse rather than better.[95] Although we hesitate to accept this finding, unless it signifies less communication between doctors and nurses, we think we gain a new perspective on the relation between age and performance when we are told that hospitals that employ a higher proportion of doctors who have been in practice for many years are also hospitals characterized by a greater laxity in coordination and control.[96]

Characteristics of Clients

So far, we have been concerned with the distribution of technical quality among providers. Much less is known about its distribution among clients, although this should be a matter of the greatest importance to public policy.[97]

Differences in the quality of care provided to different categories of persons may arise in one of two ways. Different people may have different degrees of access to different kinds of practitioners and institutions. This is a form of social differentiation that we seem willing to tolerate, even when we regard it as unfortunate. We are less able to contemplate the second possibility: that patients with similar needs for technical care will be treated differently when seen by the same practitioner, or cared for in the same institution, unless the difference is only in the amenities of care. This reluctance may partly explain our unwillingness or inability even to study the subject, with the result that there is very little known about it. More is known about a third factor that influences the quality of care, namely, the ability or willingness of clients to participate in influencing the recommendations of the physician and in carrying them out. This paper, however, does not include studies of patient participation and compliance.

The variability in the quantity and quality of provider care already noted must have its counterpart among the people who use these providers. We can expect to see, therefore, corresponding differences among those who reside in different geographic areas or who are clients of different hospitals and practitioners. The clients of any given set of practitioners can also be expected to vary a great deal in the quality of care they receive.[98]

As to the association between client attributes and the quality of care received, there are snippets of information about the effects of place of residence, age, sex, race, occupation, having insurance, and indexes of socioeconomic status.

It is reasonable to expect that rural residents experience the adverse consequences of reduced access to care, particularly to care by more highly specialized physicians and those in the larger, university-affiliated hospitals. For example, the improper use of an antibiotic has been shown to be more frequent in rural areas, even when physician specialty status has been taken into account.[99] Surgical procedures are less often performed for residents of less highly urbanized areas.[100] But if the possibility of unnecessary intervention is considered, being less subject to surgery may not necessarily be a bad thing. At least one study has noted an association of urban residence with more frequent appendectomies and higher fatality from appendicitis.[101]

The evidence concerning the possible effect of age and sex is fragmentary and inconclusive. On the one hand, there appears to be no consistent association between the age of the patient and the quality of either hospital care or office care in Hawaii.[102] On the other hand, the quality of nursing services in a selected group of urban hospitals has been observed to be somewhat better for younger males than for younger females, and better for older females than for older males.[103] In one study abroad, females were found to be more subject to appendectomy, and the surgery more often yielded normal tissue, but this could possibly be explained by the greater difficulty of diagnosing appendicitis in females.[104]

Comparisons based on differences in race are equally sparse and inconclusive. There was no association between ethnic origin and the quality of hospital care in Hawaii, nor was the quality of hospital care, at least in its conformity to technical standards, influenced in a consistent manner by whether the patient received care from a physician of similar or disparate ethnic origin.[105] Hawaii could be atypical in this regard. Other studies have found that surgical operations are fewer among nonwhites,[106] that nonwhites may be receiving nursing care of lower quality,[107] and that when surgery is done, it is more often performed by resident staff than by surgeons with more experience or higher qualifications.[108] One cannot conclude, of course, that the care provided by resident staff is necessarily inferior. In one study, house staff were found to perform quite well,[109] whereas in another study their performance was reported to be rather poor.[110]

Occupational differences are interesting partly because occupation is an important indicator of socioeconomic status (as is, unfortunately, ethnic origin) and partly because the use of services by physicians and members of their families may be used as a standard of care.[111] It has been noted, for example, that the wives of physicians are much more likely to have had a hysterectomy than are women in general.[112] This may also mean, however, that the wives of physicians are more exposed to unnecessary surgery. Hysterectomies are known to be frequently proposed and performed when not completely justified.[113] A study in the German city of Hannover shows that white-collar workers have more appendectomies but that the tissue removed is less often acutely inflamed.[114] Much more to the point is the observation that persons connected with medicine or nursing may experience higher risk because of the much greater readiness to subject them to appendectomies that prove not to have been justified.[115]

These observations suggest that greater access to care may have adverse as well as beneficial consequences. This principle appears to apply when coverage by private health insurance or by a governmental program improves the ability to pay for care. It has been observed that such coverage decreases underuse of the hospital but at the same time increases overuse.[116] Appendectomies for patients whose hospital stays were financed by Blue Cross

Plans appeared to yield normal or questionable tissue in a higher proportion of cases.[117]

In some studies, the outcomes of care have been used to tell us something about the influence of social and economic factors on the quality of care and its consequences. It has been reported, for example, that patients with higher incomes are less likely to suffer postoperative morbidity or death, even when many extraneous factors that might account for the finding are corrected for.[118] Mothers assigned to lower socioeconomic categories on the basis of average house rents have been shown to experience higher rates of preventable maternal mortality, the difference being largely attributable to failure of the expectant mother to obtain suitable care.[119] The proportion of perinatal deaths considered preventable is larger when the birth takes place in a municipal hospital rather than a voluntary one, or when the mother and child are cared for in a ward rather than the private service of a hospital.[120] When the organization of care is improved, there may be an associated improvement in prenatal care and a reduction in neonatal mortality, the relative improvements being greater for those who are ordinarily disadvantaged. But the disadvantage is not completely remedied.[121] Even approximately equal access to reasonably equal care does not necessarily result in equal enjoyment of health.

That does not mean, of course, that we must abandon hope; it only means that we must try harder, and on a wider front.

Notes

This paper is based on the epilogue to the author's book *The Methods and Findings of Quality Assessment and Monitoring: An Illustrated Analysis*, published by the Health Administration Press. Copyright to the book is held by the Regents of the University of Michigan. The work was supported by the Commonwealth Fund, the Carnegie Corporation of New York, the Milbank Memorial Fund, the W. K. Kellogg Foundation, and the National Center for Health Services Research. The views expressed are those of the author; they do not in any way represent his sponsors.

1. A. Donabedian, *Explorations in Quality Assessment and Monitoring*, vol. 1: *The Definition of Quality and Approaches to Its Assessment* (Ann Arbor, MI: Health Administration Press, 1980).

2. Ibid.; A. Donabedian, *Explorations in Quality Assessment and Monitoring*, vol. 2: *The Criteria and Standards of Quality* (Ann Arbor, MI: Health Administration Press, 1982).

3. A. Donabedian, *Explorations in Quality Assessment and Monitoring*, vol. 3: *The Methods and Findings of Quality Assessment and Monitoring: An Illustrated Analysis* (Ann Arbor, MI: Health Administration Press, 1985).

4. P. A. Lembcke, "Measuring the Quality of Medical Care Through Vital Statistics Based on Hospital Service Areas, 1: Comparative Study of Appendectomy Rates," *American Journal of Public Health* 42 (1952): 276-286; C. E. Lewis, "Variations in the Incidence of Surgery," *New England Journal of Medicine* 281 (1969): 880-884; J. Wennberg and A. Gittelsohn, "Small Area Variations in Health Care Delivery," *Science* 182 (1973): 1102-1108; A. M. Gittelsohn and J. E. Wennberg, "On the Incidence of Tonsillectomy and Other Common Surgical Procedures," in *Costs, Risks, and*

Benefits of Surgery, ed. J. P. Bunker, B. A. Barnes, and F. Mosteller (New York: Oxford University Press, 1977); J. R. Griffith, J. D. Restuccia, P. J. Tedeschi, P. A. Wilson, and H. S. Zuckerman, "Measuring Community Hospital Services in Michigan," *Health Services Research* 16 (1981): 135-160.

5. H. Stockwell and E. Vayda, "Variations in Surgery in Ontario," *Medical Care* 17 (1979): 390-396.

6. J. P. Bunker, "Surgical Manpower: A Comparison of Operations and Surgeons in the United States and in England and Wales," *New England Journal of Medicine* 282 (1970): 135-144; E. Vayda, "A Comparison of Surgical Rates in Canada and in England and Wales," *New England Journal of Medicine* 289 (1973): 1224-1229; K. McPherson, J. E. Wennberg, O. B. Hovind, and P. Clifford, "Small-Area Variations in the Use of Common Surgical Procedures: An International Comparison of New England, England, and Norway," *New England Journal of Medicine* 307 (1982): 1310-1314.

7. O. L. Peterson, L. P. Andrews, R. S. Spain, and B. G. Greenberg, "An Analytical Study of North Carolina General Practice, 1953-1954," *Journal of Medical Education* 31, pt. 2 (December 1956): 1-165; K. F. Clute, *The General Practitioner: A Study of Medical Education and Practice in Ontario and Nova Scotia* (Toronto: University of Toronto Press, 1963).

8. B. S. Hulka, F. J. Romm, G. R. Parkerson, Jr., I. T. Russell, N. E. Clapp, and F. S. Johnson, "Peer Review in Ambulatory Care: Use of Explicit Criteria and Implicit Judgments," *Medical Care* 17, suppl. (March 1979): 1-73.

9. M. A. Morehead, *Quality of Medical Care Provided by Family Physicians as Related to Their Education, Training and Methods of Practice* (New York: Health Insurance Plan of Greater New York, 1958).

10. C. B. Lyle, D. S. Citron, W. C. Sugg, and O. D. Williams, "Cost of Medical Care in a Practice of Internal Medicine: A Study in a Group of Seven Internists," *Annals of Internal Medicine* 81 (1974): 1-6.

11. D. D. Wright, R. L. Kane, G. F. Snell, and F. R. Wolley, "Costs and Outcomes for Different Primary Care Providers," *Journal of the American Medical Association* 238 (1977): 46-50.

12. J. M. Eisenberg and D. Nicklin, "Use of Diagnostic Services by Physicians in Community Practice," *Medical Care* 19 (1981): 297-309.

13. S. A. Schroeder, A. Schliftman, and T. E. Piemme, "Variation Among Physicians in the Use of Laboratory Tests: Relation to Quality of Care," *Medical Care* 12 (1974): 709-713.

14. D. K. Freeborn, D. Baer, M. R. Greenlick, and J. W. Bailey, "Determinants of Medical Care Utilization: Physicians' Use of Laboratory Services," *American Journal of Public Health* 62 (1972): 846-853.

15. H. A. Weeks, *Tightness of Organization Related to Patterns of Patient Care* (Ann Arbor: University of Michigan, School of Public Health, Bureau of Public Health Economics, n.d.); J. F. Sparling, "Measuring Medical Care Quality: A Comparative Study," *Hospitals* 36 (Mar. 16, 1962): 62-68; 36 (Apr. 1, 1962): 56-57, 60-61.

16. J. C. Doyle, "Unnecessary Hysterectomies: Study of 6,248 Operations in Thirty-Five Hospitals During 1948," *Journal of the American Medical Association* 51 (1953): 360-365.

17. J. P. Bunker, W. H. Forrest, Jr., F. Mosteller, and L. D. Vandam (eds.), *The National Halothane Study: A Study of the Possible Association Between Halothane Anesthesia and Postoperative Hepatic Necrosis* (Bethesda, MD: National Institutes of Health, National Institute of General Medical Sciences, 1969); Stanford Center for Health Care Research, "Comparison of Hospitals With Regard to Outcomes of Surgery," *Health Services Research* 11 (1976): 112-127; W. R. Scott, W. H. Forrest, Jr., and B. W. Brown, "Hospital Structure and Postoperative Mortality and Morbidity," in *Organizational Research in Hospitals,* ed. S. M. Shortell and M. Brown (Chicago: Blue Cross Association, 1976); W. R. Scott, A. B. Flood, and W. Ewy, "Organizational Determinants of Services, Quality and Cost of Care in Hospitals," *Milbank Memorial Fund Quarterly: Health and Society* 57

(1979): 234-264; A. B. Flood and W. R. Scott, "Professional Power and Professional Effectiveness: The Power of the Surgical Staff and the Quality of Surgical Care in Hospitals," *Journal of Health and Social Behavior* 19 (1978): 240-254; A. B. Flood, W. Ewy, W. R. Scott, W. H. Forrest, Jr., and B. W. Brown, "The Relationship Between Intensity and Duration of Medical Services and Outcomes for Hospitalized Patients," *Medical Care* 17 (1979): 1088-1102; A. B. Flood, W. R. Scott, and E. Wayne, "Does Practice Make Perfect? 1: The Relation Between Hospital Volume and Outcomes for Selected Diagnostic Categories," *Medical Care* 22 (1984): 98-114; A. B. Flood, W. R. Scott, and E. Wayne, "Does Practice Make Perfect? 2: The Relation Between Volume and Outcomes and Other Hospital Characteristics," *Medical Care* 22 (1984): 115-125.

18. New York Academy of Medicine, Committee on Public Health Relations, *Maternal Mortality in New York City: A Study of All Puerperal Deaths 1930-1932* (New York: Oxford University Press, for the Commonwealth Fund, 1933).

19. M. A. Morehead et al., *A Study of the Quality of Hospital Care Secured by a Sample of Teamster Family Members in New York City* (New York: Columbia University, School of Public Health and Administrative Medicine, 1964); L. S. Rosenfeld, "Quality of Medical Care in Hospitals," *American Journal of Public Health* 47 (1957): 856-865; S.-O. Rhee, "Relative Influence of Specialty Status, Organization of Office Care and Organization of Hospital Care on the Quality of Medical Care: A Multivariate Analysis" (doctoral dissertation, University of Michigan, 1975); S.-O. Rhee, "Factors Determining the Quality of Physician Performance in Patient Care," *Medical Care* 14 (1976): 733-750.

20. B. C. Payne, T. F. Lyons, E. Neuhaus, M. Kolton, and L. Dwarshius, *Method for Evaluating and Improving Ambulatory Care* (Ann Arbor, MI: Health Services Research Center, 1978); M. A. Morehead, R. S. Donaldson, and M. R. Seravelli, "Comparisons Between OEO Neighborhood Health Centers and Other Health Care Providers of Ratings of the Quality of Health Care,"

American Journal of Public Health 61 (1971): 1294-1306.

21. W. A. Ray, C. E. Federspiel, and W. Schaffner, "Prescribing of Chloramphenicol in Ambulatory Practice: An Epidemiologic Study Among Tennessee Medicaid Recipients," *Annals of Internal Medicine* 84 (1976): 266-270.

22. R. H. Brook and K. N. Williams, "Evaluation of the New Mexico Peer Review System, 1971 to 1973," *Medical Care* 14, suppl. (December 1976): 1-122.

23. Gittelsohn and Wennberg (note 4).

24. R. J. Nickerson, T. Colton, O. L. Peterson, B. S. Bloom, and W. W. Hauck, Jr., "Doctors Who Perform Operations: A Study on In-Hospital Surgery in Four Diverse Geographic Areas," *New England Journal of Medicine* 295 (1976): 921-926, 982-989.

25. Peterson et al. (note 7); Morehead (note 9).

26. Morehead (note 9).

27. Ibid.; Peterson et al. (note 7).

28. Ibid.

29. A. W. Childs and E. D. Hunter, "Non-Medical Factors Influencing Use of Diagnostic X-Ray by Physicians," *Medical Care* 10 (1972): 323-325.

30. Brook and Williams (note 22).

31. B. C. Payne, T. F. Lyons, L. Dwarshius, M. Kolton, and W. Morris, *The Quality of Medical Care: Evaluation and Improvement* (Chicago: Hospital Research and Educational Trust, 1976); Morehead et al. (note 19).

32. Ibid.

33. R. L. Riedel and D. C. Riedel, *Practice and Performance: An Assessment of Ambulatory Care* (Ann Arbor, MI: Health Administration Press, 1979); Payne et al. (note 20).

34. S. G. Kohl, *Perinatal Mortality in New York City: Responsible Factors* (Cambridge, MA: Harvard University Press, for the Commonwealth Fund, 1955).

35. S.-O. Rhee, R. D. Luke, T. F. Lyons, and B. C. Payne, "Domain of Practice and the Quality of Physician Performance," *Medical Care* 19 (1981): 14-23; Rhee, "Relative Influence of Specialty Status" (note 19); Payne et al. (note 20); Payne et al. (note 31).

36. New York Academy of Medicine (note 18); Morehead et al. (note 20).
37. Rhee, "Relative Influence of Specialty Status" (note 19); Rhee, "Factors Determining the Quality of Physician Performance" (note 19).
38. G. V. Fleming, "Hospital Structure and Consumer Satisfaction," *Health Services Research* 16 (1981): 43-63.
39. H. S. Luft, J. P. Bunker, and A. C. Enthoven, "Should Operations Be Regionalized? The Empirical Relation Between Surgical Volume and Mortality," *New England Journal of Medicine* 301 (1979): 1364-1369; Flood et al. (note 17), parts 1 and 2.
40. New York Academy of Medicine (note 18).
41. American College of Obstetricians and Gynecologists, Committee on Maternal Health, *National Study of Maternity Care: Survey of Obstetric Practice and Associated Services in Hospitals in the United States* (Chicago: American College of Obstetricians and Gynecologists, 1970).
42. Eisenberg and Nicklin (note 12).
43. Childs and Hunter (note 29).
44. Brook and Williams (note 22).
45. Peterson et al. (note 7); Clute (note 7).
46. Morehead (note 9).
47. Payne et al. (note 20); Payne et al. (note 31).
48. Rhee, "Factors Determining the Quality of Physician Performance" (note 19).
49. Riedel and Riedel (note 33).
50. Peterson et al. (note 7).
51. Ibid.
52. Clute (note 7).
53. Morehead (note 9).
54. Ibid.
55. Payne et al. (note 20).
56. Hulka et al. (note 8).
57. Childs and Hunter (note 29).
58. United Steelworkers of America, Public Relations Department, *Special Study on the Medical Care Program for Steelworkers and Their Families* (Pittsburgh: USA, 1960).
59. Sparling (note 15).
60. R. B. Fitzpatrick, D. C. Riedel, and B. C. Payne, "Appropriateness of Admission and Length of Stay," in *Hospital and Medical Economics: A Study of Population, Services, Costs, Methods of Payment, and Controls*, vol. 1, by W. J. McNerney et al. (Chicago: Hospital Research and Educational Trust, 1962).
61. A. Donabedian, "An Evaluation of Prepaid Group Practice," *Inquiry* 6 (1969): 3-27; M. I. Roemer and W. Shonick, "HMO Performance: The Recent Evidence," *Milbank Memorial Fund Quarterly: Health and Society* 51 (1973): 271-317; H. S. Luft, "Assessing the Evidence on HMO Performance," *Milbank Memorial Fund Quarterly: Health and Society* 58 (1980): 501-536.
62. Riedel and Riedel (note 33).
63. Peterson et al. (note 7).
64. Clute (note 7).
65. Payne et al. (note 31).
66. Ibid.
67. Rhee, "Relative Influence of Specialty Status" (note 19); Rhee, "Factors Determining the Quality of Physician Performance" (note 19).
68. Morehead (note 9).
69. Ibid.
70. Peterson et al. (note 7).
71. L. Gordis, "Effectiveness of Comprehensive-Care Programs in Preventing Rheumatic Fever," *New England Journal of Medicine* 289 (1973): 331-335.
72. S. Shapiro, L. Weiner, and P. M. Densen, "Comparison of Prematurity and Perinatal Mortality in a General Population and in the Population of a Prepaid Group Practice Medical Care Plan," *American Journal of Public Health* 48 (1958): 170-187.
73. J. D. Quick, M. R. Greenlick, and K. J. Roghmann, "Prenatal Care and Pregnancy Outcome in an HMO and General Population: A Multivariate Cohort Analysis," *American Journal of Public Health* 71 (1981): 381-390.
74. Morehead et al. (note 19).
75. Sparling (note 15).
76. J. Fine and M. A. Morehead, "Study of Peer Review of Inhospital Patient Care," *New York State Journal of Medicine* 71 (1971): 1963-1973; Morehead et al. (note 19); Rhee, "Relative Influence of Specialty Status" (note 19); Rhee, "Factors Determining the Quality of Physician Performance" (note 19).
77. L. Lipworth, J. A. H. Lee, and J. N. Morris, "Case-Fatality in Teaching and Non-Teaching Hospitals 1956-59," *Medical Care* 1 (1963): 71-76.
78. Kohl (note 34).
79. American College of Obstetricians and Gynecologists (note 41).

80. Stanford Center for Health Care Research, *Study of Institutional Differences in Postoperative Mortality* (Springfield, VA: U.S. Department of Commerce, National Technical Information Service, 1974); Scott et al., "Hospital Structure" (note 17).
81. Luft et al. (note 39).
82. M. I. Roemer, A. T. Moustafa, and C. E. Hopkins, "A Proposed Hospital Quality Index: Hospital Death Rates Adjusted for Case Severity," *Health Services Research* 3 (1968): 96-118.
83. M. E. W. Goss and J. I. Reed, "Evaluating the Quality of Hospital Care Through Severity-Adjusted Death Rates: Some Pitfalls," *Medical Care* 12 (1974): 202-213.
84. Kohl (note 34).
85. Morehead et al. (note 19).
86. Stanford Center for Health Care Research (note 80).
87. Roemer et al. (note 82).
88. Morehead et al. (note 19).
89. D. Neuhauser, *The Relationships Between Administrative Activities and Hospital Performance,* Research Series 28 (Chicago: University of Chicago, Center for Health Administrative Studies, 1971).
90. Morehead et al. (note 19).
91. Rhee, "Relative Influence of Specialty Status" (note 19).
92. B. S. Georgopoulos and F. C. Mann, *The Community General Hospital* (New York: Macmillan Co., 1962); S. M. Shortell, S. W. Becker, and D. Neuhauser, "The Effects of Managerial Practices on Hospital Efficiency and Quality of Care," in *Organizational Research in Hospitals*, ed. S. M. Shortell and M. Brown (Chicago: Blue Cross Association, 1976); Scott et al., "Hospital Structure " (note 17); Scott et al., "Organizational Determinants" (note 17); Flood and Scott (note 17); Neuhauser (note 89).
93. Scott et al., "Hospital Structure" (note 17); Scott et al., "Organizational Determinants" (note 17); Shortell et al. (note 92).
94. Scott et al., "Hospital Structure" (note 17); Flood and Scott (note 17).
95. Flood and Scott (note 17).
96. Scott et al., "Organizational Determinants" (note 17).
97. L. Wyszewianski and A. Donabedian, "Equity in the Distribution of Quality of Care," *Medical Care* 19, suppl. (December 1981): 28-56.
98. R. H. Brook, *Quality of Care Assessment: A Comparison of Five Methods of Peer Review* (Washington, DC: Department of Health, Education, and Welfare, Public Health Service, Health Resources Administration, Bureau of Health Services Research and Evaluation, 1973).
99. Ray et al. (note 21).
100. C. Bombardier, V. R. Fuchs, L. A. Lillard, and K. E. Warner, "Socioeconomic Factors Affecting the Utilization of Surgical Operations," *New England Journal of Medicine* 297 (1977): 699-705.
101. Lembcke (note 4).
102. T. F. Lyons and B. C. Payne, "The Quality of Physicians' Health Care Performance: A Comparison Against Optimal Criteria for Treatment of the Elderly and Younger Adults in Community Hospitals," *Journal of the American Medical Association* 227 (1974): 925-928; T. F. Lyons and B. C. Payne, "Quality of Physicians' Office-Care Performance: Different for Elderly Than for Younger Adults?" *Journal of the American Medical Association* 229 (1974): 1621-1622.
103. E. Janzen, "Quality Nursing Care Assurance: Initial Survey" (paper presented at the American Public Health Association annual meeting, New Orleans, Oct. 23, 1974).
104. S. Lictner and M. Pflanz, "Appendectomy in the Federal Republic of Germany: Epidemiology and Medical Care Patterns," *Medical Care* 9 (1971): 311-330.
105. S.-O. Rhee, T. F. Lyons, and B. C. Payne, "Patient Race and Physician Performances: Quality of Medical Care, Hospital Admissions and Hospital Stays," *Medical Care* 17 (1979): 737-747.
106. Bombardier et al. (note 100).
107. Janzen (note 103).
108. L. D. Egbert and I. L. Rothman, "Relation Between the Race and Economic Status of Patients and Who Performs Their Surgery," *New England Journal of Medicine* 297 (1977): 90-91.
109. Morehead et al. (note 19).
110. Kohl (note 34).

111. J. P. Bunker and B. W. Brown, Jr., "The Physician-Patient as an Informed Consumer of Surgical Services," *New England Journal of Medicine* 290 (1974): 1051-1055.

112. Ibid.

113. P. A. Lembcke, "Medical Auditing by Scientific Methods: Illustrated by Major Female Pelvic Surgery," *Journal of the American Medical Association* 162 (1956): 646-655; E. G. McCarthy, M. L. Finkel, and H. S. Ruchlin, *Second Opinion Elective Surgery* (Boston: Auburn House, 1981); Doyle (note 16).

114. Lictner and Pflanz (note 104).

115. J. G. R. Howie, "The Place of Appendectomy in the Treatment of Young Adult Patients With Possible Appendicitis," *Lancet*, 1968, pp. 1365-1367.

116. Fitzpatrick et al. (note 60).

117. Sparling (note 15).

118. Flood and Scott (note 17).

119. New York Academy of Medicine (note 18).

120. Kohl (note 34).

121. Shapiro et al. (note 72).

27

Relating Quality Assurance to Credentials and Privileges

Benjamin Gilbert

Benjamin Gilbert, J.D., M.P.H., is the attorney for the North Carolina Memorial Hospital, and Clinical Assistant Professor, Department of Health Policy and Administration, School of Public Health, University of North Carolina, Chapel Hill.

The legal principle that a hospital owes a direct duty to its patients to monitor the quality of care provided by its medical staff has gained acceptance only within the past 20 years. Until recently, a hospital was seen as a mere workshop for physicians, and the scope of a hospital's corporate duties toward patients was restricted to furnishing safe physical facilities and equipment and employing competent support personnel. This limited view of corporate duties persisted under the belief that a hospital was not equipped to actively supervise or control the means or methods by which independent contractor physicians treated their patients. Although it may still be true, in a practical sense, that a hospital cannot control physician performance with individual patients, today's hospital plays a much more active role in the overall quality of care provided to its patients.

This more active role in quality of care has been a result of changes in both the public's perception of hospital functions and actual changes in the organization and operation of hospitals. Acknowledgement of these changes and responsibilities and recognition of their legal consequences were heralded in the landmark case *Darling* v. *Charleston Community Memorial Hospital.*[1]

> The conception that the hospital does not undertake to treat the patient, does not undertake to act through its doctors and nurses, but undertakes instead simply to procure them to act upon their own responsibility, no longer reflects the fact. Present-day hospitals, as their manner of operation plainly demonstrates, do far more than furnish facilities for treatment. (citation omitted) . . . The Standards

for Hospital Accreditation, the state licensing regulations and the defendant's (hospital's) bylaws demonstrate that the medical profession and other responsible authorities regard it as both desirable and feasible that a hospital assume certain responsibilities for the care of the patient.[2]

The *Darling* case specifically addressed whether, in addition to the negligence of the treating physician, the hospital could also be negligent for breach of its independent legal duties to the patient. In its decision, the court held that the hospital did have an affirmative duty to the patient to scrutinize the quality of care rendered by the physician and could be held liable for negligence in monitoring the care provided by the physician. The hospital's failure to supervise and monitor adequately the medical care provided by the physician constituted a breach of its corporate duties and rendered the hospital liable for the patient's injuries.

Following *Darling*, a body of case law developed that defines the parameters of a hospital's independent responsibility for the quality of care provided by, and the competence of, its staff physicians. Recognizing the difficulties involved in assessing the day-to-day medical decisions and patient interactions of physicians, few courts have required hospitals to supervise the actual medical treatment rendered by physicians. Courts are, however, increasingly requiring hospitals to monitor, at least retrospectively, the competence of staff physicians and the quality of care rendered by them. Hospital liability, in relation to the negligent acts of a staff physician, arises when the hospital knew or should have known, through information acquired during credentialing or periodic monitoring, that a physician was not qualified or competent to exercise clinical privileges as granted.

Retrospective monitoring of physician competence, by definition, depends in large part on the availability of accurate and complete physician performance information. The legal responsibility for assuring physician competence rests ultimately with a hospital's governing body. In practice, actual monitoring of physician performance and the quality of care is delegated to medical staff committees. Ideally, these committees should analyze physician performance information and help the hospital evaluate a physician's competence at either initial selection or throughout a physician's tenure on the medical staff. All too often, however, the performance information gathered by these committees is neither coordinated nor shared in such a way as to enable the hospital to assess a physician's competence conscientiously.

This article will present recent court decisions that delineate the current scope of monitoring duties owed by a hospital to its patients. A discussion of these cases will identify the legal necessity of thorough analysis and integration of all physician performance information gathered by the various arms of the hospital. In addition, this article will identify what physician performance information, at a minimum, should be gathered and analyzed to meet a hospital's corporate duty for the quality of patient care.

Case Law Identifying Monitoring Duties

Three leading court decisions illustrate the duty assigned to hospitals to review the credentials and performance both of applicants for medical staff membership and of physicians already on the medical staff.

Granting Privileges to Applicants

In *Johnson* v. *Misericordia Community Hospital*, a physician was found negligent for nerve and artery damage and permanent paralysis resulting from hip surgery on the plaintiff.[3] In addition to the physician's negligence, Misericordia was also held liable for its own negligence in failing to ascertain the physician's professional competence before appointing him to its medical staff with orthopedic privileges.

In March 1973, the physician applied for orthopedic privileges on the medical staff of Misericordia. In his application, he stated that he was on the active staff of Family Hospital with orthopedic privileges and held consultant privileges at Northwest General Hospital and New Berlin Community Hospital. He stated that his privileges had never been suspended, diminished, revoked, or not been renewed, and that he was requesting privileges only for those surgical procedures for which he was qualified for certification. In another part of the application form, the physician failed to answer any of the questions pertaining to his malpractice insurance.

Upon his own endorsement, the physician was appointed to the medical staff with orthopedic privileges and was elevated to the position of chief of staff. It was not entirely clear when he was actually appointed to the medical staff or at what meeting his application was considered. What was clear was that Misericordia did not investigate the application before appointing him to the medical staff.

Had Misericordia or any of its committees investigated this physician's application, it would have found, contrary to his representations, that

- his privileges had been suspended and restricted at Family Hospital;

- he had never been associated with Northwest General Hospital or New Berlin Hospital;

- he had been denied privileges at St. Anthony's Hospital; and

- he had been demoted to the courtesy staff and all privileges were ultimately revoked at Mt. Sinai Hospital.

A review of his associations with various local orthopedic surgeons and hospital personnel would have revealed that they considered his competence as an orthopedic surgeon suspect. Furthermore, it was readily ascertainable that this physician was neither board certified nor board eligible in orthopedic surgery. Finally, a review of county court files would have revealed that seven malpractice suits had been filed against the same physician prior to his appointment at Misericordia.

In its decision, the court stated that the hospital's failure to exercise that degree of care, skill, and judgment exercised by the average hospital in approving an applicant's request for privileges constituted corporate negligence. The court concluded that had the hospital required a completed application from the physician and verified the accuracy of his statements, the hospital would have known that he was not competent to exercise his clinical privileges as granted. At a minimum, the court reasoned, a hospital should require a completed application for medical staff membership and verify the accuracy of the applicant's statements, especially in regard to medical education, training, and experience. Additionally, a hospital should

- solicit information from the applicant's peers, including those not referenced in the application, who are knowledgeable about the applicant's education, training, experience, health, professional competence, and ethical character;

- determine whether the applicant is currently licensed to practice and whether the licensure has been or is currently being challenged; and

- inquire whether the applicant has been involved in any malpractice action or experienced denial, reduction, or termination of professional organization membership or hospital medical staff privileges.

Reviewing Privileges of Current Staff Physicians

In addition to ascertaining a physician's competence at the point of initial appointment to the medical staff, a hospital must also monitor a physician's performance and competence throughout his association with the hospital and take appropriate corrective action if information indicates that the physician is no longer competent to exercise the range of privileges granted. Two cases illustrate a hospital's continuing duty to monitor the quality of care provided by, and the competence of, staff physicians.

In *Purcell* v. *Zimbelman*, Tucson General Hospital was held liable for a patient's injuries resulting from surgery.[4] The court determined that the hospital knew or should have known of the surgeon's prior incompetence in treating a comparable medical condition.

The surgeon initially diagnosed the plaintiff as suffering from either diverticulitis or cancer of the colon and scheduled him for exploratory surgery to determine the exact nature of his ailment. During surgery, the physician discovered a cancerous lesion on the plaintiff's rectosigmoid colon and performed a procedure called a Babcock-Bacon proctosigmoidectomy. As a result of the surgical procedure, the plaintiff suffered from a loss of sexual function, loss of a kidney, a permanent colostomy, and urinary problems.

At trial, expert medical testimony established that given the location of the plaintiff's lesion, the surgeon should have performed an anterior resection rather than a Babcock-Bacon protosigmoidectomy. Further, the trial court admitted testimony concerning two patients who were treated by the same surgeon at Tucson General Hospital prior to the plaintiff. The surgeon suspected that these patients were also suffering from either diverticulitis or cancer of the colon, and in both cases he did not perform an anterior resection, which would have been the correct procedure. Both patients developed complications and sued the surgeon and Tucson General Hospital before the surgeon's treatment of the plaintiff. It was also brought out at trial that two other patients sued both the surgeon and Tucson General Hospital prior to the plaintiff's surgery for care they received at the hospital.

The court found that evidence of these four lawsuits against both the surgeon and Tucson General Hospital was admissible to prove that the hospital should have known not only of the surgeon's apparent incompetence with regard to the procedure performed on the plaintiff and the type of ailment involved, but also of his general incompetence as a member of the medical staff. The hospital's department of surgery routinely reviewed two of the cases but took no action against the surgeon and did not recommend that the hospital's board of trustees take any action. In light of the four lawsuits, a routine surgical review did not satisfy the hospital's duty of assuring the surgeon's continued competence. The hospital should have had some mechanism in place to make a coordinated and thorough review of the surgeon's competence and clinical privileges, especially when a pattern of bad clinical outcomes became apparent. The failure to undertake such a review, when available information indicated that the surgeon was not competent to treat the condition in question, constituted a breach of the hospital's independent duty to the patient.

Elam v. *College Park Hospital* [5] expands on the holding of *Purcell* and addresses more specifically the necessity of thorough integration and coordination of physician performance information. *Elam* also suggests how closely courts will scrutinize the effectiveness of peer review activities in identifying deficient practice and in taking corrective action against incompetent physicians.

In this case, the plaintiff claimed that her podiatrist negligently performed surgery intended to correct bilateral bunions and bilateral hammertoes. She also claimed that College Park Hospital negligently failed to assure the competency and quality of care rendered by the podiatrist. As evidence of the hospital's negligence, the plaintiff asserted that the podiatrist had been the defendant in three prior malpractice actions, that College Park Hospital knew of one of the lawsuits four and one-half months before her surgery, and that prior peer review of this podiatrist's cases had not resulted in any corrective action being taken.

The hospital asserted that its medical care evaluation committee, set up in accord with Joint Commission on Accreditation of Hospitals (JCAH) standards, had routinely reviewed the podiatrist's charts and never had a reason to consider him incompetent or unqualified to practice podiatric surgery. The hospital did admit that it had received notice of one malpractice suit four and one-half months prior to the plaintiff's surgery.

The court, reversing summary judgment in favor of the hospital, found that the hospital's inaction after learning of the earlier malpractice suit could result in liability for the hospital. Even though the hospital had complied with JCAH standards for initial selection of the podiatrist, and had in place a peer review mechanism, the hospital was unable to document that an investigation of the podiatrist's clinical competence followed notice of the malpractice claim against him. The hospital's difficulties in this case can be traced directly to its failure to ensure that relevant physician performance information was coordinated in such a way to enable a thorough review of the podiatrist's competence. The court did not actually determine that College Park Hospital was independently liable for the plaintiff's injuries resulting from surgery, only that the hospital's conduct raised issues that should have been addressed by a jury. For example, the court asserted that a jury should address whether the hospital should have conducted an investigation upon notice of the malpractice suit, whether the peer review committee had conducted its periodic review of the podiatrist in a non-negligent manner, and whether the committee would have recommended revocation or suspension of privileges following review. The case was remanded to the trial court for determination of these factual issues.

Information That Hospitals Should Analyze When Granting or Reviewing Privileges

Table 27-1 presents some of the information that courts are requiring hospitals to collect and analyze to meet their independent duty for the quality of care rendered by their medical staffs. The information contained in Table 27-1 can serve as a starting point for evaluating a physician's application for initial or continued hospital privileges.

Application for Initial Privileges

Licensing boards, residency training programs, and specialty boards may be contacted to verify an applicant's professional credentials and to ascertain whether any disciplinary action has been taken against the applicant or is being considered. Licensing boards may also have information concerning an applicant's disciplinary status at other hospitals. In several states, the chief executive officer of a health care facility is required to report disciplinary action taken against a practitioner, including revocation, suspension, or limitation of a physician's privileges in that institution.[6]

Other hospitals at which an applicant has privileges may be contacted directly to ascertain the applicant's current status at those hospitals. A properly drafted authorization for release of confidential information, signed

Table 27-1. Checklist for Review of Medical Staff Privileges.

Information That Hospitals Should Collect and Analyze When Granting Medical Staff Privileges

Hospitals should be assured that the applicant has

- a valid license;
- completed a residency program;
- board certification status;
- no disciplinary actions by other hospitals, professional societies, specialty boards pending;
- good standing at current hospitals;
- adequate malpractice insurance in force; and
- satisfactory recommendations covering professional performance, clinical skills, ethical character, and ability to work with others.

Hospitals should be aware of the applicant's

- malpractice claims history;
- privileges at other hospitals;
- high risk areas of practice and need for probationary privileges;
- previous drug and alcohol problems; and
- physical and mental health status.

Information That Hospitals Should Collect and Analyze When Renewing Medical Staff Privileges

Hospitals should be assured that the applicant has

- a valid license;
- no disciplinary actions by other hospitals, professional societies, specialty boards pending;
- adequate malpractice insurance in force;
- exhibited satisfactory professional performance and clinical judgment;
- complied with bylaws, rules, and regulations; and
- satisfactory physical and mental health.

Hospitals should be aware of the applicant's

- malpractice claims situation;
- patterns of adverse clinical outcomes; and
- use of privileges previously granted.

by a physician in an application for medical staff membership, will enable the chiefs of staff, chief executive officers, or clinical department chairmen of other hospitals to supply information concerning an applicant's professional performance, clinical skills, ethical character, and ability to work with others. The chief executive officer of another hospital can also verify the scope of an applicant's privileges at that hospital.

An applicant's malpractice history may be obtained from the applicant's insurance carrier, and the applicant's current limits of coverage may be verified by securing a copy of the applicant's certificate of insurance. In addition, an applicant's malpractice experience may be ascertained from court documents that are public records and are therefore open for inspection and review.

Reappointment and Renewal of Privileges

When evaluating a physician's application for reappointment and renewal of clinical privileges, a detailed record of professional performance should be available from various sources within the facility. Clinical departments should be able to identify aberrant death rates and complication rates, by physician, from morbidity and mortality reports and peer review activities. A clinical department chairman should also be able to evaluate, by comparing privileges actually used with privileges granted, whether a physician has maintained skill levels and is competent to continue to exercise the range of privileges requested. Several hospital committees should also be gathering information that may be used to evaluate physician performance and competence. For example, the pharmacy and therapeutics committee should be surveying drug utilization practices; the tissue or pathology review committee should be verifying physicians' preoperative diagnoses with pathology evaluations; the utilization review committee should be monitoring utilization of hospital resources and facilities; and the medical records committee should be identifying incomplete, inadequate, or delinquent medical records.

Hospital Liability for Denying, Revoking, or Modifying Clinical Privileges

In exercising its corporate duty to use reasonable care in evaluating a physician's credentials and competence, a hospital must balance the public's interest in quality of care against a physician's interest in practicing his profession within that hospital. When a hospital denies, revokes, or modifies a physician's medical staff membership or clinical privileges, the hospital must do so in accord with its bylaws and with the constitutional or common law requirements of due process.

A physician's property interest in practicing his profession will generally invoke the application of constitutional due process to the actions of a public hospital in medical staff matters.[7] Courts have also fashioned common law rules, essentially equivalent to constitutional standards, for the medical staff actions of private, nonprofit hospitals,[8] and one commentator argues that with regard to medical staff appointments and clinical privileges, both public and private hospitals must adhere to the same standards of fairness.[9]

Whether of common law or constitutional origin, due process involves both substantive and procedural fairness. Substantive due process requires that rules or standards for medical staff membership and clinical privileges bear a rational relationship to professional standards of patient care,[10] to the legitimate objectives of the hospital,[11] or to the character and ethical behavior of an applicant.[12] Procedural due process requires that the process by which the substantive rules are applied be fundamentally fair. Minimal requirements of procedural due process include written notice of the reasons for denial, revocation, or modification of privileges; a hearing by a relatively impartial hearing body; an opportunity to produce and refute evidence and witnesses; written notice of the hearing body's decision; and an opportunity for the physician to appeal.[13] Standards and procedures that are neither arbitrary nor capricious and that provide for a fair review of reasonable criteria will be given great deference by the courts.[14]

Conclusion

As courts continue to assign liability to hospitals for negligence in selecting medical staff members and monitoring their clinical performance, the coordination and evaluation of all relevant physician performance information must assume a high priority for hospitals. Courts are requiring not only that credentials and peer review committees be in place, but that they play an active role in the initial and continuing evaluation of the competence of members of the medical staff. While striving to meet their corporate duty to evaluate and monitor the quality of care provided by their medical staffs, hospitals' actions in denying, revoking, or modifying staff membership or clinical privileges will also be evaluated by courts for compliance with due process guidelines. When hospitals apply reasonable criteria in a procedurally fair manner, courts will afford deference to decisions in medical staff matters.

Notes

1. *Darling* v. *Charleston Community Memorial Hospital*, 33 Ill.2d 326, 211 N.E.2d 253 (1965), *cert. denied* 383 U.S. 946 (1966).
2. *Darling* v. *Charleston Community Memorial Hospital*, 211 N.E.2d at 257.
3. *Johnson* v. *Misercordia Community Hospital*, 99 Wis.2d 708, 301 N.W.2d 156 (1981).
4. *Purcell* v. *Zimbelman*, 18 Ariz.App. 75, 500 P.2d 335 (1972).

5. *Elam* v. *College Park Hospital*, 132 Cal.App.3d 332, 183 Cal.Rptr. 156, as modified by 133 Cal.App.3d94A (1982).
6. *See, eg,* N.C. Gen. Stat. 131E-87.
7. *See, eg, Sosa* v. *Board of Managers*, 437 F.2d 173 (5th Cir. 1971).
8. *See, eg, Silver* v. *Castle Memorial Hospital*, 53 Haw. 475, 497 P2d 564, *cert. denied*, 409 U.S. 1048 (1972).

9. Southwick AF: The physician's right to due process in public and private hospitals: Is there a difference? *Medicolegal News* 9:4-10, Feb 1981.
10. *See*, eg, *Klinge* v. *Lutheran Charities Association of St. Louis*, 523 F.2d 56 (8th Cir. 1975); *Moore* v. *Board of Trustees of Carson-Tahoe Hospital*, 88 Nev. 207, 495 P.2d 605 (1972); *Campbell* v. *St. Mary's Hospital*, 252 N.W.2d 581 (Minn. 1977).
11. *See* eg, *Guerrero* v. *Burlington County Memorial Hospital*, 70 N.J. 344, 360 A.2d 334 (1976); *Wilkinson* v. *Madera Community Hospital*, 144 Cal.App.3d 436, 192 Cal.Rptr. 593 (1983); *Adler* v. *Montefiore Hospital*, 452 Pa. 60, 311 A.2d 634 (1973).
12. *See*, eg, *Battle* v. *Jefferson Davis Memorial Hospital*, 451 F.Supp. 1015 (S.D. Miss. 1976); *Huffaker* v. *Bailey*, 273 Ore. 273, 540 P.2d 1398 (1975); *Bricker* v. *Sceva Spears Memorial Hospital*, 111 N.H. 276, 281 A.2d 589 (1971).
13. *See*, eg, *Silver* v. *Castle Memorial Hospital*, supra, note 8; *Ascherman* v. *San Francisco Medical Society*, 39 Cal.App.3d 623, 114 Cal.Rptr. 681 (1974); *Christhilf* v. *Annapolis Emergency Hospital Association Inc.*, 496 F.2d 174 (4th Cir. 1974).
14. *See*, eg, *Unterthiner* v. *Desert Hospital District*, 33 C.3d 285, 188 Cal.Rptr. 590, 656 P.2d 554 (1983).

28

An Integrated Approach to Liability

Edie Siler

Edie Siler, R.N., B.S.N., is the Infection Control Nurse, Mercy Medical Center, Denver.

For two decades the increase in proportion of monetary allocation to health services has exceeded the rise in the gross national product. Hospital costs have accelerated out of proportion to other health care costs. For hospitals to operate with effectiveness and efficiency, a maximum effort needs to be given to overcoming the new administrative difficulties and challenges of today's health care industry.

For effective utilization of human resources, hospital administrators should devise a system that would meld preexisting functions that focus on review of specific aspects of care into an organized facility-wide program. The purpose of such a system would be to describe and monitor those areas of accountability, liability, and quality of care.

In most hospitals today there are three specific departments, quality assurance (QA), infection control (IC), and risk management (RM), that have similar goals and purposes. If these three areas conduct their activities independently and their information is not integrated, the results are fragmentation, duplication of efforts, and excessive costs. Each department provides and uses similar information and each should be feeding into and drawing from a central data base. The activities of an integrated trio should provide a central data base from which potential problems and/or problematic patterns and trends in patient care and facility management can be identified. Within the triad, the lines of authority and accountability should be clearly defined so that appropriate and timely actions can be taken to resolve problems. The benefits of such an integrated trio should be the minimizing of financial loss as well as the prevention of harm to visitors, employees, and patients.

QA activities for hospitals were mandated by the Joint Commission on Accreditation of Hospitals (JCAH) in its 1979 standards. The implementation of such standards is based on the assumption that a QA activity will include the following steps:[1]

1. Identification of the problem
2. Assessment and problem resolution
3. Establishment of clinically valid criteria
4. Selection of assessment methodology
5. Identification of problem cause
6. Implementation of corrective actions
7. Evaluation of problem resolution

Problems identified through QA activities are ranked on the basis of their importance to patient care, frequency of occurrence, and impact on the health of those affected.[2]

IC activities became formalized and popular in the United States approximately 10 to 15 years ago. The JCAH added its support by expanding the definition and responsibilities of IC activities in its standards of 1976. The reason for an IC program can be quickly explained by reviewing the economic impact of nosocomial or hospital-related infections. Nosocomial infections are acquired by 2% to 15% of all inpatients. In the United States every year approximately 1.7 million hospitalized patients acquire an infection. If the average additional stay is 4 days at a cost of $600 per day, the annual costs would be 1 billion dollars.[3] In today's marketplace and with the limited resources available, this figure is staggering. Moreover, it does not include the additional potential losses due to malpractice liability suits or the sequelae associated with increased morbidity or mortality.

By definition, IC is a cluster of activities designed to minimize the frequency and optimize the management of hospital-related infections. The elements of a program include (1) policies and procedures pertaining to the detection and management of infections, (2) a comprehensive and concurrent screening system to promptly detect all deviations from defined levels of care, and (3) a response mechanism that concurrently corrects the problem by pattern analysis and provides feedback for the growth and development of the system.[4] To implement a successful IC program the strategies used must include scientific approach, research methodology, and rational procedures for planned change. The value of a central data base to identify, explore, and evaluate issues affecting patient care is clear.

Industry has successfully controlled liability for several decades through the use of procedures and techniques of RM. In health care facilities most proposals for designing RM programs are relatively new and have not been fully implemented or tested.

RM can be defined as the minimization of adverse effects of accidental loss at the least possible cost.[5] Ideally, the goal of an effective RM program is to identify all of the risks that an institution faces and to eliminate problems that may result in harm to the organization, its staff, and most important, its public. The obvious procedural steps are assessment, monitoring, and problem solving. From data gathered on a facility-wide basis, the specific functions of a RM program would include the following:

1. Identification and correction of problems in the delivery of care

2. Identification and correction of problems related to environmental safety

3. Identification and investigation of individual undesirable events

4. Claims management.[6]

In today's health care facilities it may seem difficult to justify the associated costs of developing a new program. However, it is not a question of developing a new program, but rather of changing the emphasis or reorganizing the existing activities. RM philosophy can be easily applied to existing functional elements. Most RM activities will fall within four basic categories: (1) prevention—any program or activity within the hospital that fosters and encourages personal as well as quality technical care; (2) correction—activities that not only remedy existing problem situations but seek out and solve hidden or potential problems; (3) documentation—activities used to review the documentation and quality of services provided; and (4) education—activities used to teach, maintain, and improve the quality of care delivered.[7]

The methodology used in all three specialties includes setting of standards via a system for sampling and data collection; procedures for validation of suspected problems, and a systematic approach to problem solving. Even though the functions of all three areas are similar, differences exist that are significant enough to preclude the collapse of one into the other. The primary focus and motivation of each department are different and each function demands expertise in separate areas. QA requires individuals with clinical expertise. IC requires individuals with expertise in epidemiology as well as infectious disease and clinical matters. RM requires individuals with managerial expertise. The overlap area is loss prevention and safety for visitors, employees, and patients. The purposes and functions are complementary to one another and an integrated approach may provide new solutions by establishing an optimal communication link.

The managerial incentives for developing an integrated system are threefold; professionalism or ethics, the safety or protection of visitors, employees, and patients, and efficiency or cost and resource conservation. An integrated system is illustrated in Fig. 28-1.

An integrated approach will (1) reinforce the importance of all three separate departments; (2) prevent duplication of efforts in collecting and analyzing data; (3) provide a systematic approach for problem verification, tracking of patterns and trends, following up on patient complaints, and preventing recurrences; (4) provide an opportunity to share resources such as legal, consultation, and data sources; (5) provide professional knowledge and

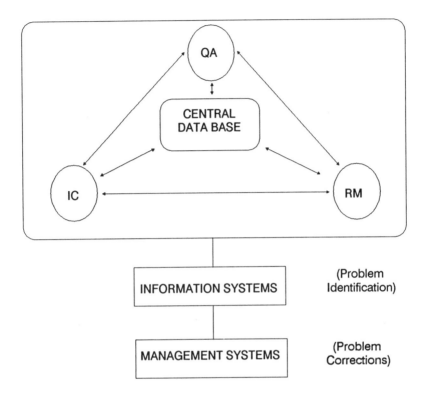

Figure 28-1. Integrated Systems Model.

skills to accomplish and influence behavior change; and (6) establish mechanisms whereby corrective actions can be made effective.

QA, IC, and RM, from a loss-prevention perspective, address the hospital's greatest risk—professional liability. The three departments cannot perform optimally alone. To realize their fullest potential they must develop in concert to provide maximum achievable health benefits in a safe environment and in the most cost-effective manner possible.

The health care delivery system is changing rapidly. The institutions of today are becoming more complicated, diversified, sophisticated, and dynamic. As resources become more scarce, each segment must tighten its belt and justify its existence. In today's arena, hospitals with programs that offer only paper compliance will not only be unable to justify their existence, but they will be financially destroyed. Risk is a potential in any hospital, and it is therefore vital to have a strong QA/IC/RM program to prevent loss of dollars and to properly care for patients.

Notes

1. Meisenheimer, C.: Incorporating JCAH standards into a quality assurance program. *Spring*, pp. 1-8, 1983.
2. Donaldson, M. and K. Keith: Planning for program effectiveness in quality assurance. *Evaluation and the Health Profession*, 6:233-244, 1983.
3. Daschner, F.D.: Practical aspects for cost reduction in hospital infection control. *Infect Control*, 5:32-35, 1984.
4. Fifer, W.: Infection control as a quality control in an integrated hospital quality assurance program. *Am J Infect Control*, 9:120-122, 1981.
5. Collins, P.: The integration of QA and risk management. *Tex Hosp*, May 1983, pp. 30-31.
6. Kessler, P. and J. Eric: *The risk management primer*. Chicago: Care Communications, Inc., 1981.
7. Brown, B.: Risk management. *Am J Infect Control*, 9:82-86, 1981.

29

Developing Patient Risk Profiles

Walter J. Jones, Buddy Nichols, and Astrid Smith

Walter J. Jones is Assistant Professor of Political Science, Memphis State University, and Director, Institute of Governmental Studies and Research, Memphis.

Buddy Nichols is President of United States Security Insurance Companies Group, Memphis.

Astrid Smith, R.N., is Risk Control Director, United States Security Insurance Companies, Memphis.

Today's hospital risk managers face many internal and external pressures demanding a reduction in claim costs. Adding to that pressure is the recent change in the reimbursement system for federally subsidized patients, which rewards hospitals that are cost efficient. Administrators may not consciously want to diminish the quality of care, but in their zeal to be more efficient, suboptimal care can be the result. Thus, the risk manager's job is to help increase efficiency while maintaining a high quality of patient care.

The job suggested is not an easy one. It requires a great deal of data collection and analysis, which in itself can be difficult. Hospital risk mangers have constantly struggled to find more quantitative methods of analyzing risk exposures. Generic screening of medical records, quality assurance methodologies, in addition to more conventional loss control techniques such as incident reporting forms and product safety committees have been utilized. But in the complex and highly professional world of medicine, none of these methods is free from a certain amount of criticism, suspicion, or outright rejection.

In particular, there has been a great deal of skepticism with regard to the incident reporting system in hospitals. The usual complaints center around the proposition that only minor incidents are documented on incident reporting forms while more severe incidents go unrecorded. It is our contention, however, that all incidents can be tabulated using the incident reporting

Printed by permission from *Risk Management,* 32(6) June 1985, pp. 28, 30, 32. Copyright 1985 by Risk Management Society Publishing, Inc. All rights reserved.

system if you include all sources of information in the report. These sources include telephone calls, on-site visits, and any other method you might use to find out about an incident. By using every credible method to gather information you can draw a more accurate picture of where your risk exposures lie.

The incident reporting system, however, is not the only method of risk reduction that should be utilized. Occurrence screening, safety committees, and all other strategies of risk reduction should be evaluated and, where applicable, implemented. Reliance upon one method as the sole approach to achieving risk control is in itself disastrous.

Patient Risk Profiles

Once sufficient information is collected, certain risk profiles can be developed. These profiles identify the individuals most susceptible to hospital mishaps and can be applied to newly admitted patients. Risk avoidance recommendations can then be provided to the patient care team (physicians, nurses, and ancillary staff) for implementation. If this basic risk control application effectively identifies and reduces risk, the profiles will necessarily change over time and be modified. This is an obvious manifestation of the dynamics of risk management.

A significant beginning in this area has been made with the first-phase completion of the Patient Risk Profile Research Project, carried out by U.S. Security Insurance Companies and Memphis State University. It involved an analysis of approximately 1,000 incident reports filed over a three-month period at a large metropolitan hospital in the Southeastern United States. All of the information provided in each report was coded and placed into the Memphis State University computer system. Various cross tabulation, correlation and regression analyses were then performed, and the statistical results assessed.

For the purpose of analysis, incidents were separated into two categories: regular and medication. Patient falls, treatment and testing errors, miscellaneous patient incidents, and incidents involving visitors were categorized as regular incidents. Medication incidents included wrong medications, wrong dosages, medication administered to the wrong patient, duplications, omissions, wrong routes and wrong rates. These data were related to more than a dozen independent variables, including patient sex, age, race, diagnostic category and medication number; and such nonpatient factors as incident time and location. A number of statistically and substantively significant results were obtained.

To begin with, we found that the age of a patient is the single most important determinant of incident involvement for both medication and regular incidents. Overall, only 36.3 percent of hospital patients were age 60 or older, but they were involved in 56.5 percent of regular and 55.1 percent of medication occurrences, as shown in Table 29-1. Obviously, as a higher proportion of

Table 29-1.

Age Group	% Total Patient Population	% Total Regular Incidents	% Total Medication
1−20	5.7%	3.7 %	2.4%
21−40	24.7	18.7	17.1
41−60	33.3	21.2	25.4
61−70	14.4	22.0	27.2
71−80	14.4	22.4	21.0
81 +	7.5	12.1	6.9
Total	100.0% (n = 189)	100.1% (n = 619)	100.0% (n = 350)

the American population enters the 60-and-older age category in coming decades, the need to intensify hospital supervision of this incident-prone group can only increase.

Measuring Diagnostic Status

The diagnostic status of a patient was also related to incident involvement. Individuals suffering from endocrine, nutritional or metabolic disorders were significantly overrepresented in both regular and medication incidents. These patients comprised only 1.6 percent of the total, but accounted for 5.7 percent of regular incidents and 6 percent of medication incidents. On the other hand, patients suffering from digestive disorders were underrepresented in the incident totals. These patients accounted for 10.3 percent of all patients but only 8.4 percent of regular and 6.9 percent of medication accidents.

People in some diagnostic categories were more likely to suffer from one type of incident rather than the other. For example, nervous disorder patients were disproportionately linked to regular incidents; they made up only 4.9 percent of the total patient population but accounted for 9.3 percent of the regular incident cases. Any useful predictive profile for incidents would have to include diagnostic status as an important factor.

A third variable that correlated to both regular and medication incidents was incident time. Almost 40 percent of all incidents took place from 6 a.m. to noon. In particular, the time period from 10 a.m. to 11 a.m. featured more medication incidents than any other one-hour interval, and almost twice as many regular incidents.

There were a number of important findings in the research project that pertained only to regular incidents. Patient falls were the most commonly reported regular incidents, representing 39.3 percent of the total. These occurred more frequently with patients who had less restrictive activity orders (that is, they had "up" privileges with or without assistance). Individuals were usually alone at the time the fall occurred.

Most strikingly, the age and medication number of the patients were strongly related to the type of regular incident occurring. The older the patient was, the more likely he or she was to become involved in a fall. Patients who received single or multiple medication also suffered a high proportion of falls, see Tables 29-2 and 29-3. Conversely, treatment and procedure incidents were more likely to transpire with younger, nonmedicated patients.

A somewhat different set of variables proved significant with respect to medication incidents. The largest contributing factor to all medication errors was the failure to follow hospital policies and procedures. The most common medication error was that of omitted medication, which accounted for 40 percent of these incidents. It should come as no surprise to find that the majority of medication incidents (52.7 percent) are multiple medication cases, which makes the frequency of medication omissions more understandable, though obviously still not acceptable.

More specifically, it was found that medication errors tend to come from a very small number of medication types. More than half (56.7 percent) of the incidents were produced by anti-infective, central nervous system (CNS), and electrolytic/caloric/water balance agents (see Table 29-4). Central nervous system drugs were usually linked to incidents of wrong medication or wrong dosage, while electrolytic, caloric, and water balance substances were more frequently involved in the wrong rate of intravenous administration.

Reducing the Risks

The above findings will be explored further and refined in the second phase of the research project. But how should hospital risk managers respond at this stage to information of this nature? We believe that there are several steps that can be taken to minimize the frequency of incidents, given the above analysis.

1. To begin with, it is important to communicate to physician, nursing and pharmacy staffs that there are positive relationships between a patient's age, multiple medications, and the time of day, with the likelihood that he or she will suffer a fall. Falls make up the largest number of hospital incidents. They are also potentially quite costly—physically to the patient and financially to the hospital. It is therefore necessary for risk managers to emphasize to hospital personnel that they must minimize the occurrence of falls through preventive measures and constant vigilance. In particular, it is important to stress the need for hospital personnel to be used as a deterrent to patient falls by providing assistance with walking.

2. In a related fashion, risk managers should urge hospital personnel to check patient rooms frequently and offer assistance, particularly during the high risk period of 6 a.m. to noon.

Table 29-2.

Incident Type	Patient Age					
	1–20	21–40	41–60	61–70	71–80	81+
Fall	33.3%	25.2%	25.0%	37.3%	59.4%	69.6%
Treatment	14.3	17.8	11.2	14.3	4.7	8.7
Procedure	19.0	26.2	22.4	15.1	10.9	8.7
Other	33.3	30.8	41.4	33.3	25.0	13.0
Total	99.9% (n=21)	100.0% (n=107)	100.0% (n=116)	100.0% (n=126)	100.0% (n=128)	100.0% (n=69)

Table 29-3.

	Medication Number		
Incident Type	**None**	**Single**	**Multiple**
Fall	26.8 %	64.6 %	66.1%
Treatment	13.6	1.5	7.9
Procedure	26.6	6.2	4.7
Other	33.0	27.7	21.3
Total	100.0 % (n=418)	100.0 % (n=65)	100.0 % (n=127)

Table 29-4.

Medication Type	% of Total Medication Incidents
Anti-Infective	18.7%
CNS	19.0
Electrolytic/Caloric/Water	19.0
Cardiovascular	11.4
Autonomic	3.5
Blood Form./Coagulants	4.4
Gastrointestinal	4.8
Hormones/Synthetic Subs.	9.2
Other	9.8
Total	100.0 % (n=315)

3. Hospital administrators and risk managers should work together to review current policies and procedures in medication administration so that they can determine their feasibility and applicability. The evidence collected indicates that many omissions and other classifications of medication incidents (particularly with multiple medication cases) could be avoided through better planning. Again, some additional preliminary efforts can eliminate much physical discomfort and financial expense.

4. Additionally, hospitals should encourage the utilization of controllers or volumetric pump devices in intravenous medication administration. This would insure more accurate rates of flow of intravenous therapy, thus further reducing the number of intravenous medication incidents.

The Patient Risk Profile Research Project is still incomplete, thus its findings will undoubtedly be expanded and refined in the coming months. In any event, enough has been done to help risk managers locate and identify risks so they can not only save money, but also improve the quality of patient care in the process.

30

PRO Objectives and Quality Criteria

Paul L. Grimaldi and Julie A. Micheletti

Paul L. Grimaldi, Ph.D., is Director, National Health Care Practice, Coopers and Lybrand, New York City.

Julie A. Micheletti, B.S., R.N., is Manager, National Health Care Practice, Coopers and Lybrand, New York City.

Under Medicare's prospective pricing system (PPS), peer review organizations (PROs) are required to determine whether hospitals comply with federal admission, procedure, and quality objectives. Although the presently contracted objectives may change, hospitals need to begin preparing for review now.

Each PRO's specific objectives are contained in its contract with the U.S. Department of Health and Human Services. The contract identifies the specific DRGs, diagnoses, procedures, and providers targeted for focused review. A hospital may obtain a copy of its PRO's contract from the PRO itself or from the federal government under the Freedom of Information Act.

Admission and Procedure Objectives

As federally required, the PROs will try to (1) reduce admissions for procedures that can be performed safely and effectively in an ambulatory surgical setting or on an outpatient basis, (2) reduce inappropriate or unnecessary admissions or invasive procedures for specific DRGs, and (3) reduce inappropriate or unnecessary admissions or invasive procedures by specific practitioners or hospitals.

Table 30-1 capsulizes selected admission and procedure objectives of PROs in California, Florida, and New York. As the table reveals, some of the specific objectives are similar. Differences in PROs' specified objectives may stem from the variance in perceived overutilization problems from state to state. Sometimes, the desired numerical reductions reflect the excess of state utilization rates over national averages or local use rates over state use rates. For example, based on findings for hospitals in two Florida counties, the PRO

Reprinted by permission from *Hospitals,* Vol. 59, No. 3, February 1, 1985, pages 64-67. Copyright 1986, American Hospital Publishing.

Table 30-1. Selected PRO Admission and Procedure Objectives.

Objective	California Medical Review, Inc.	Florida Professional Foundation for Health Care	New York Empire State Medical, Scientific, and Educational Foundation, Inc.*
Outpatient care	Reduce by 1,237 the number of unnecessary admissions for arthroscopy; reduce by 11,706 the number of colonoscopies and upper gastrointestinal endoscopies; reduce by 960 the number of dilatation and curettage procedures; reduce by 1,290 the number of breast biopsies; reduce by 1,033 the number of carpal tunnel release procedures; reduce by 229 the number of lymph node biopsies and excisions; reduce by 260 the number of bronchoscopies; reduce by 1,401 the number of cervix procedures; reduce by 27,544 the number of cataract extractions; reduce by 5,239 the number of inguinal hernia repairs.	Reduce by 51,064 the number of unnecessary admissions for DRG 39 (lens procedures) by concentrating on cataract removal, lens insertion, and lens replacement; reduce by 1,267 the number of unnecessary admissions for DRG 6 (carpal tunnel release) that can be performed on an outpatient basis; reduce by 2,023 the number of unnecessary admissions for DRG 225 (foot procedures) by focusing on tarsal tunnel release, bunionectomies, and other relevant procedures that can be performed on an outpatient basis.	Reduce by 7,460 the number of unnecessary admissions for 52 procedures such as septoplasty, packed cell transfusion and fiberoptic bronchoscopy that could be performed as outpatient procedures.
Specific DRGs	Reduce by 3,832 the number of medically unnecessary admissions for DRG 127 (heart failure and shock) and by 974 the number of medically unnecessary admissions for DRGs 89 and 90 (simple pneumonia and pleurisy with or without Age > 69 and/or CC).	Reduce by 2,216 the number of unnecessary intravenous pyelograms performed on patients with principal diagnosis of hypertension; reduce by 4,231 the number of nonindicated unnecessary thyroid scans and uptakes.	Objective is not applicable.

Table 30-1, continued.

Objective	California Medical Review, Inc.	Florida Professional Foundation for Health Care	New York Empire State Medical, Scientific, and Educational Foundation, Inc.*
Specific providers	Reduce by 678, 285 and 89 the number of inappropriate admissions in 3 specific hospitals; reduce by 15 the number of unnecessary chemonucleolysis procedures in one specified hospital; reduce from 1.75% to .4% the number of unnecessary short-stay admissions in 1 hospital; reduce by 14 the number of readmissions of patients with 6 or more admissions in 1 hospital.	Reduce by 9,607 the number of inappropriate or unnecessary admissions within defined DRGs in 24 hospitals where at least 20 percent of the admissions had an average stay significantly below average.	Reduce by 39,235 the number of selected one- and two-day stays that would not be expected to require hospitalization.

*Waivered state.

Source: Health Care Financing Administration and waivered states.

concluded that 51,064 lens procedures could be shifted to an outpatient setting. Similarly, hospitals, physicians, diagnoses, and procedures slated for intensified review may have utilization patterns that exceed state or national averages.

Because recent research suggests that a substantial proportion of surgery performed on an inpatient basis may be unnecessary or could be done in another setting, preadmission review will be a key PRO function. PROs have identified the types of Medicare patients earmarked for preadmission review. Hospitals must agree to such review subject to payment denials for inappropriate admissions.

Among the most popular procedures slated for a change from inpatient to outpatient settings are lens procedures (DRG 39), carpal tunnel release (DRG 6), and foot procedures (DRG 225). Inpatient surgical and invasive interventions that will be widely reviewed include herniorrhaphies, major joint procedures, hysterectomies, cholecystectomies, and esophagogastroduodenoscopies.

Some of the most common medical conditions to be scrutinized are back problems, chronic obstructive pulmonary disease, kidney or urinary tract infections, cerebrovascular disorders, and "suspect" diagnoses such as dehydration, epistaxis, and lumbosacral pain. In the case of medical back problems, certain PROs seem convinced that at least a few patients could be treated at home with bed rest until the definite need for inpatient hospitalization was established.

Quality Review

The federal government requires PROs to pursue the following five quality objectives:

- Reduce unnecessary readmissions due to substandard care during the prior admission
- Ensure the provision of medical services which, when not performed, have significant potential for causing serious patient complications
- Reduce avoidable deaths
- Reduce unnecessary surgery or other invasive procedures
- Reduce avoidable postoperative or other complications.

In many states, PROs are taking aim at acute myocardial infarction, coronary bypass graft surgery, aminoglycoside therapy, transurethral prostatectomy, and urinary tract infections.

However, variations abound (see Table 30-2). Florida's PRO, for example, wants to eliminate at least 90 percent of the unnecessary intravenous pyelograms performed on patients with a principal diagnosis of hypertension (DRG 134). New Mexico's PRO wants to *increase* by 50 percent the number of intravenous pyelograms performed for patients with a principal diagnosis of urinary tract infection (DRGs 320 to 322).

Criteria

The quality objectives are accompanied by treatment protocols that indicate the types of tests, procedures, or steps to be performed under certain circumstances (see Table 30-3). Some of these criteria may have been applied under professional standards review organization programs. The criteria, currently at various levels of specificity, are likely to change over time because of technological and treatment innovations. Many PROs may follow New Hampshire's lead; that state's PRO seeks hospital input when formulating quality criteria.

In some states, hospitals are required to develop PRO action plans to implement PRO policies. Oregon, for instance, requires hospitals to submit

Table 30-2. Selected PRO Quality Objectives.

Objective	California Medical Review, Inc.	Florida Professional Foundation for Health Care	New York Empire State Medical, Scientific, and Educational Foundation, Inc.*
Readmissions	Reduce by 2,010 the number of unnecessary readmissions within 7 days resulting from substandard care during the prior hospital admission.	Reduce by 1,049 the number of readmissions due to substandard care for patients undergoing a major joint procedure.	Reduce by 4,610 the number of unnecessary readmissions resulting from substandard care during the prior admission.
Under-utilized services	Assure the provision of medical services for diagnoses such as diabetes mellitus, chest pain, diarrhea, dehydration, and lower abdominal pain.	Improve preoperative care for patients undergoing a thoracotomy by increasing by 2,363 the times a diagnostic preoperative bronchoscopy is done.	Reduce by 9,244 the incidence of postoperative complications for elective surgical procedures due to the lack of preoperative services; reduce by 1,724 the mortality rate due to postoperative complications following elective surgical procedures.
Avoidable deaths	Reduce by 720 the number of avoidable deaths in instances where one of the following resuscitative procedures was performed: arterial puncture, Swan Ganz catheterization, tracheotomy or tracheostomy, endotracheal intubation, pulmonary wedge monitoring and cardiopulmonary resuscitation.	Reduce by 120 the number of avoidable deaths due to septicemia by improving compliance with developed criteria.	Reduce by 514 the number of avoidable deaths from pneumococcal, aspiration, or bacterial pneumonia.
Unnecessary surgery/ invasive procedures	Reduce by 3,721 the number of invasive procedures performed unnecessarily such as radical mastectomy, colonoscopy, and retrograde pyelography.	Reduce by 2,894 the number of contraindicated hemiorraphies in poor risk patients.	Reduce by 1,350 the incidence of unnecessary colonoscopies.

Table 30-2, continued.

Objective	California Medical Review, Inc.	Florida Professional Foundation for Health Care	New York Empire State Medical, Scientific, and Educational Foundation, Inc.*
Postoperative complications/ procedures	Reduce by 50 the number of cases where reoperation occurs within 72 hours.	Reduce by 2,708 the number of hospital-acquired urinary tract infections caused by urinary catheter insertion.	Reduce by 156 the incidence of avoidable pulmonary embolisms occurring as a postoperative complication for orthopedic procedures involving hip, femur, pelvis, or lower extremity joints; reduce by 50 the number of avoidable deaths due to the postoperative complication of pulmonary embolism for elective admissions.

*Waivered state.

Source: Health Care Financing Administration and PRO contracts.

written plans for the provision of physical therapy and diagnostic services for patients with hip fracture surgery. Hospitals with high mortality rates for elective aortocoronary bypass procedures in Arizona must develop a process to correct the problem. New Mexico's PRO requires that treatment plans for patients with decubitus ulcers be telephoned to the PRO within three days of admission.

Quality criteria for given conditions or procedures may vary among states due to differences in identified problems. Infection problems have been attributed to inadequate isolation practices (Nevada); inappropriate perioperative management and administration of prophylactic antibiotics (West Virginia); suboptimal compliance with urinary catheter procedures (Florida); and breach of infection control procedures in catheterization technique (Oregon).

As for aminoglycoside therapy, problems have been ascribed to insufficient lab monitoring (Georgia); insufficient renal function studies (Kansas); inadequate performance or peak and trough levels, infrequent BUN and creatinine levels, and improper monitoring of nephrotoxicity (Louisiana); and lack of physician understanding of the importance of effective medication levels and close monitoring (Utah).

Table 30-3. Quality Criteria for the Clinical Management of Pulmonary Embolism (New York PRO).

Objective: to reduce the incidence of pulmonary embolism as a postoperative complication following specified orthopedic procedures and to reduce avoidable deaths.

Preventive management. For patients defined as susceptible to pulmonary embolism, this includes at least one of the following:
- Aspirin, 10 grains p.o. q.d. or 300 mg. p.o. q.d. or greater
- Anticoagulant medication where baseline prothrombin time is below 16 or the activated PTT is less than 60mm Hg.
- Thromboembolitic stockings or ace wraps to lower extremities
- Elevation of lower extremities without popliteal pressure

Postoperative assessments. For patients recovering from specified orthopedic surgery, the following are required:
- Daily physician evaluation including patient interviews for complaints, chest examination, physician examination for symptoms of phlebitis or thrombophlebitis, review of vital signs, review of all lab values including all coagulation studies, and review of any radiology examinations
- Once per shift nursing evaluation for dyspnea, chest pain, hemoptysis, syncope, unexplained or sudden onset

of anxiety, calf tenderness or pain, edema or swelling of an extremity, positive Homan's sign, increased warmth of the calf to touch, and vital signs
- Documentation in the medical record of the physician's action plan if the physician is notified by nursing that questionable signs or symptoms exist

Suspect pulmonary embolism management protocols. The following are required if one or more abnormalities are evidenced:
- Chest x-ray
- Arterial blood gases
- Electrocardiogram
- Perfusion lung scan
- Pulmonary angiography (where indicated)

Discharge management. The procedures outlined below should be followed for patients who have had a postoperative pulmonary embolism:
- Medical record documentation that the patient is scheduled for a follow-up appointment
- Prescription for a supply of oral anticoagulant medication
- Medical record documentation of patient teaching regarding the use of the drug, its dangers, and that it should not be taken with vitamin K diet therapy or vitamin K supplement

Interdepartmental Cooperation

Hospital personnel must familiarize themselves with their PRO's review objectives and quality criteria. Close working relationships are imperative to ensure full compliance with the PRO's activities and to minimize its denials of Medicare payment.

Physicians, the admitting department, and surgical staff must know the types of Medicare patients designated for preadmission review and any criteria precisely defining whether surgery should be performed on an inpatient basis or on an outpatient basis (e.g., cataract surgery). The utilization review (UR) department should be notified promptly of these patients. The quality assurance department should be informed of situations where concurrent review is warranted.

Nurses, UR, and quality assurance should coordinate efforts to screen tests and procedures their PRO has cited to increase or decrease. For example, the nursing staff, pharmacy, and clinical laboratory need to integrate procedures to conduct accurate and expeditious drug level assays for aminoglycoside therapy patients.

Appropriate hospital committees should ascertain whether clinical management protocols for certain diseases or procedures need to be modified to satisfy PRO quality criteria. New standing orders may have to be developed. To treat patients with congestive heart failure, for instance, standing orders may be needed for electrolytes, chest x-rays, low-sodium or salt-free diets, and daily weights or accurate intake and output. In some cases, the nursing staff or emergency room physicians may need authority to generate orders and maintain the patient.

Documentation

It is essential that the performance and/or timing of tests, procedures, or services specified in PRO quality criteria be documented accurately and completely in the medical records. Medical records should contain information explaining why PRO criteria were not followed in certain instances. The hospital's quality assurance committee should be informed of general and specific situations where PRO criteria are inapplicable.

Physicians should document, *prior* to their occurrence, explicit reasons for surgical interventions that are subject to PRO retrospective review. Designated nurses could be given the responsibility of preauditing and documenting reasons for performing on an inpatient basis procedures targeted for outpatient settings. In all cases, physicians and medical record staff must be apprised of the exact information needed for PRO review.

To comply with PRO initiatives, medical record personnel may have to capture and code more information than is required for DRG assignment. The Minnesota PRO, for instance, requires certain hospitals to submit a complete list of all patients who receive hyperalimentation. Also, insofar as PROs (e.g., Wisconsin's) will review certain ICD-9-CM codes, physicians and medical record personnel must be aware that particular "nonspecific" diagnoses and codes may trigger a PRO review.

The medical record department may not in the past have collected some of the information PROs now will require for review purposes. This may have resulted in the PRO's baseline information exaggerating the type and extent of particular problems (e.g., not reporting intravenous pyelograms or thyroid scans). Corrective policies must be implemented and appropriate reporting forms revised or developed.

Malpractice

PRO review objectives and quality criteria seem to add new dimensions to the malpractice environment. First, the identification of the precise types of suspected medical practice problems may enable providers to develop more effective risk management and quality assurance programs. Second, quality criteria may be viewed as community medical standards against which *documented* treatment plans will be compared in order to evaluate the provider's culpability. The absence of PRO-required tests or timely services may help to resolve legal decisions in the plaintiff's favor.

Conclusion

The PRO program has the potential to introduce greater standardization into medical practice and to reduce the costs of overutilization. Effective hospital responses to the program will transform utilization review programs into utilization management programs. Medical staff support and involvement are essential for these programs to be successful.

Human Resources and Change

Selection 31, "Hospital Personnel Management in the Late 1980s: A Direction for the Future" by Stephen A. Robbins and Jonathon S. Rakich, traces the evolution of personnel administration in hospitals and offers a model for the future. The authors note a significant upgrading of the role, process, and influence of hospital human resource managers. In selection 32, "Hospital Union Election Activity 1974-85," written by Edmund R. Becker and Jonathon S. Rakich, union election activity by hospital ownership, size, geographic area, and type of union is discussed. The data indicate a substantial lessening of such activity in recent years.

Selection 33, "Adapting Theory Z to Nursing Management" by Marlene K. Strader, focuses on motivating nurses. Opportunities for achievement, recognition, and advancement are important. The author also advocates implementation of quality circles in nursing service as a means to facilitate collaborative and participative management. Selection 34, "Becoming a Healthcare Change Master," written by Rosabeth Moss Kanter, discusses forces of change external to the health care organization, the importance of capitalizing on the need to change, and how innovative organizations adapt.

335

31

Hospital Personnel Management in the Late 1980s: A Direction for the Future

Stephen A. Robbins and Jonathon S. Rakich

Stephen A. Robbins, M.B.A., J.D., is Director of Operations, Western Michigan Region, Sisters of Mercy Health Corporation, Lansing, Michigan.

Jonathon S. Rakich, Ph.D., is Professor of Management and Health Services Administration, The University of Akron, Ohio.

Introduction

A hospital's success is largely dependent on the quality and work efforts of its employees; therefore, the personnel administration function is critically important to the efficient and effective operations of such organizations. Yet, environmental forces affecting health services delivery are causing changes that will alter the personnel administration function in the future and the organization's view of its human resources.

The purpose of this article is to describe hospital personnel administration of the future, namely its approach, role, and process. To do so, personnel administration activities are categorized; the contemporary perspective toward human resources is described; and four models of hospital personnel administration are longitudinally presented, with the last—the matrix model—representing our view of the future, the late 1980s and early 1990s.

Hospital Personnel Management

Personnel management is composed of the wide range of activities, programs, and policies related to acquisition and retention of human resources in a hospital as well as their eventual exit from it. Conceptually, these activities can be viewed from a time flow incorporating multiple phases as shown in Fig. 31-1.

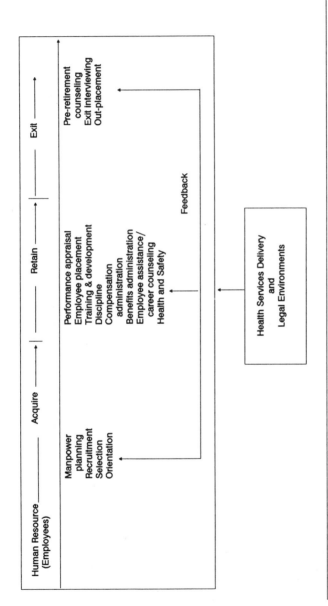

Figure 31-1. Hospital Personnel Management Activities.

Personnel management in hospitals is different today from twenty years ago, not only in terms of role and process but, more importantly, in terms of an approach and philosophy toward human resources. The evolution has not been smooth, but it has been progressive.

A Contemporary Perspective

Today, progressive hospitals embrace the "human resources perspective" that describes their approach to personnel management. This perspective embodies the following attributes:

- Employees are the principle component in accomplishing organizational objectives.

- An employee's value is measured not only in terms of the costs of employing them, but in terms of the investment in training and development and on-the-job experience.

- Organizations and employees have reciprocal obligations to and interest in each other; they both gain from these relationships.

- Employer and employee share goals that make for greater employee identification and involvement with the organization.

- There is a managerial attitude receptive to changing, modifying, and evolving organizational arrangements and job design to accommodate and capitalize on the interests and needs, abilities, and skills of employees, as opposed to force-fitting them into rigid structure/task slots.

- There is a permeating climate of mutual respect, positive interaction, and desire to improve organizational effectiveness and efficiency; that is, individual organizational work results by improving employee quality of work life.[1]

Models of Hospital Personnel Management

By examining the evolution of personnel administration in hospitals, it is possible to highlight implications of the human resources perspective as it exists now and to predict changes to come. To do so, four evolutionary models are presented. For the sake of convention and description, they are labeled the 1) personnel; 2) labor relations; 3) human resource; and 4) matrix models. Fig. 31-2 describes them and suggests time frames when each model was the prevailing trend.

Time	Pre-1965	About 1965-1975	About 1975-1985 (The present)	Post-1984 (The Future)
Attribute	*Simple Personnel Model*	*Labor Relations Model*	*Human Resource Model*	*Matrix Model*
Approach to personnel management	Benign neglect Indifference	Containment of external forces	Human resources perspective (emphasis on people as the most important resource)	Modified human resources perspective
Role	Record keeping	Cope	Intervention (for change)	Intervention (for organizational survival)
Process	Simple functional (not integrated)	Fully-functional	Integrative functional	Creative functional
Organizational philosophy about employees	Neutral (employees are just another resource)	Conflict and confrontation	Collaborative-cooperative (organization and employees have mutual interests)	C o m p e Participative i t i v e
Predominant strategy	Inactive compliance	Reactive	Proactive	Innovative
Influence on organizational policy	Minimal	Increasing	Enhanced	Greater
Acceptance by managers and staff	Minimal	Necessary	Enhanced	Greater

Figure 31-2. Hospital Personnel Management Models.

Simple Personnel Model (pre-1965)

The unsophisticated and uncomplicated pre-1965 personnel model reflected its environment. In many respects the need for an activist, influential personnel administration department did not exist, certainly not to the degree it does today. The pre-Medicare 1965 environment was stable; there was relatively abundant manpower and few cost pressures.

Until demand for health services fundamentally changed in the mid-1960s, many hospitals had rudimentary personnel systems and paid relatively low wages. There was little or no attention given to the impact of organizational structure and work systems design on employees. Performance appraisal systems, job descriptions, and job specifications were archaic, seldom updated, and often not based on systematic job evaluation. Compensation systems were rudimentary, perhaps arbitrary, and at times inconsistent. As a result, inconsistencies existed among departments, and wages were set on the basis of a perception of relationships between jobs (or, even worse, political power).

Training and development programs, although present, focused primarily on job-oriented skills rather than on the development of individuals. Recruitment and selection activities were *ad hoc* and relatively unsophisticated before enactment of equal employment opportunity and other nondiscrimination legislation.

As the model shows, the predominant strategy of personnel departments during the era was inactive compliance. Personnel managers were neither activists nor innovators. Their role was simply record keeping, and the approach to personnel administration was benign neglect or indifference.

Labor Relations Model (About 1965-1975)

The late 1960s and early 1970s were turbulent years for hospitals in general and personnel management departments in particular. Among the external influences affecting personnel administration in hospitals were:

- Enactment of Medicare and Medicaid programs (1965) and a resultant increase in demand for services. Hospitals responded by increasing the number of employees. Improved personnel record systems were necessary for purposes of cost allocation and reimbursement.

- Application in 1967 of federal minimum wage laws and overtime to hospitals affected wage administration systems.

- Enactment of the 1964 Civil Rights Act mandated equal employment opportunity and had a significant effect on selection, testing, performance appraisal, promotion, demotion, equal pay for equal work, and nondiscrimination in matters of employment.

- Enactment of other federal legislation such as OSHA forced attention on safety in the work environment, and ERISA in 1974 affected benefits administration.

- In the late 1960s and early 1970s, hospitals fell victim to market forces as certain categories of trained manpower became scarce, particularly RNs and technologists. With the boom in technology, specialized and more skilled personnel were required. Therefore, manpower planning, recruitment, compensation, and training and development activities were affected. Inflation, increased demands for services, and technological advances gave impetus to rising healthcare expenditures that resulted in voluntary and imposed efforts to contain manpower costs.

- Increased unionization in hospitals began in the late 1960s and was supported with passage of the 1974 Hospital Amendments to the Taft-Hartley Act. As unions focused organizing efforts on hospitals, labor relations became a dominant theme.

The effect of all these external changed was to increase the importance of personnel administration in hospitals and force upgrading of programs and systems.

The perceived threat of unionization of hospitals or its actuality permeated the era. This led to two outcomes. First, organizational acceptance of centralized personnel administration was viewed as necessary, thus increasing its influence on organization policy. Second, the organizational philosophy regarding employees turned from neutrality to one in which the underlying theme was conflict and confrontation.

During the era of the labor relations model, the character of the personnel administration department changed significantly. Departmental professionalism was upgraded, programs were expanded, and influence on organizational policy was increased. It became evident that systematic and well-designed programs for acquiring and retaining employees were necessary. This evolution was driven by reaction to external influences and events, and the approach was basically containment of them.

Human Resource Model (1975-1985): The Present

For the preponderance of hospitals, the human resource model describes the present. For a select few—those in transition to the matrix model—it represents the immediate past. All the same factors and environmental forces that led to evolution of the labor relations model also facilitated development of the human resource model. In the mid to late 1970s it became evident to managers that the adversary, conflict, containment, and reactive attributes of the labor relations model were inappropriate. Furthermore, the intensification of cost pressures, the reality of resource constraints, and the increase of federal intervention forced managers to focus attention on more effective utilization of existing human and other resources. As a result, progressive hospitals began to recognize the importance of their employees.

Embodied within this concept is the human resources perspective. The role is one of interventionist, with personnel administration responsible for initiating and facilitating organizational change throughout the hospital, not only focusing on acquisition and retention activities. While the generic scope of acquisition and retention activities was part of the fully-functional labor relations model, such activities were often mechanical, reactively set in place with little thought for a synergistic, organization-wide outcome and direct relationship to organizational goals.

The human resource model goes beyond this. In terms of process, it seeks to integrate the fully-functional manpower acquisition and retention activities with the structure-tasks-people components of the hospital to yield a particular organizational climate.

Other attributes of the model include an organizational philosophy based on a collaborative and cooperative relationship between management and employees in contrast to the conflict and adversary relationship in the labor relations model. The predominant strategy is proactive to serve as an impetus for organizational change. Finally, personnel administration in this model has experienced enhanced influence on organizational policy and acceptance by other organizational components.

Thus, the human resource department is instrumental and proactive in monitoring and improving the employment climate. This includes employee needs assessment, attitude surveys, and identifying employee satisfaction and dissatisfaction (assessing morale). Interventions to change structure and task design occur so that quality of work life is improved and that more effective resource utilization results, giving both the employee and the organization a chance to accomplish objectives together.

Performance appraisal systems yield information for compensation changes. These systems are also integrated with programs of positive behavior modification to improve employee performance. Training and development not only focus on skills enhancement and technological upgrading but also on addressing social skills such as coping with a job, reducing stress, and fostering interpersonal relationships.

Career counseling based on aptitude and interest assessment is performed to enable people to develop to their fullest potential. While the payback to the organization may not seem tangible, this activity provides an important safety valve to the frustrated or unhappy employee. It also serves long-range manpower planning by upgrading employees' skills in areas in which manpower is in short supply, builds loyalty to the hospital because those helped tend to have a sense of obligation to the organization, and demonstrates to others the philosophy that employees are valued and respected as individuals with individual needs.

Integrated with other retention activities are employee assistance programs designed to preserve and, if necessary, salvage human resources.

The direct and indirect costs of alcoholism and drug abuse in lost time, low productivity, and human wreckage are staggering. Providing treatment without recrimination to the employee who comes forward seeking help makes sense from the human resources perspective. Corollary programs include marital and financial counseling and health awareness and fitness. They are good investments in the organization's human resources.

As suggested earlier, programs consistent with the human resources perspective reflect the culmination of societal value changes throughout the 1960s and 1970s. However, to state that changing values alone explain the motivation behind this evolution ignores the fact that hospitals must recognize basic positive financial implications of their actions.

There is a realization that quality, quantity, and cost of human resources have a significant impact on the hospital's financial viability. Hence, productivity underlies the increased attention paid to the people component of hospitals. It is believed that through collaborative and cooperative efforts, the hospital's goals can be achieved while currently recognizing the needs, values, and aspirations of employees.

Matrix Model (post-1985): The Future

Health services delivery is presently in transition. It is undergoing traumatic change, the scope of which has not been seen since the enactment of Medicare and Medicaid in 1965. A culmination of forces ranging from federal policy initiatives to corporate and other client activism set in place in the early 1980s is beginning to substantially alter the system. The result is that personnel administration is now evolving out of the human resource model into a new era.

In the healthcare industry, today's predominant theme is survival and growth in a hostile, market-driven environment. Characteristics of this new environment include:

- The partial dismantling of federal regulation and active encouragement of a pro-competitive environment.

- Emergence and growth of alternate forms of delivery and organizations such as HMOs; nontraditional competitors such as emergicenters, surgi-centers, and preferred provider organizations; and growth of multi-institutional arrangements among both not-for-profit and for-profit hospitals.

- Increasing cost consciousness and activism by consumers, third-party payors, and large employers, the latter having formed coalitions to enhance their market power vis-á-vis hospitals.

- Changing beneficiary financial obligations with increases in copayments and deductibles, both of which alter health service consumption patterns.

- Medicare's fundamental, revolutionary alteration to the third-party payor reimbursement system in which reimbursement to hospitals is shifting to one increasingly output based, regardless of inputs consumed. As other third-party payors adopt fixed output-based pricing (i.e., DRGs), hospitals will be at greater risk.

The effect of all of these changes leads to two outcomes. First, revenue constraints require hospitals to emphasize productivity improvement. Second, there is increased risk. Hospitals that do not adjust to the new environment are unlikely to survive in their present configuration, if at all. These two outcomes are working to materially affect personnel administration for the future.

Whatever plans a hospital adopts to respond to these changes in the environment, senior management must study the state of its own personnel function and its current philosophy to determine if the department is prepared to fulfill its part in supporting the plans. While the matrix personnel function is designed for this purpose, a personnel department operating at a lower end of the development line can be either a hindrance to success or an outright barrier to change.

We have certainly seen a parallel in other industries where productivity gains, adaptation to new technology, and changes in job structure were necessary for survival, but the human resources function and philosophy were inadequately developed to facilitate the change. From autos to steel, meat packing to the airlines, the typical scenario is one where a troubled management has to respond quickly, then attempts to work with the employees, fails, dictates to the employees, fails, and finally reduces the scope of operations, pulls out of an area, closes facilities, or goes bankrupt.

Eleventh-hour attempts to upgrade the human resources function are generally unsuccessful. When done under the pressure of an emergency, there is understandable skepticism, resistance, and resentment on the part of the employees.

Hospitals are not in a position to relocate their operations the way a manufacturing plant can. The alternative for a hospital is failure. Thus, it is even more critical that today's hospital be proactive in positioning its human resources department to adapt to this new environment.

The new model of personnel administration that is envisioned is labeled the matrix model. As presented in Fig. 31-2, the matrix model incorporates many of the attributes of the human resource model, yet blends in these risk-survival factors. Its approach will be a modified human resources perspective providing a base on which a participative-competitive organization philosophy about employees is overlaid.

The key evolutionary differences between the matrix model and the human resources model stem from the need to deal with the risk-survival issues. In multihospital settings this means the creation of a new corporate level human resources office with responsibilities to coordinate and direct the overall program as a matrix responsibility to the hospital. As policies, benefits and wage systems become more centralized and standardized, their impact will be greater and therefore a new attention to quality will result in an overall upgrading of the entire human resource function.

This should also bring about cost savings through such obvious outcomes as the ability to be more sophisticated and efficient in benefits administration, larger self-insurance pools, or the enhanced economic clout in buying insurance coverage. In addition, more cost savings from uniform and effective organizational policies will result.

Another marked difference in structure will involve the human resource department assuming a role in productivity enhancement. The matrix department will be called on for advice and support in changing work methods, standards, and staffing practices. In larger hospitals management engineering may fall under the human resources department as a logical extension of its matrix role.

We believe that the emphasis will always be on people as the most important resource, but it will be affected by the predominant criterion of productivity improvement. To the extent that the human resources perspective yields improvements in productivity, it will be embraced and maintained. However, its emphasis will erode—become modified—if and when organizational survival becomes paramount.

The organizational philosophy about employees will become increasingly participative, yet competitive. Employees will have opportunities to participate in organizational and work systems design, to the extent that results lead to productivity improvement; they will participate in the fruits of such efforts, perhaps through incentive programs. Concurrently employees will also be at risk in terms of employment security as hospitals alter their character to cope with competition.

Hospitals that are successful in these efforts will be ones that are able to rechannel displaced employees. Elements of this may include active intrusion into new markets with programs requiring differing human resource skills; retrenchment of existing programs and services (and thus, personnel) to survive the onslaught of aggressive competition and sustain the organization; corporate reorganizations; and joining with other organizations via such means as merger or acquisition in which the autonomy of the hospital may or may not be retained. All of these scenarios will change personnel administration.

The matrix model will have to function under multiple modes: a single hospital setting that may be expanding or contracting or a multi-institutional arrangement in which activities will be centralized beyond the single institutional level. In all cases, the role will be interventionist with the purpose of designing and implementing programs to ensure organizational survival. The process will be creative—functional—and will incorporate the integrative aspects of the human resource model in ways not previously considered. For example, employee piecework and incentive systems may be instituted in production type departments, lessened job security may be partially mitigated by bonus and stock option programs, and transfers of personnel among member facilities of multi-institutional systems may be commonplace.

The predominant strategy will incorporate the proactive character of the human resource model, but it will also have to be innovative. The risk-survival issues caused by the wrenching change in this turbulent environment will raise employees' apprehensions and fears. Innovative methods for design and integration of personnel administration acquisition and retention programs will be required to overcome both.

Through the 1980s and into the 1990s, the influence of personnel administration on organizational policy is expected to increase, with that manager's authority and responsibility even greater than in the human resource model. The emphasis on productivity improvement as a survival strategy must primarily focus on the hospital's human resources because personnel expenditures account for a majority of hospital operating costs. Similarly, the acceptance of personnel administration by other managers and staff is expected to be even greater, significantly more than the enhanced acceptance under the human resource model.

Future Trends

The matrix model of hospital personnel administration is a derivation of the human resource model. Its base is the human resources perspective, which is conditioned, modified, and limited by productivity improvement considerations. On top of this base is the participative-competitive organizational philosophy attribute that is inherent in the risk-survival environment.

Some hospitals—particularly for-profit, multi-institutional chains—can be currently described as moving toward this model. In fact one reason we have termed our model a matrix comes not only from the diverse factors affecting it but because of its multiple reporting relationships in the multihospital system which will dominate healthcare in the future. The matrix model human resources function will have accountabilities to both its individual institution and its corporate parent. Since the matrix model is the view of the future (1985 and beyond), it is useful to present a potpourri of future trends that are envisioned as likely to occur.

Acquisition and Manpower Utilization

There will be changes in the marketplace of labor. With manpower shortages in the health services field having already virtually disappeared (at least for the foreseeable future), hospitals will be relating to the labor market accordingly. The inference is that employee concerns about job security will increase while supply of labor and other resources adjust to the diminished demand caused by the continued expansion of prospective pricing and competition.

Employers are likely to increase the mix of part-time, temporary, and on-call employees in order to "swing" labor with demand. This may have a negative impact on the collaborative-cooperative character of the human resources perspective and organizational commitment by employees.

As multi-institutional systems grow and capture several facilities in single geographic areas, a new labor force will appear that works for the corporate parent and that can be shifted between the parent's various facilities in a given geographic market. This will facilitate a trend toward standardization among a "multi" group, less loyalty to one specific facility, increased identification with the corporate parent, and cost-effective utilization of manpower not previously achievable.

Through the 1960s and 1970s, hospitals experienced increasing specialization of their labor forces. This led to inefficiencies incompatible with the new marketplace. A trend reversing this specialization is likely beginning in the technical area. For example, "super techs" may be cross-trained to perform EKGs, EEGs, echocardiograms, and ultrasounds, etc., resulting in a smaller force of more widely trained, flexible technicians. In some instances, RNs will be picking up some of these duties on the floor. The encroachment will be followed in nontechnical areas also; but, where unions are in place, it will meet with significant resistance. Some breakdown of licensure barriers is foreseen, especially with regard to an erosion of nurse and physician practice acts nationwide.

The Link to Personnel Management

The issue of productivity in health services is expected to play a major role in developing and shaping personnel management. To date, they have not been closely linked, but this will change. Management engineering will be merged into personnel administration's acquisition and retention programs. The outcome will be a more technically oriented and capable, more powerful role for personnel administration. It will oversee the use and application of labor resources in a similar manner to the way the director of finance oversees the application and use of funds. As an offshoot, computer systems will support this activity and grow in usage. Data bases that are now dispersed and nonintegrated will have to be emerged.

Retention

There will be changes in compensation systems. A combination of scarce labor supply and high inflation caused automatic, across-the-board increases to drive the hospital wage system of the 1960s and 1970s. This trend for the moment has stopped; however, it is believed that even if appreciable inflation re-emerges, other factors will prevent widespread cost-of-living increases from once more becoming part of hospital wage practices.

This new environment includes the change in the supply of labor (catching up and surpassing demand), cost-containment pressure, increasing sophistication of hospital compensation systems, and the fact that the prior movement was fueled by the overall low levels of compensation in healthcare. Today, for example, most housekeepers are better paid in hospitals than their hotel/motel counterparts.

Many hospitals will implement innovative appraisal and incentive compensation systems. Productivity improvement will be the driving force. In investor-owned (for-profit) hospitals, stock options, bonuses, and profit sharing are emerging as strategies to reward senior management. This trend is expected to continue to grow, perhaps spreading in some derivative form to other employees and to not-for-profit hospitals. As employees assume some of the share of risk, so too will they correspondingly share in the gain.

Consolidations Will Affect Personnel Management

A major change will be centralization of the personnel function into a new matrix hierarchy. It will be staffed by highly talented professionals and technocrats responsible for overseeing the operation of several hospital personnel management departments. Policies and practices will be set at a higher organizational level, resulting in greater standardization of acquisition and retention activities along with enhanced effectiveness among subsidiary hospitals.

A second implication is that career paths for a large number of professional and managerial employees (and personnel managers in particular) will be possible within one large organization composed of subsidiary entities. In the past, managerial promotion possibilities were relatively limited in single, stand-alone hospitals. A move up often meant a move out.

Now, promotions and transfers will be encouraged and supported by corporate style career pathing methods. This will also tend to build a corporate culture and identification new to health services delivery. Major corporate entities will be able to support innovative, long-term developmental programs such as the "corporate college" concept already in place in several of the major hospital chains. It will not be unusual to have middle and senior managers transferred among subsidiaries, as is done in the industrial sector.

Labor Relations/EEO: Important, But Not Dominant

No reversal is seen in the trend toward less labor relations activities. Unions grew strong quickly in hospitals, but they have become less and less of a factor and will continue to diminish in importance. For unionized hospitals threatened with survival, givebacks and a greater flexibility in work practices are likely to occur. Unions that do survive and prosper will have to take a posture of working closely with management to allow cost- and market-competitive advantages to occur.

This will mean a major reorientation for unions, and many of them may leave the healthcare field. Multi-institutional systems are unlikely to acquire or affiliate with hospitals that have union problems; therefore, access to capital will become a problem for these institutions, multiplying the changes for their failure and increasing the need to stay union-free.

EEO, affirmative action, and other similar programs have reached a mature state; while their influence will remain strong, growth is not expected. There are some advocates for expansion of the laws, but their influence is limited and their chance of effecting change small. Issues such as sexual preference and comparable worth will lead attempts at any new developments, but any new law (legislation or case law) will be so diluted that it will have minimal impact.

Physician-Hospital Relationships Will Change

In the early 1990s, a totally new phenomenon will revolutionize the hospital structure. Due to the oversupply of physicians and the squeeze placed on their incomes, more and more of them will seek refuge in closer affiliations with hospitals. As physicians' dependence on hospitals grows, their influence on the system will decrease; large numbers of them will become employees.

Physicians are now still largely treated as members of an outside body of "the medical staff " and come under the purview of the hospital CEO for some purposes while acting as independent members of the medical staff for others, such as professional activities. Their relationship with the personnel administration department is usually nonexistent. This will change. It is expected that the hospital's control and influence over physicians will grow, with personnel administration taking a major role in acquisition and retention of them.

Conclusion

Productivity improvement and concern about resource allocation and use are increasingly becoming a part of hospital managers' psyches; the present hostile and competitive environment requires it. Soon it will be indelibly etched on a whole generation of hospital managers; there will be a long-lasting residual effect. However, care must be exercised not to totally discard the human resources perspective in favor of one antithetical to it. To do so would ignore the fact that employees are a hospital's most important asset.

We believe the matrix model represents a posture which addresses the dilemma. It acknowledges the risk-survival attributes of the present health services environment. The human resources perspective can be retained as long as the underlying theme is productivity improvement through employees, not the abuse of them. Similarly, if employees are to share some of the competitive risk, they should also have opportunities for greater participation in organizational and work systems design. To the extent that they positively contribute to the accomplishment of the hospital's goals, so should they participate in the fruits of such efforts.

Note

1. Jonathon S. Rakich, Beaufort B. Longest, Jr., and Kurt Darr, *Managing Health Services Organizations* (Philadelphia, PA: W.B. Saunders Co., 1985), pp. 428-429.

32

Hospital Union Election Activity 1974-85

Edmund R. Becker and Jonathon S. Rakich

Edmund R. Becker, Ph.D., is Project Director and Research Associate, Department of Health Policy and Management, School of Public Health, Harvard University, Cambridge.

Jonathon S. Rakich, Ph.D., is Professor of Management and Health Services Administration, The University of Akron, Ohio.

Introduction

With the enactment of the Nonprofit Hospital Amendments to the Taft-Hartley Act (THA) in August 1974, Congress brought the nation's private (nongovernmental), nonprofit hospitals under the jurisdiction of the National Labor Relations Board (NLRB). This action affected more than 1.5 million hospital employees in more than half the nation's 7,000 hospitals that were not previously covered under any federal labor legislation. Several studies have explored the impact of union election activity in the hospital industry during the 1970s (Adamache and Sloan 1982), but relatively little work has been done to provide an overview of union election activity in the 1980s. This study seeks to fill this gap by analyzing NLRB *Monthly Election Reports* for the health care industry for a 65-month period January 1980 through May 1985. Combining this election information with data on hospital characteristics from the 1984 American Hospital Association (AHA) Annual Survey of Hospitals, this study gives a summary of union activity in the hospital industry for the first half of the 1980s. In addition, this investigation combines the recent data with earlier work on union activity that appeared in the *Health Care Financing Review* and summarized union election activity from NLRB *Monthly Election Reports* and AHA data for the 65-month period August

An earlier version of this paper was presented at the Midwest Decision Sciences Institute Meeting April 24, 1986. The research for the 1974-79 period was covered in part by Grant No. 18-P-97090/4 from the Health Care Financing Administration. The opinions expressed are those of the authors and do not necessarily reflect the opinions of the Health Care Financing Administration.

Reprinted from *Health Care Financing Review*, Vol. 9, No. 3, Spring 1988.

1974 through December 1979 (Becker, Sloan, and Steinwald 1982). Together these two studies give a comprehensive overview of union election activity in the hospital industry from 1974 to 1985.

The analysis begins with a brief background on the history of labor law and the hospital industry. Then the NLRB election results from 1974 through 1979 are summarized. Election information for hospitals and area characteristics for the 1980-85 period are analyzed and compared with the 1974-79 period. Union and election characteristics are similarly compared, and union elections and victories are examined by period and year. Finally, the summary and conclusions are presented.

Background

The Wagner Act of 1935, also known as the National Labor Relations Act (NLRA) implemented landmark federal legislation that protected the worker's right to organize and collectively negotiate with employers. It is the major federal statute governing labor relations in the United States. The NLRA outlined employers' responsibilities and rights in the bargaining process. For example, the NLRA identified unfair labor practices (i.e., interference, coercion, discrimination against union members, not bargaining in good faith) and specified the general nature of how the employers should interact with union representatives once the union was recognized. In addition, the NLRA established the National Labor Relations Board (NLRB) and provided the NLRB with broad powers to oversee the nation's union election activities and resolve unfair labor practices. The NLRA initially included all private hospitals, both nonprofit and profit. Government hospitals, however, were excluded.

In effect, many have argued that passage of the NLRA signaled a fundamental change in public policy and, consequently, power relations in the workplace. Furthermore, the NLRA gave government, as a regulator, a direct role in labor relations (Begin and Beal 1985).

In 1947, the NLRA was amended by the Taft-Hartley Act (THA) to redress imbalances in the original legislation. While reaffirming the original intentions of the NLRA and the rights of employees to organize, THA identified unfair labor practices on the part of employees and expanded the role of the NLRB to cover these activities. THA also elaborated on the nature and composition of the bargaining unit. For example, some of the provisions in THA specify that supervisors cannot be part of the bargaining unit, security guards must be in separate bargaining units, professional and nonprofessional workers should generally not be combined in the same bargaining unit, and a 60-day notice of the contract termination or modification must be given by the parties involved.[1]

One provision in the THA (Section 2.2), however, specifically excluded from its definition of employer " . . . . any corporation or association operating a hospital if no part of the net earnings inures to the benefit of any private shareholder or individual. . . ." (Rakich, Longest, and Darr 1985). Also excluded in this section of THA were any government-owned corporations. As a result, most of the nation's hospitals were now excluded from coverage by the NLRA, and only proprietary hospitals remained covered by THA. Nevertheless, at the NLRB's discretion, jurisdiction was not extended to proprietary hospital employees under THA until 1967 (National Labor Relations Board 1978).

NLRA coverage was modified in 1962 when President Kennedy signed Executive Order 10988 authorizing collective bargaining in the federal services. Federal hospitals were now afforded protection by labor law regulation. In return for the right to organize, federal hospital bargaining units established under E.O. 10988 must agree not to strike. However, nonprofit and government hospitals were still not covered by any federal legislation. With the enactment of the Nonprofit Hospital Amendments to the Taft-Hartley Act, also known as the National Labor Relations Act NLRA, in August 1974, Congress finally brought the nation's private (nongovernmental), nonprofit hospitals back under the jurisdiction of the National Labor Relations Board.

When private, nonprofit hospitals were excluded from NLRA coverage in 1947, states were free to fill the legislative vacuum. However, most states opted not to take a position. By 1974, only 12 states had enacted laws to regulate hospital union activity.[2] Moreover, the provisions and coverage for union activity in these states varied considerably. As a result, the vast majority of hospital health care employees were not covered by the NLRA until the 1974 legislation (U.S. Department of Labor 1979).

Since these changes in 1974, health care analysts and policymakers have focused considerable attention on the health care industry in an effort to understand how union election activity will influence the delivery and costs of health care (Becker, Sloan, and Steinwald 1982). Although evidence indicated that only 27.4 percent of all U.S. hospitals were unionized in 1980 (Beker, Sloan, and Steinwald 1982), one study predicted that by 1990, 65 percent of the nation's hospitals would have a signed union contract (Feldman, Lee, and Hoffbeck 1980). If correct, this increase could have a dramatic impact on hospital costs that for fiscal year 1984 exceeded $160 billion (Levitt, et al. 1985) and are projected to exceed $213 billion by 1988 (Arnett, et al., 1986). Sloan and Steinwald (1980), for example, found that a hospital that acquired an active union (one willing to strike or engage in other job actions) reported short-run labor costs 12 to 15 percent higher than those hospitals without an active union. Given that, in general, labor costs constitute 55 percent of a hospital's total budget,[3] the consequences of increased unionization in the hospital industry could be significant. But how have the unions fared since the passage of the 1974 amendments?

Union Election Results: 1974-79

In an earlier study, Becker, Sloan, and Steinwald (1982) found that 16.2 percent of U.S. nongovernment hospitals had elections during the period August 1974 through December 1979. Of these elections, unions won 48.6

percent. Seventy-one percent of the 1,025 elections occurred in three of the nine U.S. Census Divisions: Mid-Atlantic, East North Central, and Pacific, with these three census divisions representing 70.7 percent of the 498 union victories in the period.

Other findings from the earlier study can be summarized as follows:

- For-profit hospitals had the lowest percentage of union elections (8.6 percent) among the various forms of hospital ownership, but exhibited the highest union victory rate (57.0 percent).

- The percentage of hospitals with an election increased with hospital bed size. Elections increased from a low of 7.8 percent for hospitals with a bed size of less than 100 beds to a high of 33.0 percent, for hospitals with more than 400 beds.

- Unions had lower victory rates (32.0 percent) in right-to-work states[4] and higher victory rates (56.3 percent) in states where employees had been offered state protection prior to the 1974 changes to Taft-Hartley.

- Of the various employee organizations, independent unions and the Service Employees International Union were involved in the highest percentage of union elections (52.0 percent) between 1974 and 1979 with the independent unions winning the largest percentage of elections, 61.7 percent.

- Professional and/or technical unions were involved in the largest number of elections, 43.9 percent, and had a win rate of 57.1 percent. Departmental unions had the highest win rate (69.2 percent), and the combined professional and office unions had the lowest (33.3 percent).

- Finally, there was a short-lived spurt in hospital union election activity immediately after the 1974 amendments were enacted. The number of elections peaked in 1977 at 237 elections and fell to 145 elections in 1979. In absolute numbers, union victories peaked with 113 victories in 1975, or 22.7 percent of all the victories for the 1974-79 period. The number of victories fell to 70 in 1979, or 14.1 percent of the victories for the 1974-79 period.

Union Elections Results: 1974-85

Hospital and Area Characteristics

Union election results for the two 65-month time periods, August 1974 through December 1979 and January 1980 through May 1985, are shown in Tables 32-1 through 32-3. Data are presented on elections and election outcomes and include only nongovernmental hospitals, because government hospitals are not covered by the NLRA. Observational units are the hospital in Table 32-1, and the election in Table 32-2, and elections by year in Table 32-3. A total of 1,025 elections in 556 hospitals were reported for the 65-month period 1974-79 and 834 elections in 537 hospitals were reported for the 65-month period 1980-85.

As shown in Table 32-1, 12.8 percent of nongovernment hospitals had an election during the January 1980 through May 1985 period. This is down slightly from the 16.2 percent during the 1974-79 period. Of the 834 elections, unions won 47.6 percent. This is almost identical to the earlier rate of 48.6 percent for the 1974-79 period.

The census regions with the highest number of elections during the 1980-85 period were, in rank order, the Mid-Atlantic (303), Pacific (152), East North Central (131), and New England (92) census regions. These regions accounted for 81.3 percent of all elections during the period and 81.9 percent of all union victories. When compared with the 1974-79 period, the percent of victories to elections fell in all census areas except the Pacific and the West South Central census region where it rose from 48.5 to 52.6 and 22.2 to 50.0 percent, respectively. It should be noted that the sizable increase in the West South Central census region represents victories in only three of six hospital elections.

For the 1980-85 period, nonprofit, nonreligious hospitals were the most likely to experience an election (15.3 percent) and also the type of hospital ownership where the unions were most likely to win (49.9 percent). In both periods studied, for-profit hospitals still were the least likely among the various forms of hospital ownership to experience a union election (8.6 percent in 1974-79 and 6.4 percent in 1980-85). However, in contrast to the earlier evidence from the 1974-79 period that showed union success to be highest in for-profit hospitals (57.0 percent), it fell appreciably in the 1980-85 period to 30.3 percent, the lowest among the various forms of hospital ownership.

The number of hospitals experiencing a union election in both time periods appears to grow with bed size. However, for the latter period, it peaked at the 250-399 bed size. The less than 100 bed size category still appears to be the hospital size where unions are most likely to be victorious (52.8 percent). This victory rate has changed little since the 1974-79 period when it was 52.9 percent.

In the 1980-85 period, unions continued to avoid areas where the legal and social environment (primarily the south) were not receptive to union election activity. For example, only 33 of the 537 hospitals with elections, or

Table 32-1. National Labor Relations Board Elections and Outcomes in Nongovernmental Hospitals, by Selected Hospital and Area Characteristics: August 1974-December 1979 and January 1980-May 1985.[1]

Selected characteristic	Number of hospitals with elections		Percent of hospitals with elections[2]		Number of elections		Number of union victories		Union victories as a percent of elections	
	1974-79	1980-85	1974-79	1980-85	1974-79	1980-85	1974-79	1980-85	1974-79	1980-85
All hospitals	556	537	16.2	12.8	1,025	834	498	397	48.6	47.6
Census division										
New England	58	59	24.9	25.2	106	92	61	45	57.6	48.9
Middle Atlantic	156	172	31.4	30.5	310	303	163	149	52.6	49.2
South Atlantic	33	32	7.5	5.1	55	50	23	19	41.8	38.0
East North Central	121	93	20.1	13.0	221	131	91	51	41.2	38.9
East South Central	17	11	8.2	3.7	23	21	13	9	56.5	42.9
West North Central	27	26	6.7	5.4	51	33	25	16	49.0	48.5
West South Central	13	4	3.4	0.1	18	6	4	3	22.2	50.0
Mountain	25	22	12.5	9.2	39	32	20	14	51.3	43.8
Pacific	106	109	23.5	20.3	202	152	98	80	48.5	52.6
Puerto Rico[3]	—	9	—	20.0	—	14	—	11	—	78.6
Ownership										
Nonprofit-religious	115	83	17.7	10.6	176	135	64	63	36.4	46.6
Nonprofit-non-religious	395	403	17.6	15.3	756	623	381	311	50.4	49.9
For-profit	46	51	8.6	6.4	93	76	53	23	57.0	30.3

Bed size

Less than 100	118	112	7.8	7.7	204	159	108	84	52.9	52.8
100-249	207	202	18.5	16.8	387	333	186	159	48.1	47.7
250-399	121	117	25.8	23.0	198	181	86	76	43.4	42.0
More than 400	110	106	33.0	20.4	236	161	118	78	50.0	48.4

Right-to-work

No	509	504	21.4	19.0	950	785	474	378	49.9	48.2
Yes	47	33	4.6	2.2	75	49	24	19	32.0	38.8

Worker protection

No	268	227	11.2	7.5	453	340	176	137	38.9	40.3
Yes	288	310	27.9	26.5	572	494	322	260	56.3	52.6

[1] Data for the period 1974-79 appear in Becker, et al. (1982), Table 4.
[2] Based on census of AHA registered hospitals 1974 and 1984, respectively.
[3] Due to research design, Puerto Rico was not included in the 1974-79 study.

SOURCE: National Labor Relations Board: *Monthly Election Reports* for two 65-month periods, August 1974-December 1979 and January 1980-May 1985.

Table 32-2. National Labor Relations Board Elections and Outcomes in Nongovernmental Hospitals by Selected Union and Election Characteristics: August 1974-December 1979 and January 1980-May 1985.[1]

Selected characteristic	Number of union elections		Percent of union elections[2]		Number of union victories		Union victories as a percentage of elections	
	1974-79	1980-85	1974-79	1980-85	1974-79	1980-85	1974-79	1980-85
All hospitals	1,025	834	100.0	100.0	498	397	48.6	47.6
Employee organizations[3]								
Independent Union	[4]313	175 } 287	[4]30.5	18.5 } 30.4	[4]193	69 } 128	[4]61.7	39.4 } [5]44.6
American Nurses' Association		112		11.9		59		52.7
Service Employees	220	159	21.5	16.8	103	73	46.8	45.9
District 1199	128	139	12.5	14.7	64	71	50.0	51.1
Teamsters	68	62	6.6	6.6	21	19	30.9	30.6
Operating Engineers	51	22	5.0	2.3	24	12	47.1	54.5
State, County and Municipal Employees	45	26	4.4	2.8	17	5	37.8	19.2
United Food and Community Workers[6]	40	59	3.9	6.3	13	24	32.5	40.7
Laborers International	29	13	2.8	1.4	7	9	24.1	69.2
Communication Workers	14	10	1.4	1.1	0	1	0.0	10.0
Office Employees International	13	17	1.3	1.8	6	7	47.2	41.1
Guard Workers	10	19	1.0	2.0	6	6	60.0	31.6
Others	94	131	9.2	13.9	44	42	46.8	32.1

Type of union

Industrial	227	161	22.1	19.3	66	59	29.1	36.6
Departmental	39	52	3.8	6.2	27	29	69.2	55.8
Craft[7]	—	31	—	3.7	—	19	—	61.3
Guard	35	31	3.4	3.7	22	16	62.9	51.6
Professional and/or technical	450	372	43.9	44.6	257	199	57.1	53.5
Office, clerical and other white collar	131	70	12.8	8.4	67	35	51.2	50.0
Combined professional and office	18	10	1.8	1.2	6	3	33.3	30.0
All others	125	107	12.2	12.8	53	37	42.4	34.6

Type of election

Stipulation	597	575	58.2	68.9	293	281	49.1	48.9
Regional director-ordered	314	226	30.6	27.1	133	97	42.4	42.9
Board ordered	44	8	4.3	1.0	19	2	43.2	25.0
Consent	70	20	6.8	2.4	53	15	75.7	75.0
Expedited[8]	—	5	—	0.6	—	2	—	40.0

Nature of election

Single union	886	728	86.4	87.3	419	334	47.3	45.9
Multi union	139	106	13.6	12.7	79	63	56.8	59.4

[1] Data for the period 1974-79 appear in Becker, et al. (1982), Table 5.

[2] Percentages do not always add to 100.0 due to rounding.

[3] Total "employee organizations" for the 1980-85 period totals 944 due to multiple employee organizations seeking to represent a category of employees at the time of a single given recognition election. Data for the 1974-79 period does not use this counting method.

[4] ANA data separate from the independent union category were not available in the study covering the years 1974-79.

[5] (69 + 59) ÷ (175 + 112) = 44.6 percent.

[6] Listed as Retail Clerks International Association in the 1974-79 study. In 1979, it merged with the Meat Cutters and Butchers Union to form the United Food and Commercial Workers' Union.

[7] Due to research design, craft type of union was not used as a separate category in the 1974-79 study.

[8] Due to research design, expedited elections were not used as a separate category in the 1974-79 study.

SOURCE: National Labor Relations Board: *Monthly Election Reports* for two 65-month periods, August 1974-December 1979 and January 1980-May 1985.

Table 32-3. National Labor Relations Board Elections and Outcomes in Nongovernmental Hospitals by Year, August 1974 through May 1985.[1]

Year	Number of union elections — By year	Union elections as a percent of all union elections — By year	Union elections as a percent of all union elections — By year for all years 1979-85	Number of union victories — By year	Union victories as a percent of all union victories — By year	Union victories as a percent of all union victories — By year for all years 1974-85	Union victories as a percent of union elections
Total August 1974-May 1985	1,859		100.0	Σ895		100.0	(895 ÷ 1,859 = 48.1) 48.6
August 1974-December 1979							
Period total	1,025	99.9	55.1	498	100.1	55.6	48.6
1974[2]	74	7.2	4.0	50	10.0	5.6	67.6
1975	236	23.0	12.7	113	22.7	12.6	47.9
1976	181	17.7	9.7	87	17.5	9.7	48.1
1977	237	23.1	12.7	109	21.9	12.2	46.0
1978	152	14.8	8.2	69	13.9	7.7	45.4
1979	145	14.1	7.8	70	14.1	7.8	48.3
January 1980-May 1985							
Period total	834	99.9	44.9	397	100.0	44.4	47.6
1980	252	30.2	13.6	110	27.7	12.3	43.7
1981	214	25.6	11.5	100	25.2	11.2	46.7
1982	150	18.0	8.1	68	17.1	7.6	45.3
1983	87	10.4	4.7	48	12.1	5.4	55.2
1984	99	11.9	5.3	53	13.4	5.9	53.5
1985[3]	32	3.8	1.7	18	4.5	2.0	56.2

[1] Data for the period August 1974-December 1979 appear in Becker, et al. (1982), Table 5.
[2] August-December only.
[3] January-May only.

SOURCE: National Labor Relations Board: *Monthly Election Reports* for two 65-month periods, August 1974-December 1979 and January 1980-May 1985.

6.1 percent, were in states with right-to-work (RTW) laws. These 33 hospitals represented only 2.2 percent of the potential hospitals in these states that were eligible for elections. This is slightly lower than the 1974-79 period when 4.6 percent of the hospitals in RTW states had elections. In contrast, states in which the legal environment has traditionally been receptive to union election activity—those with laws that protected and facilitated collective bargaining in nonprofit hospitals before 1974—had election rates that were more than three times higher than states that had no such laws (26.5 percent versus 7.5 percent).

Union and Election Characteristics

Frequency distributions of NLRB union elections by union and election characteristics as well as union victory rates for both the 1974-79 and 1980-85 periods are shown in Table 32-2.

The four employee organizations that were involved in the largest share of elections in the 1980-85 period were the independent unions (employees not associated with any national union), Service Employees International Union, District 1199 of the Retail, Wholesale, and Department Store Union, and the American Nurses' Association. Together these four unions accounted for 62 percent of all hospital elections.

The independent unions had a much lower victory rate, 39.4 percent, than the national average, 47.6 percent. In part, this lower victory rate, when compared with the 1974-79 study victory rate of 61.7 percent, is attributed to the fact that we have separated the American Nurses' Association (ANA) out of this category. The NLRB did not separately distinguish elections that the ANA was involved in until 1977. Nevertheless, even if the ANA and independent union categories are combined as they were in the 1974-79 period, the independent unions (plus the ANA) had a much lower union victory rate (44.6 percent) than they did in the 1974-79 period.

Unions organized into professional and/or technical units were responsible for almost half the NLRB elections during the 1980-85 period (44.6 percent), virtually the same percentage they participated in during the 1974-79 period (43.9 percent). This was more than twice the election rate of industrial employee organizations (19.3 percent), the type of union with the second highest number of elections. Professional and/or technical units also appeared to be above the national average in their victory rates. For the 1980-85 period, professional/technical units were victorious in 53.5 percent of their elections, considerably higher than the 47.6 percent national average. This is down slightly, however, from their 1974-79 victory rate of 57.1 percent.

The NLRB distinguishes between five types of representative elections. Most common are the two kinds of consent elections. In the "agreement for consent" election, the regional NLRB director makes the final resolution in any disputes concerning the conduct of the election. In the "stipulation for certification on consent" election, the NLRB settles all disputes. The term "stipulation" in Table 32-2 is far more common than the former, termed "consent" in the table. Stipulation elections usually require a longer period of time to be resolved if disputes arise. This is typically because consent elections are not contested by the organization being unionized and therefore disputes are not as acrimonious. The fact that the NLRB is involved may appeal to unions and employers alike on 'fairness' grounds. Nevertheless, union victory rates are substantially higher in consent elections than in stipulation elections, although involvement of the NLRB is not necessarily a factor in this difference.

Union elections may also be ordered by the NLRB or by a regional NLRB director. A board-ordered election occurs when there are questions concerning the appropriateness of the bargaining unit or circumstances involving a novel issue, for example, a unique bargaining unit. The regional director may order an election when a disagreement occurs between the bargaining parties, but there are no novel issues or unique circumstances involved.

The final type of election identified by the NLRB is the expedited election. This usually occurs when an unfair labor practice is involved. In these situations the NLRB typically changes the election timeframe by moving the election forward.

There were only five expedited elections and eight board-ordered elections in the 1980-85 period. The majority of elections were stipulated, followed by regional-director ordered elections, and consent elections, respectively. Although consent elections represent only a small proportion of the elections held during this period (2.4 percent), unions won 75.0 percent of these elections. Stipulated elections (representing 68.9 percent of all elections) had the next highest union victory rate, 48.9 percent, followed by the regional director-ordered election (representing 27.1 percent of all elections) with a union victory rate of 42.9 percent.

The vast majority of elections involved only one union. Multiple elections, in which two or more unions competed with one another to represent the bargaining unit, occurred approximately one-seventh as often as single union elections. However, in spite of this difference, multiple union elections had a higher victory rate (59.4 percent) than their single union counterparts (45.9 percent). These victory rates for multiple and single union elections did not change substantially from the 1974-79 period when they were 56.8 percent and 47.3 percent, respectively.

Elections by Period and Year

Union elections and victory data by period and by year are presented in Table 32-3. The number of union elections in the 65-month 1974-79 period was approximately one-fourth higher than the 65-month 1980-85 period (1,025 and 834, respectively) as was the number of union victories (498 and 397, respectively). The overall victory rates for both periods, however, were nearly identical—48.6 and 47.6 percent, respectively.

When combining data from both periods and examining all years, several observations should be noted. The highest percentage of the 1,859 union elections in the combined 10-year and 10-month period occurred in 1980. For this year, union elections as a percentage of total elections reached a high of 13.6 percent. In 1975 and again in 1977, the percentage of elections was slightly lower, 12.7 percent. Since 1981, however, the percentage of union elections taking place has fallen dramatically. In the last 2 full years of data, 1983 and 1984, the percentages of the 1,859 elections that occurred were 4.7 and 5.3 percent, respectively.

A similar pattern appears for union victories. Of the total 895 union victories that occurred between 1974 and 1985, 12.6 percent were in 1975, 12.2 percent in 1977, and 12.3 percent in 1980. In contrast, of the total number of union victories, only 5.4 and 5.9 percent occurred in the years 1983 and 1984, respectively.

Summary and Conclusions

This study, using data from the National Labor Relations Board *Monthly Election Reports* for a 65-month period, January 1980 through May 1985, and the 1984 American Hospital Association Survey of Hospitals, has sought to update the status of union election activity in nongovernmental hospitals in the first half of the 1980s and compare that activity to the previously reported 65-month 1974-79 period. As a result, a comprehensive profile of union election activity in the hospital industry following the passage of the 1974 amendments to the Taft-Hartley Act is presented. A number of conclusions seem warranted.

First, in contrast to earlier predictions that 65 percent of all hospitals would be unionized, our evidence shows a rather dramatic decrease in the extent of union election activity in the hospital industry, especially since 1981. Our data do not permit us to estimate exactly how many hospitals were unionized by 1985 because a hospital can have more than one union. However, if we assume that the ratio of hospital elections to total elections is roughly the same as it was for the 1974-79 period (a very liberal estimate, because the "easier" hospitals were supposedly unionized first), we would calculate that slightly more than half of the 537 hospitals in our study that had elections (268 hospitals) were hospitals that were experiencing their first election. Since unions won approximately half of the elections they were involved in, this would mean that 134 hospitals acquired a union. This would represent approximately a 3.3 percent increase in the number of hospitals with unions since 1980. Adding this 3.3 percent to the 27.4 percent of hospitals that were found to have union contracts in 1980 (Becker, Sloan, and Steinwald 1982) would suggest that approximately 30.7 percent of the nation's hospitals had a union by May 1985. This is considerably lower than previous estimates. Moreover, it would imply that, without significant changes in the rate of union election activity, unions will have contracts in only about 34 percent of U.S. nongovernmental hospitals by 1990.

Second, somewhat surprisingly, union victory rates in the hospital industry have not declined substantially. For the 1974-79 period, union victory rates were 48.6 percent compared with 47.6 percent for the more recent 1980-85 period. This fact coupled with the evidence that unions are not as active in the hospital industry as in the earlier period (834 versus 1,025 elections) suggests that unions are being very selective in the hospitals they choose to unionize. Consequently, they are still able to win approximately half the elections they enter. This probably reflects the reality that the "easier" hospitals have been unionized and those remaining require considerably more time and resources if the unions are to maintain their success.

Third, the dramatic decline in the number of elections since 1981 would suggest that the hospital industry, similar to other industries, has become more resistant to union election activity and better able to oppose union organizing efforts. It would appear that the dramatic changes in the health services industry beginning in the early 1980s have had a substantial impact on hospitals. Included in these changes are the implementation of a prospective payment system for hospitals,[5] the dismantling of national health planning and its regulatory influence, and the rising competitive environment which includes health maintenance organizations, preferred provider organizations, and hospital diversification and consolidation. The net effect is that hospitals are more concerned with their productivity and costs (i.e., survival). It would appear that this hostile and turbulent environment with accompanying declines in occupancy, length of stay, hospital beds, and staff has made hospitals even more resistant to union organizing efforts. The fact that only 20 of the 834 union elections held during the 1980-85 period were consent elections (elections where the hospital did not contest holding the election) reflects the combative nature of the vast majority of these elections. Evidence has shown that where the election process is prolonged, such as in a stipulated or board-ordered election in comparison to a consent election, unions' chances for success decline substantially (Prosten 1978).

Fourth, different hospitals and area characteristics have a dramatic impact on both the likelihood of an election and the outcome of the election. In part, the regional patterns reflect the concentration of hospitals in certain areas of the country. However, considerable social influence is still apparent. For example, regions of the country that have a strong history of supporting union election activity, as evidenced by states that had legislation supporting union activity in hospitals prior to the passage of THA, are more likely to have an election and the union appears more likely to be victorious than areas where such support is lacking. The converse appears to be true in areas that traditionally have not supported union election activity. In states that have right-to-work legislation, for instance, there is a much lower likelihood of having a union election and less chance that the union will win the election. This is very similar to the pattern that appeared in the 1974-79 period.

Fifth, the majority of the union elections since 1980 took place in nonprofit, nonreligious hospitals. This same group of hospitals, when compared with nonprofit religious hospitals and for-profit hospitals, experienced the highest union victory rate of 49.9 percent. This victory rate is almost identical to the union victory rate in this form of hospital ownership during the 1974-79 period of 50.4 percent. In contrast, the most dramatic change among union victory rates in the various types of hospital ownership for the 1974-79 versus the 1980-85 period is in the for-profit hospital. During the earlier period, unions had a 57.0 percent victory rate in for-profit hospitals; in the latter period, the union victory rate in for-profit hospital ownership dropped to 30.3 percent. This may, in part, result from the acquisition of many of the free-standing for-profit hospitals by multihospital chains. The fact that most of these multihospital systems have experienced labor relations departments and a larger pool of resources available to resist organizing efforts may account for the decline in union success between the two periods.

Sixth, among the various employee's organizations, there is still considerable variation in their success rate. Independent unions, which were responsible for the largest number of elections of any group in the 1970s, still accounted for the largest number of elections in the 1980s. Their victory rate, however, has declined dramatically from 61.7 percent in the 1970s to 39.4 percent in the 1980s. This may be explained in part by the fact that the elections of the American Nurses' Association (ANA) were combined with the independent unions category in the 1974-79 period. Nevertheless, even if they are combined, the independent unions still achieved only a 44.6 percent victory rate, still considerably below their rate of victory in the 1970s.

Finally, in 1983 and 1984, the last 2 full years for which we have information, the number of union elections dropped below 100 for the first time since 1974. For the first 5 months of 1985, only 32 hospital elections had taken place. If this rate continues, it would imply that the hospital industry would experience around 77 elections in calendar year 1985. These figures are far below the 252 and 214 hospital elections that took place in 1980 and 1981, respectively. It would appear, at least for the near future, that union election activity will continue to decline in the hospital industry and unions will continue to experience considerable difficulty in organizing the hospital industry.

Acknowledgment

The authors are grateful to Levent Ersalman for his assistance in data collection and to Killard Adamache and three anonymous referees for helpful comments on an earlier draft.

Notes

1. For further information on the history of collective bargaining in the United States, see Begin and Beal, 1985.
2. States with worker protection prior to 1974 are Colorado, Connecticut, Hawaii, Massachusetts, Michigan, Minnesota, Montana, New York, Oregon, Pennsylvania, Wisconsin, and Utah.
3. Schramm (1978) points out that this is a conservative estimate. Other estimates are: Taylor (1979) found that for 1976 labor costs, excluding fringe benefits, represented 51.4 percent of total costs; Sloan and Steinwald (1980) found that, in 1974, labor costs including fringe benefits represented about 59 percent of total costs. Although all three studies

reported that labor costs were declining, they still appear to represent the major share of a hospital's expenses.

4. The right-to-work states are Alabama, Arizona, Arkansas, Florida, Georgia, Iowa, Kansas, Louisiana, Mississippi, Nebraska, Nevada, North Carolina, North Dakota, South Carolina, South Dakota, Tennessee, Texas, Utah, Virginia, and Wyoming.

5. With the passage of the Tax Equity and Fiscal Responsibility Act and the 1983 Social Security Amendments (Public Law 98-21), Federal reimbursement to hospitals for Medicare beneficiaries, with certain exceptions, shifted from a cost-based system to a prospective payment system based on diagnosis-related groups.

Bibliography

Adamache, K. and Sloan, F.: Unions and hospitals: Some unresolved issues. *Journal of Health Economics*, 1(1): 1-24, May 1982.

American Hospital Association: *Hospital Statistics*. Chicago. 1975.

Arnett, R. H., McKusick, D., Sonnefeld, S., and Cowell, C.: Projections of health care spending to 1990. *Health Care Financing Review*. Vol. 7, No. 3. HCFA Pub. No. 03222. Office of Research and Demonstrations, Health Care Financing Administration. Washington, DC: U.S. Government Printing Office, Spring 1986.

Begin, J. P. and Beal, E. F.: *The Practice of Collective Bargaining*. Homewood, IL, Richard D. Irwin, Inc., 1985.

Becker, E. R., Sloan, F., and Steinwald, B.: Union activity in hospitals: Past, present, and future. *Health Care Financing Review*. Vol. 3, No. 4. HCFA Pub. No. 03143. Office of Research and Demonstrations, Health Care Financing Administration. Washington, DC: U.S. Government Printing Office, June 1982.

Feldman, R., Lee, L., and Hoffbeck, R.: *Hospital Employees' Wages and Labor Union Organization*. Grant No. 1-R03-H503649-01 prepared for the National Center for Health Services Research. Rockville, MD, Nov. 1980.

Levitt, K., Lazenby, H., Waldo, D., and Davidoff, L.: National health expenditures, 1984. *Health Care Financing Review*. Vol. 7, No. 1. HCFA Pub. No. 03206, Office of Research and Demonstrations, Health Care Financing Administration. Washington, DC: U.S. Government Printing Office, Fall 1985.

Metzger, N.: Labor Relations. *Hospitals*. 44(3): 80-84, 1970.

National Labor Relations Board: *A Guide to Basic Law and Procedure Under the National Labor Relations Act*. Washington, DC: U.S. Government Printing Office, 1978.

Prosten, R.: The longest season: Union organization in the last decade, a/k/a How come one team has to play with its shoelaces tied together? *Proceedings of the Thirty-First Annual Meeting*. Industrial Relations Research Association Series. Dennis, B.D., ed. Chicago, Aug. 29-31, 1978.

Rakich, J., Longest, B., and Darr, K.: *Managing Health Service Organizations*. Philadelphia, PA: W.B. Saunders Company, 1985.

Schramm, C.: Regulating hospital labor costs: A case study of the politics of state rate commissions. *Journal of Health Politics, Policy, and Law*. 3(3): 364-374, 1978.

Sloan, F. and Steinwald, B.: *Insurance, Regulation, and Hospital Costs*. Lexington, MA.: Lexington Books, 1980.

Taylor, A.: Government health policy and hospital labor costs: The effect of wage and price controls on hospital wage rates and employment. *Public Policy*. 27(2): 203-225, 1979.

U.S. Department of Labor, Office of Research, Federal Mediation and Conciliation Service: *Impact of the 1974 Health Care Amendment to the NLRA on Collective Bargaining in the Health Care Industry*. Washington, DC: U.S. Government Printing Office, 1979.

33

Adapting Theory Z
to Nursing Management

Marlene K. Strader

Marlene K. Strader, Ph.D., R.N., is Assistant Professor, Southern Illinois University, Edwardsville.

While nurses are indeed concerned with salaries and staffing patterns, recent surveys and studies have indicated they are genuinely dissatisfied with work relationships and management flexibility. They hold negative perceptions of achievement, recognition, advancement or even the work itself with its lack of autonomy or advanced technology.[1] In 1978, a survey of nearly 17,000 nurses showed that most job complaints centered around leadership and management skills of supervisors, their failure to follow through on problems, isolation and overuse of authority.[2] When hospitals listen to nurses and put their ideas into action, they are rewarded with a lower turnover rate.[3]

The AMICAE (Achieving Methods of Interprofessional Consensus, Assessment, on Evaluation) project in the San Francisco Bay area indicated that nurses feel hospitals do not allow them to find job satisfaction from their work environment.[4] They seek more autonomy and participation in the decisions which affect their working environment. They also want and need support for these ideas from their nurse managers, many of whom may not clearly understand the needs of the professionals they employ.[5]

Intermittent attempts to increase salaries, implement some staffing patterns, or institute different models of nursing care have fallen short of satisfying nurses sufficiently to keep them. It would make better sense to identify the major job dissatisfiers and motivators, then develop a management style that promotes job satisfaction.

Herzberg's Basics . . .

Widely accepted in the field of management, Frederick Herzberg's Two-Factor Theory explains factors that promote job satisfaction.[6] (See Fig. 33-1.)

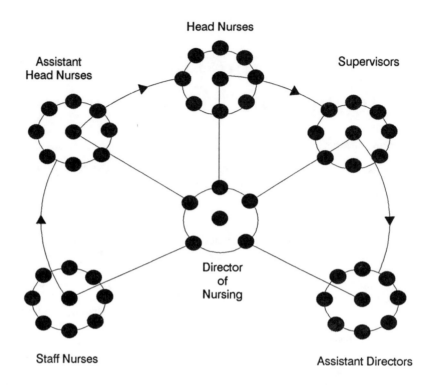

Figure 33-1. Formation of Quality Circles.

To manage employees effectively, the major satisfiers must distinctly balance or outweigh the dissatisfiers. If employees perceive that they do not, or that they hover at some neutral point, they will perform poorly and/or terminate. Since managers control the major factors in job satisfaction, it is within management's power to offset the dissatisfaction and return employees to equilibrium. Therefore, to proceed along the continuum of job satisfaction, RNs must have, for example, equitable salaries, adequate time off, productive relationships among superiors, peers and subordinates, and a management process that promotes achievement, recognition and advancement. Nurses' lower needs must be met, and they must have opportunities for fulfilling their higher quality needs.

Support Theory Z

The management approach known as "Theory Z" incorporates Herzberg's Two-Factor Theory.[7] Ouchi contends that the current Japanese edge on quality derives ultimately from this collaborative style which trusts workers and consults them on those matters which affect them and the product. The assumption is that workers have ideas which, if heard and used, will result in a more satisfied, motivated and productive workforce. The system emphasizes consensus on decisions, lifetime job security, and a strong commitment to the goals of the institution. Through these means, managers strive to intensify job commitment, lower turnover and dramatically increase productivity.

The group participation process in "Z" management is called a "quality circle." Through such groups, employees study methods to improve their product. Quality circles are thoroughly disciplined operations committed to training, group skills and a rigorous step-by-step improvement procedure.

Many managerial decisions are made in the circles. Whenever a policy or procedure change is being made, discussion continues within the circles until a true consensus has been achieved. No decision is final until every member has had a part in the decision and agrees with the outcome. Undeniably, this takes time, but once consensus has been reached, implementation is instantaneous, the net effect for productivity is increased, and job satisfaction enhanced.

In other forms of participatory decision making, when the majority wins, a dissatisfied, obstinate minority may remain. Theory Z's advocates claim that consensus resolves negative feelings: everyone feels a part of the process, has a voice in the decision, and is, therefore a winner.

Theory Z organizations encompass many factors which contribute to job satisfaction. Arriving at consensus reduces conflict among superordinates, peers, and subordinates. Z companies promote a homogeneous group through networking that binds all employees together, but still respects privacy. Achievement, recognition, and personal growth take place within the framework of a holistic concern which views workers as psychosocial beings and facilitates their personal, as well as job, development.

One cannot convert a bureaucratic organization into a consensual one overnight. A commitment to this type of management takes several years to mature. Before an institution attempts Z organization, managers must develop a meaningful philosophy which closely defines all of the Theory Z goals and establishes a supportive Z environment.

Establishing Z organizations within a typical hospital nursing structure takes six stages: 1) awareness phase; 2) formation of quality circles; 3) philosophy and policies audit; 4) career incentive creation; 5) union involvement (when applicable); and 6) evaluation.

1. Teach Awareness

In the initial phase, outline an educational program and time frame which will inform all RNs about Z management's principles and goals through seminars, workshops, or training sessions. In training programs, nurses learn decision-making approaches to consensus. Once they have become acquainted with Z theory, practice circles enable them to learn the necessary group process skills and explore the potential of this style. At the same time, these activities reinforce the nurses' sense of importance as thinking, contributing members of the institution.

2. Form Quality Circles

The development of groups called Quality Circles begins immediately thereafter and extends the awareness phase. Groups of 8 to 10 nurses are formed from each level and by department or floor. For example, each circle consists of nurses, head nurses, supervisors, assistant directors, and directors of nursing from Medical, Surgical, OR, L&D, or by floor. Start with three circles and add additional ones until all nursing personnel have a place in a circle. A circle leader is selected and this role is rotated every three months until all members have served. Each leader will interface with a higher level circle. (See Fig. 33-2.) Choose a circle facilitator from the floor or department to see that all levels of employees are continuously represented at all levels of deliberation. This should assure communication flow from the staff nurse to the administrative level.

3. Audit the Philosophy and Policies of the Institution

Review institutional philosophy and policies for their consonance with facilitating Theory Z management. Either the circles or outside consultants can conduct these reviews. Sometimes the philosophy of the hospital and/or nursing service no longer accords with what actually takes place. Deviations slip in so subtly that no one can identify where they arose in the first place. A Z management philosophy must be clear, precise, meaningful in content, reflect the reality and autonomy of nursing, and give direction to policies and practice. Nurses must be instrumental in writing the philosophy, and they must determine the related goals and objectives. They must have financial data with which to formulate feasible goals.

4. Broaden Career Paths and Create Incentives

Planning for the future in terms of career development creates incentives in increments which intensify and reinforce commitment to the institution. Purposely, Z organizations have slow evaluations and promotions. Formal evaluations should take place only after the nurse has mastered competencies for a given level over a period of time. For promotion, the nurse must reach a high level of achievement. Mentorship/internship systems to guide nurses through this can intrinsically reward competent senior nurses and help them learn how to manage wider professional responsibilities one step at a time.

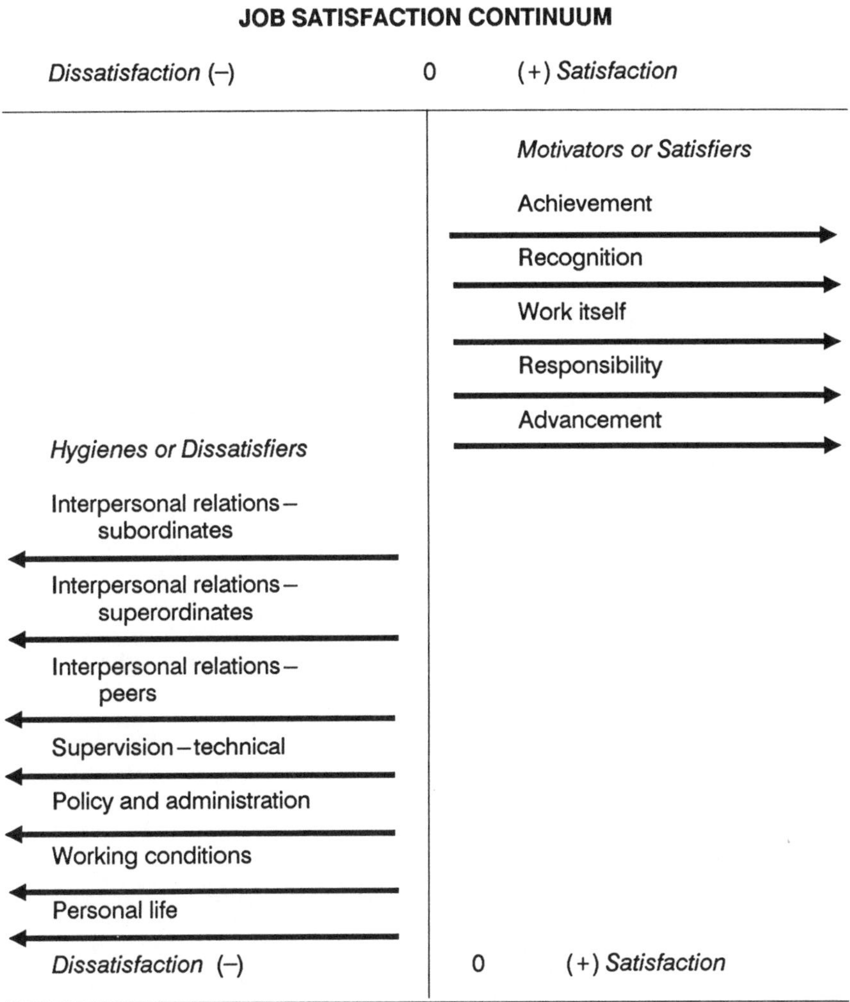

JOB SATISFACTION CONTINUUM

| *Dissatisfaction (−)* | 0 | *(+) Satisfaction* |

Figure 33-2. Herzberg's two-factor theory. Reproduced from Wayne K. Hoy and Cecil G. Miskel. *Educational Administration: Theory, Research and Practice*, with permission.

This method targets the needed support services on nurses as they expand their competence and self-confidence.

Quality circles also determine the type of incentives that would reinforce job satisfaction and encourage length of service. The Scanlon Plan has demonstrated that work groups at all levels in a company can contribute in constructive, valuable ways to an organization's well-being and competitive edge.[8] For example, nurses might decide they do not require the same benefit package at various stages of their careers. Designing a flexible benefit program could provide a cost-effective series of incentives to them. Some might elect more time off, while others might choose more upfront cash, and still others, a pension or profit-sharing package.

5. Involve the Union

A 1982 survey showed only 25 percent of U.S. nurses are represented by collective bargaining units. Fifty-one percent of these RNs declared their unionism compatible with professionalism; 41 percent said they are not. Staff nurses, the RNs most likely to join unions, comprise 59 percent of those seeing "no conflict," and 39 percent of nurse managers already think the marriage between unionism and professionalism will work out.[9]

The reasons to seek union involvement center around the same factors which cause job dissatisfaction.[10] Within an autocratic management system, unions will revert to extremes of their own hierarchy. Involving unions in decision making restores faith in management and provides the incentive to sustain a working relationship. In a decision process oriented toward consensus that has won employees' trust, the union will have no adversary role. However, for Z theory to work, the same internal changes — decisions by consensus, developing interpersonal skills, commitment to a working philosophy — must take place *within the union* as well. When the union arrives at decisions in the same manner as management does, managers have the best possible communication system through which to organize, integrate and educate nurses.

6. Evaluate the System and the Individual's Role

This phase is continuous and must monitor effectiveness of Z management. Outside consultants provide an objective source. So does using validated scales which measure group interaction and problem solving skills to determine whether all nurses meet the criteria for Z managers and/or team members. If Z theory is progressing, many nurse managers will experience some sense of loss and insecurity because their decisions are regularly challenged and others have input into planning and decision making. Productivity and job satisfaction need to be evaluated to see if the system is working. Employees are skeptical about participation just for show. They want to see how much their efforts are influencing working conditions and outcomes. They need to see that they will be rewarded.

Participation needs constant renewal for the sake of both Quality Circles and the organization. Recent surveys have shown that after about 18 months of intense activity, groups experience a form of burnout. Periods of intensity need to alternate with periods of distance to give people a chance to renew their energies. New circles need to form or rev up just as old circles begin to drop out. Those who are left out of one round of activity can know that they will be included in future organizational dynamics.[11]

Critics of Z theory disclaim it as faddish and state it will not work in a society impatient for immediate success. However, one study showed improved morale, decreased alienation and greater incentives for unified productivity when Quality Circles were introduced.[12] From their research, Likert and his colleagues concluded that, in general, the closer a management profile approaches the participative, the greater the likelihood of superior performance and job satisfaction.[13]

Providing nurses with the systematic input and initiative they are demanding, quality circles and management by consensus in a trusting environment are steps in that direction.

Theory Z's concept particularly suits both the aspirations of employed professionals and the institutions in which they deliver their services. It establishes regular channels through which discreet — even diverse — technical perspectives and interests can negotiate united efforts. In one direction, these efforts work to target pertinent resources upon patient populations and, within them, each patient's needs. In the other direction, Z management constantly draws upon the background and current experience of its multifaceted workforce to conserve service capacity and to renovate and expand it. Although originally designed to suit certain industrial needs, Z management may prove even more productive in the service enterprises which hospital nursing operations quintessentially represent.

Notes

1. Everly, G.S. and Falcione, R.L., "Perceived Dimensions in Job Satisfaction for Staff Nurses," *Nursing Research*, 25: September/October: 346-348; Link, C.R. and Settle, R.F., "Financial Incentive and Labor Supply of Married Professional Nurses and What Can Be Done About It," *Nursing Research*, 29:July-August: 238-243; Colavecchio, Ruth, "Direct Patient Care: A Viable Career Choice?", *The Journal of Nursing Administration*, July/August, 1982, 17-22; Aiken, Linda H., "Nursing Priorities for the 1980's: Hospitals and Nursing Homes," *American Journal of Nursing*, 81:2:324-330; and Prescott, P. A., *et al.*, "Supplemental Service Agencies: Who Uses Them? Who Does Not?", *American Journal of Nursing*, 82:11:1714-1717.
2. Godfrey, M.A., "Job Satisfaction — Or Should It Be Dissatisfaction? Part I," *Nursing '78*, 8:4:89-100.

3. Seybolt, J.W. and Walker, D.D., "Attitude Survey Proves to Be a Powerful Tool for Reversing Turnover," *Hospitals*, 54:5:77-80; and Araujo, Marianne, "Creative Nursing Administration Sets Climate for Retention," *Hospitals*, 54: 5:72-76.
4. Colavecchio, *loc. cit.*
5. Kanter, R.M. and Stein, B.A. *Life in Organizations*, (New York: Basic Books, 1979).
6. Herzberg, Frederick, *et al.*, *The Motivation to Work*, (New York: Wiley, 1959).
7. Ouchi, William, *Theory Z: How American Business Can Meet the Japanese Challenge* (Massachusetts: Addison-Wesley, 1981).
8. *Ibid.*
9. Lee, Anthony A., "A Wary New Welcome for Unions," *RN*, November, 1982.
10. *Ibid.*

374 *Management Functions*

11. Kanter, R.M., "Dilemmas of Management Participation," *Organizational Dynamics*, Summer, 1982.
12. Moore, R.C., *et al.*, "On the Scene: Quality Control Circles at Barnes Hospital," *Nursing Administration Quarterly*, 6:3:23-46.

13. Likert, Rensis, *New Patterns of Management* (New York: McGraw-Hill, 1967).

34

Becoming a Healthcare Change Master

Rosabeth Moss Kanter

Rosabeth Moss Kanter is the Class of 1960 Professor, Harvard Business School, Cambridge, Massachusetts.

Management fads can be dangerous. Techniques are borrowed with little thought for what is truly essential. Changes are introduced and resources wasted.

Yet, despite often disastrous results, people and organizations continue to seek change and innovation. Why?

- *New technology*: While technology may be a solution and an innovation, it can also be a problem. Unless people know how to innovate and take advantage of the opportunities created by technology, it is often wasted.

- *The politics of raw material*: This country is vulnerable to the actions of foreign governments for critical sources of supply such as energy. What is needed is the flexibility to handle volatile situations that are almost never under our total control.

- *Government regulations*: Regulation is present not only in healthcare, but also in airlines, trucking, telecommunications, and financial services. The demand is for people who can move with agility and speed when a new problem is created or when a new opportunity opens up.

- *Demographic shifts*: The burgeoning elderly population and the aging baby boom generation mean consumers who are more fickle, less brand loyal, and more likely to demand quality and value for their dollar.

- *The new labor force*: Its members are more rights conscious and expect a voice in decisions at work. They want not a job, but a career, and they view it as a matter of entitlement. More healthcare professionals are becoming employees, but employees are wondering why they can't be consultants and entrepreneurs.

The Meaning Behind Change

What do these trends say? In an effective organization the mean time between surprises must be less than or equal to the mean time between decisions. If there are more surprises — and they happen at increasingly frequent intervals, close to or far below the mean time to make decisions — then the organization is in trouble. Organizations must act faster than what's thrown at them — not only to respond quickly and effectively, but also to be the source of surprise for someone else.

Today, effective management of change means less bureaucracy and red tape. It means the ability to act fast in a rapidly changing environment. And it means the capacity to innovate — to both encourage the development of new ideas and to act on ideas that will impact and shape the environment.

But what makes a healthcare organization — or any organization for that matter — capable of implementing change?

Tuning In and On

Effective organizations tune into their environments. That's because innovation and change always begin with need. Somebody's got a problem; someone isn't fulfilled. Innovation almost never starts with solutions.

The ultimate question is not, "What have we got that we can force people to take?" but, "What do people need that we can supply?" Unfortunately, even the most elaborate market research is very present oriented.

No one in America, for example, rose up and said, "I want a personal desk top computer." It would have never showed up on a market research survey. But the founders of Apple Computers turned first to their own needs and then those of their close friends to gauge their market. When they sold 50 computers, they knew they could move ahead.

And when Honda executives contemplated entry into the U.S. motorcycle market, they immersed themselves not in arm's length surveys, but in people's needs. They understood the customer and the market by looking at people in their total life context — not just that narrow part of the person that intersects with the organization.

Expanding Horizons

Successful organizations tune into their environments, but they also know how to enlarge them. They know that change is triggered by those who have contact with professionals outside their own field. So they look to those who will not only enhance their knowledge base, but who will also challenge and criticize their ideas.

In many ways, successful organizations think like kaleidoscopes. By twisting, turning, and shifting their points of view, they perceive alternative realities. And they begin to realize that by putting the pieces together in a different way, they can obtain even better results.

Innovative organizations expand their environments, carrying people far away from the home office to a totally unrelated experience. Instead of shutting others out from their environment, they send managers to meetings in fields other than their own so that the clash of ideas enlarges their perspective and gives them a sense of new possibilities. Other executives have people work on four or five projects simultaneously, because by moving on to a second project, they get new insights into the first.

In it all is an element of creativity, and what is creativity, after all, but play and irreverence? It's playing with ideas and using irreverence against tradition. In fact, CEOs often convey their commitment to creativity through somewhat irreverent, outrageous symbolic acts — from assembling a parade of elephants on the beach to getting on a horse and riding through a town to promote a new service.

Communicated Vision

Organizations act on ideas because a single person made those ideas compelling and easy to follow. It's why venture capitalists say, "Back the person, not the idea." Creativity isn't getting hundreds of ideas; it's having a few ideas that someone believes in enough that they're willing to take the lead in making them happen.

Leaders communicate the essence of their change with a clear vision, dream, and direction. It is vision — and the leader who can articulate that vision — that helps people in the organization accept uncertainty.

Much resistance to change is no more than fear of the unknown. Vision substitutes for that fear and gives people the confidence to stand up and say, "I have a dream, and I want to be part of it."

Seeking Support

But no change can be achieved without coalitions of backers and supporters. Many innovations failed because innovators neglected to get their coalitions together in advance of the project launch. Just as entrepreneurs must find venture capital, innovators must locate people within the organization with the power to propel their ideas. Often this involves going outside the organization for people to support the idea or building informal, one-on-one connections internally.

No matter what the strategy, there is a definite art and rhythm to coalition building. In the words of a favorite computer company, it starts with planting seeds — not with surprises. If you spring new ideas on people and give them little chance to react, they will often reject the ideas outright. But with advance warning, ideas have time to blossom and grow.

In one company, idea promoters typically wander around the organization asking for budgetary support, venture partners, task force members, personnel, or information systems assistance. By making early commitments, others in the organization begin to care if the project succeeds or fails. And by finding out how people react to their ideas, promoters can take the first step in plugging up potential holes.

In addition to building coalitions, organizations must build teams that identify with the innovation and feel a sense of ownership. Change is work; it requires people to think, learn, and invest time. Few people will act on new ideas by themselves; they count on the contributions of others and on being part of a team.

But not matter how strong an organization's teams are, no innovation will reach completion without perseverance. Often, the only difference between success and failure is time — how long people stay with an idea. Some organizations succeed with ideas that others gave up on too early in the game. Innovation always requires longer time horizons.

Middles are especially difficult because almost all innovations look like failures in the middle. With new projects, it's often difficult to meet deadlines and budgets. And in some organizations, accuracy of forecasting is valued above results — division managers don't get credit if they bring in higher revenues than predicted.

Political problems also abound in midstream. Most people refuse to spend their political capital by saying no to a good idea at the beginning. Instead, they wait until the project is hovering in midair and then they attack. An innovation is rarely threatening until it looks like it's going to be a success.

Managing the change process is more than having a vision or dream and letting others do it. It's during the rough spots that the innovator has to be even closer to the process, following through and staying involved.

A Matter of Culture

It's the organization's corporate culture that makes it easier to guide innovations. That culture has several dimensions:

- *The structure of jobs* — High innovation organizations have broader assignments and fewer job classifications, and they give people larger pieces of responsibility. At a Procter and Gamble Company plant, for example, work teams get responsibility for an entire area of production, and people are paid by the number of skills they master. Costs are half those in comparable plants, quality is higher, and there is greater flexibility to take on new assignments.

- *A culture of pride* – High innovation organizations also have a culture of pride rather than a culture of mediocrity or inferiority. For change to occur, they need to be receptive to new ideas and willing to work side by side. Gaining their respect begins with the belief that this is not only a good organization, but that our people get better all the time.

- *An investment in people* – High innovation organizations invest more in training and development. In very concrete ways, they declare that their people are getting better every day. In contrast, low innovation organizations operate with a poor organizational image and believe that if you've been there more than two years, you must be a turkey. Often high technology companies put people through as many as 20 interviews to ensure quality recruitment. Elaborate recognition systems – awards, merit badges, and trophies – are positive because they both motivate people and publicize achievements.

In high innovation companies, awards are not just payoff oriented; they're investment oriented. Often these awards are given before the fact in the form of opportunity, challenge, or a budget for a special project. At Data General, for example, they call it the pinball principle: "If you win, you get a free game." That's important because entrepreneurial professionals and inventors often work not for the payoff, but for the challenge.

- *Information flow and access* – People need the tools to act on their ideas and that's why high innovation organizations have a freer flow of information, more open communication, and easier access to data. Typical are advanced warnings about strategic directions and shifts in plans as well as increased communications between divisions. But in low innovation companies, people tend to treat information as a weapon.

- *Support and collaboration* – High innovation organizations install mechanisms to create networks, from encouraging mobility from area to area, to bringing people together across departments, to inviting speakers.

- *Resources* – Often it helps to have money, equipment, and time decentralized so that people can have extra resources to invest. Sometimes it can involve a small pool of money – not necessarily at the top, but lower down in the organization—so that others can help seed projects and introduce innovations.

A New Culture

The factors discussed above are parts of an integrated culture. Territories overlap and are not neatly divided. Communication knits the organization together. Information flows easily. People have access to each other. This is a culture which encourages innovation.

But the enemy of innovation is segmentation. Departments are divided from other departments. Peoples' careers take them through only one path. No one has an obligation or commitment to care about others. Only the CEO pulls it all together, and it's difficult to get power tools because people refuse to share information and to collaborate.

But healthcare executives can make a choice to create high innovation organizations. They can:

- create more receptivity to new ideas through special programs.

- encourage faster approvals and reduce red tape by decentralizing resources.

- bestow more praise and recognition.

- provide more advanced notice of changes.

- generate more open communication.

- build resources for experimentation.

- promote an attitude that the organization is always learning.

Taking these initiatives converts change from a threat to an opportunity. The difference rests in how the change is managed. Change will always be a threat if it's done to people, if it's imposed and forced. "They're making me do it," the employees will cry. But change is an opportunity if it's accomplished by people. Then it is their opportunity to become heroes, to be involved in something larger than themselves. Few things can be more liberating for management and more encouraging of change and innovation.

Part III

Environmental Factors and Ethics

Introduction

For several decades the health services system has been in flux. Chronic financing and access problems seem to be impossible for providers, consumers, and politicians to solve. There is a sense among the population that health care is a right, but there is no agreement on how that right should be perfected, although government remains an indispensable element. After a hiatus of 15 years, Congress is again considering health insurance proposals, though of more modest scope. The most likely result will be coverage for catastrophic illness. Many states are adopting or considering programs to aid the uninsured by expanding Medicaid, by reimbursing providers directly for care, by imposing requirements on employers and existing private insurers, or by developing new initiatives such as comprehensive health insurance associations, also known as risk pools.

It is increasingly apparent that consumer confidence in health services organizations is diminished. This lack of confidence extends to hospitals and nursing homes and has even penetrated the inner sanctum—the practice of medicine. Medicine continues to command more respect than other professionals, but consumer's high regard of physicians has lessened considerably, and their work is increasingly seen as a business. This loss of confidence is compounded by expectations of positive, even miraculous, results in any encounter with the health services system.

Concerns about need and access are not new. In 1932, the Committee on the Costs of Medical Care reported numerous problems in delivering and financing health care.[1] Reading that report now gives one an eerie feeling—despite its age it could be a summary of current problems. Shortcomings have existed for over 50 years. Contextual and perceptual changes exacerbate them.

Critics argue that free enterprise can neither define the mission of a health care system nor solve access and financing problems. Thus, for many, federal government must be the prime mover in any solution. Such involvement is not necessarily undesirable, but there is ample evidence available from analogous services (e.g., social welfare and education), from within the health services system itself (e.g., the end-stage renal disease program), and from experience in other countries (e.g., England), that large-scale government involvement also causes problems. Government participation offers no panacea; it simply exchanges one set of problems for another, and the second may be no less amenable to solution than the first.

Yet to be answered is the question of how medical education should be financed. In the past, all payors unquestioningly paid the higher costs of care provided in teaching hospitals. Now, however, both public and private sources are reluctant to bear the costs of medical education. Government subsidies are the solution suggested most often. As of now, there is no consensus.

And what of regulation? During the 1970s federal government undertook a sustained effort to control acute care hospitals by regulating the supply and costs of services and facilities. State governments added controls such as certificate of need and rate review. In the 1980s competition became the watchword. This change was enthusiastically adopted, especially at the federal level. However, among hospital managers only just accustomed to the security offered by a regulated environment, one almost free of aggressive competition, the change was received apprehensively. Then diagnosis-related groups (DRGs) were implemented by a Congress eager to save costs in a Medicare program seemingly out of control. Other third-party payors are adopting DRGs or variants and applying similar cost-cutting measures to most patients.

Where we should go from here is unclear. Efforts will continue to include in DRGs those physicians' services rendered in hospitals, and such a policy is likely to be adopted eventually. The basic purpose is to further reduce Medicare costs. Reports that acute care hospitals earned average margins of 12 to 15 percent on Medicare patients in 1984 and 1985 will also spur reductions in DRG payments. It has been suggested that a capitation-based program is the natural, evolutionary next step. In the meantime, attention has been directed to a concept called the "prudent buyer" or "buying right," wherein consumers actively participate in selecting and purchasing medical services as well as engage in prevention. It is thought that these activities will bring to bear market forces, and inefficient and ineffective providers will be driven out. Such developments will result in greater challenges for hospital managers. There is little doubt that, despite many changes, especially the unbundling of services previously concentrated in them, acute care hospitals will continue to be the flagship of the health care delivery system.

Government and Health — The Constitution

Significant government involvement in health care is a recent phenomenon. No evidence of federal concern with public or personal health is found in the U.S. Constitution, which drew heavily on a view of nature supported both by Christian tradition and by seventeenth-century science. The Constitution is based on the philosophy of John Locke, who postulated that by nature men are born equal and have a right to life, freedom, and the fruits of their labor. However, there is the difficulty that each person is a judge of his or her own rights, and that some refuse to accept their obligations. To defend their natural rights, therefore, human beings have to give up their natural condition and form a political society that will protect these same rights.[2] The autonomous states agreed to relinquish some powers to a central authority; thus, the Constitution is concerned with how federal government is organized and what its limits are regarding states and citizens.[3] Another reason for ratifying the Constitution was to provide economic stability among the states. The first ten amendments, the Bill of Rights, were added when it was found that a specific statement was needed to protect liberty rights.

"Natural rights" in eighteenth-century thought meant liberty. The Constitution makes no mention of what were later identified as distributive (benefit or claim) rights, that is, rights associated with income maintenance, housing, food, and health care. Those who speak of a "right" to health care or of other distributive rights are implicitly arguing a natural rights philosophy.* There is often an implied or even explicit assumption that distributive rights may be granted on the same basis as liberty rights. This is not the case. Distributive rights require society's productivity to guarantee them. The allocation varies with the distributive right involved and the extent of the entitlement (e.g., food stamps versus housing subsidies), but the economic effect can be significant. Besides the obvious qualitative distinction, liberty rights require far fewer societal resources. Further, liberty rights exercised by one group does not make them less available for another.

Education is a distributive right, but like health care it is not mentioned in the Constitution. It is useful to compare education, which was considered by the Constitutional Convention, and health care, which was not. One constitutional scholar notes that federal aid to educational institutions was proposed during the convention, but the matter was not pursued.[4] Thus, the Constitution provides no guidance for federal involvement in education, and control of it was left to the states.[5] This view was consistent with the distrust of central government exhibited by the Founding Fathers.

Similarly, no mention of health and medicine is found in the Constitution or in the debate surrounding its adoption by the Constitutional Convention.[6,7] The amendments ignore them, too. Constitutional justification for federal in-

---

* The "right to health care" must be distinguished from a "right to health." Society can attempt to guarantee access to health care, but "health" depends on so many components beyond society's ken (e.g., genetic makeup and life-style), that it cannot be guaranteed.

volvement in public health and medical care has come from the commerce and general welfare clauses. The commerce clause was initially used to legitimize federal involvement in quarantine legislation. The general welfare clause has been used to justify broad federal involvement in health, education, and welfare activities. It is found in Article 1, Section 8, clause 1:

> The Congress shall have Power to lay and collect Taxes, Duties, Imposts and Excises, to pay the Debts and provide for the common Defence and General Welfare of the United States . . .

The general welfare clause has been interpreted as a limitation on the federal power to "lay and collect Taxes," rather than a distinct power.[8] This view was expressed by James Madison in Federalist paper no. 41 and reiterated in a letter from Madison to Andrew Stevenson in 1830.[9] An opposite school of thought advanced the view that the general welfare clause was a distinct power. This concept was accepted by the Supreme Court when it upheld the constitutionality of the Social Security Act of 1935.

One can conclude that had health care been discussed when the Constitution was adopted, it would have been left to the states, as was education. At the time, responsibilities for public health were already exercised by state and local governments through the police power, a power not delegated to federal government, and local governments had organized and financed health care for the indigent.

Curative Medicine and Public Health

Eighteenth-century curative medicine had little to offer, and it would be another 100 years before it became efficacious. Public health had not advanced much further theoretically or technologically. However, unlike curative medicine, public health had developed general principles that were exercised by a monarch or other governmental authority. Sovereign power over sanitation can be traced to Hammurabi, during whose reign (2123-2080 B.C.) a code of laws was promulgated.[10] A similar tradition appears in the Old Testament's sanitary laws. The ancient Greeks and Romans recognized the value of sanitary measures, and there is evidence they used health officials.[11] The principle that the sovereign is responsible for protecting and promoting public health was found in England. Thus, when the New World was colonized, there was precedent for government involvement in public health. "As early as 1648 . . . Massachusetts Bay Colony passed an Act for Maritime Quarantine, and various other health laws were promulgated by different colonies before the Revolution."[12] Little was known about communicable diseases, but empirical evidence showed that separating the ill (or those who might become ill) from the healthy prevented the spread of the disease.

The early years of the republic were a time during which were delineated the powers that the states, through the Constitution, had granted to federal government and divided among its three branches. *Gibbons v. Ogden* (1824) was a landmark Supreme Court decision in terms of future federal government intervention in health matters, especially quarantine.[13] The nation's first 150 years showed diverse government efforts regarding health care, but most personal health services were provided, organized, and financed privately. The federal government's role evolved slowly and was virtually unchanged until the 1930s.

Evolution of Federal Involvement

Pre-Medicare and Medicaid (1965)

By 1900, government was involved in what may be characterized as opposite ends of a public and personal health care continuum. At one end was public health: quarantine, immunization, and sanitation. Local and state governments carried this burden. At the other end were special beneficiaries: military personnel, veterans, Indians, and merchant mariners. For all of these groups the federal government provided care. In the first decade of the twentieth century this involvement was delineated further.

The rapid strides being made in health care were unavailable to many early in this century. The rejection of large numbers of World War I draftees for medical reasons, many of whose problems could have been remedied or prevented, dramatized the discrepancy. In a sense, these preinduction physical examinations were the first national health survey. Evidence of congressional interest in another specialized group, mothers and children, is found in the 1922 Sheppard-Towner Act. Documentation of unmet needs and problems in organizing and financing medical care was reported by the Committee on the Costs of Medical Care in 1932. This evidence mounted with a formal national health survey during the 1930s. Mobilization and the conduct of World War II further emphasized unmet health needs.

The Great Depression, followed by American involvement in World War II, provided unique circumstances that permitted and encouraged the federal government's entry into areas that had been state, local, or private enclaves. Primarily, the question was one of money. Passage of the Sixteenth Amendment in 1914 gave the federal government the power to collect substantial revenue through personal and corporate income taxes, while state and local governments clung to far less lucrative sales and property taxes.

The states' inability to cope with the Depression was forcefully noted by Justice Cardozo in the *Steward Machine Company* case, one of three decisions that held the Social Security Act of 1935 constitutional. Thus, as areas of need became manifest, federal assistance seemed appropriate. Traditional groups—veterans, Indians, and merchant mariners—continued to receive care. However, during a 15-year period beginning in the mid-1930s, federal government provided financial support in more diverse ways. Its role in medical research, after a small start at the National Institutes of Health during the

1930s, became preeminent in the 1940s and 1950s. Passage of the Hill-Burton Act in 1946 continued and increased federal activity in health facility construction begun in the 1930s.[14] Programs to educate health care personnel were enacted in the 1950s. In 1965, Medicare and Medicaid began to pay for large numbers of beneficiaries.

No general policy was developed by federal government prior to its involvement. Need and circumstance dictated participation. Nonetheless, a policy can be identified from successful and unsuccessful legislation. Economic and political factors affected its rapidity and direction, but each acceptance recognized a duty to provide an entitlement. Once adopted, programs were incrementally expanded to improve benefits.

Post-Medicare and Medicaid

The enactment of Medicare and Medicaid in 1965 was a significant policy shift. They were the federal government's first major financing of health services. Rising costs have made federal government increasingly concerned with hospital efficiency. This concern was evidenced in the early 1970s health planning legislation and in efforts to control the use of services through utilization review. There is increasing pressure from all levels of government and consumers to control costs.

The federal government first sought to regulate acute care hospitals with passage of the Comprehensive Health Planning Act of 1966. Inadequate sanctions made it unsuccessful. More stringent requirements were enacted in P.L. 93-641, the National Health Planning and Resources Development Act of 1974. Amendments further controlled unnecessary expenditures by encouraging states to enact certificate-of-need laws. Congress legislated a short-lived effort to control rapidly rising health care costs in the Economic Stabilization Act of 1971. Portions of P.L. 92-603, the Social Security Amendments of 1972, were directed at acute care hospitals: the establishment of professional standards review organizations (PSROs) and limits on capital expenditures.

Laws regulating financial and market activities of hospitals were the most important and direct. Ominously, it seemed, not-for-profit hospitals lost some of their favored status in Congress. They were included with business enterprises in health and safety laws (Occupational Safety and Health Act of 1974) and labor relations laws (Taft-Hartley Act Amendments of 1974). Since that shock decade of the 1970s when paranoia was pervasive, hospital managers have responded effectively to external pressures. Congressional initiatives of the 1980s have focused on controlling costs and encouraging interhospital competition. Examples include the Medicare and Medicaid Amendments of 1980 (cost containment and cost efficiency); the Tax Equity and Fiscal Responsibility Act (TEFRA) of 1982, which established professional review organizations (PROs) to replace PSROs (same basic purpose, but with more emphasis on quality and efforts at cost control, e.g., limits on payments for hospital inpatient operating costs and payments to hospital-based radiologists and pathologists); the Social Security Amendments of 1983, which established a prospective payment system (PPS) based on DRGs; and the Medicare and Medicaid Budget Reconciliation Amendments of 1984, which provided incentives for physicians to accept assignment, limits on PPS rate increases, and numerous other provisions.

The discontinuation of federal health planning in 1986 caused significant changes. Some states have funded health systems agencies (HSAs), but many have closed. Other support for health planning has come from private business and third-party payors, who view it as integral to cost containment. Provider performance statistics are suggested as a substitute for health planning and a way to control health care costs that have chronically risen faster than general inflation. This is also consistent with the current emphasis on market forces. Recently, the Health Care Financing Administration (HCFA) began releasing mortality data on hospitals that receive payment from it. In addition, over 30 states have created data base commissions to collect data from providers and share it with employers, insurers, and health maintenance organizations (HMOs). These developments add a new and very important dimension to competition in health services.[15]

Of all the changes in the last decade, the politicization of health services ranks among the most important. Hospitals were cast into an arena where they were both uncomfortable and ill-prepared. Historically, hospitals had provided an almost sanctified service, one that transcended political boundaries. They took pride in being apolitical, but politicization made the old approach risky. Hospitals had to become involved, and this put them in a position of having friends and enemies. It is likely that in the future they will not enjoy the same level of public respect. To do nothing, however, would leave them mute in the decision-making process, and ultimately in the outcome.

Responsiveness, Cost Control, and Regulation

Generally, hospitals have been accountable to the community only if they chose to be. Data are sketchy, but responsiveness seems to be greater when service areas are clearly defined. In the past, most charges of unresponsiveness came from metropolitan areas, usually when the hospital's constituency changed. This problem has lessened. Some hospitals use consumer advisory groups; others include consumers on governing bodies. To the extent that it exists, public financing will demand public accountability—at least by proxy through those who authorize expenditure of public monies.

Deregulation removes a significant barrier between providers and consumers. Providers need not look to a regulator for continued existence; rather, in a competitive market, consumers are the focus. Deregulation, however, does not remove the demands made of providers by third-party payors concerned with costs, and cost control causes interventions in the physician-patient relationship that may not benefit the patient. Whether acute care hospitals will be more responsive to the funding constituency or the service constituency is as yet undetermined. Historically, and by analogy to other programs, it is likely to be the funding constituency. Desire to serve is invariably tempered by the demands of economic survival. It is here that ethics, especially in the provider-patient relationship, are a major consideration.

Hospitals are unique service enterprises, yet they are amenable to considerations of efficiency, effectiveness, and cost consciousness. In addition to organizational changes, they will be involved in new delivery and financing arrangements, such as surgicenters, HMOs and independent practice arrangements (IPAs), hospices, and wellness programs. Multihospital systems, joint ventures, shared services, contract management, and mergers offer great potential for savings and increased effectiveness. Despite these advantages, however, such activities should be undertaken cautiously. Information about joint ventures, for example, suggests a failure rate as high as 70 percent.[16] It was predicted that by 1990 virtually all hospitals would be part of a not-for-profit or an investor-owned system, but that prediction now seems improbable. Nonetheless, the trend is toward fiercer price and nonprice competition, and financially weak free-standing hospitals will close.

A leader in cost saving will be the investor-owned and -managed hospital, where the profit motive provides a powerful incentive. Despite their rapid growth during the late 1960s and the 1970s, national investor-owned acute care hospital systems have passed their zenith and are retrenching. The primary reason is the change in reimbursement. Hospital payments for Medicare beneficiaries are now diagnosis related, and the high profit margins of the cost-reimbursed system of the first 20 years of Medicare are gone.

Juxtaposed against pressures for cost control, many of them federal, are the efforts of the Federal Trade Commission and the Justice Department, both of which enforce federal laws prohibiting activities that diminish competition. Previously, these regulators scrutinized organizations such as the American Medical Association and the American Dental Association, but they have been less active recently. The anticompetitive effects of mergers, joint ventures, and shared services are unclear, and legally acceptable relationships are ill-defined. The death of federal health planning eliminates the HSA imprimatur, and this protection is no longer available to hospitals that engage in cooperative activities, for example. More efforts to ensure competition are likely. Because of the predictability and probable efficiency it would bring to the field, a federal law exempting cooperative arrangements from the antitrust laws would be welcome.

Policy and tax questions have been raised about the large numbers of not-for-profit hospitals that engage in for-profit ventures, both independently and in cooperation with the medical staff organization (MSO). Early in 1987 Congress and some states investigated the for-profit activities of hospitals, largely in response to business associations, which protested the unfairness of tax-subsidized competition. A basic change in the tax treatment of for-profit activities of not-for-profit organizations is likely.

The New Environment for Hospitals

Role Changes

Acute care hospitals face paradoxes and contradictions. Government regulation is cited as a way to reduce costs, but it also limits freedom of action. Concomitantly, there are expectations of initiatives to reduce costs and demands to make patient care more efficient. Hospitals are urged to expand access and their range of services, both of which usually result in higher costs. They are told to be humanistic and show compassion, but at the same time they are expected to be more cost conscious and businesslike. Measuring the results only in dollars further highlights the paradox. These demands may come from different sources; nonetheless, hospitals are put in awkward, contradictory, and often untenable positions.

An important question facing hospitals is whether they will, or can, continue to be the hub of the health services system. Traditionally, hospitals have cared for the sick and injured. To a lesser extent they educated medical personnel and conducted clinical research. Prevention and health promotion were down the list. On the basis of this historical central role it is suggested that hospitals should coordinate the greater health services system. A question to be asked is whether acute care hospitals are prepared to provide prevention and health education—essential elements in any comprehensive health care system.

Emphases on the social, environmental, psychological, and genetic dimensions of health highlight the problem. Reviewing the trend in the compulsive psychological diseases is instructive. In the early 1970s alcoholism was redefined as a disease—no longer a character defect, but something for which the individual was not accountable. Drug abusers, compulsive gamblers, and child and spouse abusers may well receive similar designations. It would be short-sighted for acute care hospitals to treat only the physical and psychological manifestations of these problems and ignore the social elements. Conversely, these new emphases demand different organizational arrangements and personnel, as well as changes in management requirements and governance. The historical institutional and inpatient orientation of hospitals, as opposed to programmatic and outpatient emphases, may cause inadequate responsiveness in an environment where adaptability is key. As an unintended consequence of efforts to meet the challenges of this new role, hospitals may be less able to deliver high-quality acute inpatient care. One solution would be for acute care hospitals to organize a vertically integrated health services system that is also integrated in a backward and forward fashion. This would be a substantial change for most hospitals, and it is possible that some would not be responsive or as able to provide such services as would a categorical new entity.

All aspects considered, however, it is desirable that hospitals become comprehensive centers for all types of health services. Whether this occurs, and whether it is successful, depends on how willing and able the hospital is to provide a leadership role and to respond to community needs and expectations. Many initiatives are being undertake by hospitals. Among the newest is adult day care. As the over-75 population grows, so too does the number of families who cannot personally give care, but are able to pay for it. Many communities lack facilities to provide adult day care; by providing such care hospitals can both fill excess capacity and delivery needed services. There are opportunities, but also risks for acute care hospitals that undertake enterprises where the medical model is inapplicable. The continuing care retirement community is an example where there have been problems.

The problem of slow response to changes in the marketplace was highlighted in a 1986 American Hospital Association study, which concluded that hospitals perform outpatient surgery in the same settings and with the same pricing policies they had in 1980.[17] The study found that 87 percent of hospitals perform outpatient procedures in inpatient surgical suites. Only 12 percent use freestanding facilities, and less than 1 percent have formed joint ventures with physicians to provide ambulatory surgery. Few were found prepared for the transition to prospective pricing in ambulatory services. Despite this finding, another study showed that the ambulatory care center (ACC) market is changing from one dominated by physicians to one in which hospitals and nonphysician corporations control almost 60 percent of ACCs.[18] Hospitals are diversifying broadly to establish extended care units, contract-managed physical therapy services, hospital-based podiatric and occupational therapy services, sleep centers, wellness and stress management programs, and geropsychiatric units.

Managed care and managed care health programs (MCHPs) result from commercial innovation rather than government action and represent a major shift in health services delivery that affects both hospitals and MSOs. The generic term for financing and/or delivery activities that are not a part of the traditional fee-for-service system is *alternative delivery system* (ADS). Included in ADS are competitive medical plans (CMPs, a model for Medicare patients), HMOs, preferred provider arrangements (PPAs), IPAs, and private health plan options (PHPOs). Technically, the IPA is a physician economic unit. Some HMOs are organized using an IPA for delivery of physician services, and their number has increased rapidly since 1984. ADS's compete directly with hospitals for certain patients, but may cooperate in other activities. Red flags have been raised suggesting that managed care may be detrimental to the patient because it stresses minimizing services provided. A major safeguard is the hospital's quality assurance program.

Prospective Pricing

Few environmental changes have as great potential to affect hospitals as does prospective pricing. The implications of prospective pricing on hospital efficiency are obvious, and the Medicare prospective pricing system (PPS) provides the first look at it. More subtle will be its effect on medical staff and patients. It is increasingly common for MSO members to be measured against the costs they generate for the hospital, and there is early evidence that in the near future "economic" criteria for hospital privileges will be included in the medical staff bylaws. To date the most apparent foci of prospective pricing have been length of stay and use of diagnostic procedures. PPS highlights diagnostic skills, and there is implicit or explicit pressure to select the most serious diagnoses. Computer software programs have been developed to assist in this regard. Research has shown that hospitalized patients are sicker and require more nursing care, and that they are being discharged "sicker and quicker." Despite earlier discharge, however, there is no evidence that patients are at increased risk. The ripple effect of earlier discharge affects skilled nursing facilities, home health care, and family members. It is suggested that PPS is a deliberate government strategy to position hospital management between physician and patient in order to reduce costs. A further implication is that physicians will have to adjust to making less money, being less powerful, having less authority, and commanding less respect.[19]

Administrative and biomedical ethics were matters of concern in hospitals long before PPS, but the current emphases on cost reduction and efficiency highlight their importance. The organizational philosophy must emphasize protecting and furthering the patient's interests. Managers' personal ethics must stress their role as moral agents, all of whose decisions affect others—hospital managers are not morally neutral technocrats. Guiding principles in an organizational philosophy *and* in a personal ethic should include the autonomy of the patient, beneficence (a positive duty to do good), non-maleficence (a duty not to inflict harm), and justice. Hospitals implement their organizational philosophy and derivative principles through managers who develop the staff's attitude, policies, procedures, and environment. Much work remains to be done if hospitals are to develop an internal environment reflecting these principles.

Health Insurance

There is a general attitude that health care ought to be available to all—that health care is a right. But an increasingly sophisticated electorate realizes that the costs to the taxpayer of this desirable goal will be stupendous. Comprehensive, universal, and compulsory national health insurance (NHI), an issue to which much attention was paid in the late 1960s and early 1970s, has yet to emerge as a major issue of the 1980s. The country's conservative political mood has reinforced a concern about health services cost increases that can be traced to the late 1970s and early 1980s. The costs of Medicare primarily, but also of Medicaid, have given politicians cause for caution. The United States' experience with health services cost inflation is similar to that of Sweden and West Germany, where, despite greater control, cost containment has been equally difficult. Implementing NHI absent effective controls courts disaster. The nub of the problem is a fact of political life: Always eager for reelection, politicians are reluctant to eliminate or reduce entitlement programs, despite the costs.

In late 1986, Secretary of Health and Human Services Otis Bowen released a plan to provide catastrophic coverage for Medicare beneficiaries. For a premium of about $5.00 per month, liability for services covered would be no greater than $2,000 per year.[20] Despite initial opposition, the Reagan administration endorsed the plan. The proposal was received in Congress, where several similar bills were introduced by Democrats who pledged to make it a top priority on the legislative agenda. Other issues in Congress affecting hospitals are Medicare deficit reduction reforms (e.g., setting rate increases for hospital payments, refining the payment methodology for capital costs, and reducing payment adjustments to teaching hospitals); Medicare quality-of-care issues; and access to health care.

Competition

It is intriguing to speculate about the potential effects of hospital competition. It is the high-stakes game, and there are far more pitfalls than in the predictable, safe environment of regulation. As yet there is no consensus as to what constitutes acceptable competition in the health field. Health services organizations and individual practitioners are testing the limits of consumer and ethical acceptability. It is far from clear what will happen if traditional economic concepts of competition and marketing are applied in a field with so many features that distinguish it from commercial enterprise. Intent focus on preserving, protecting, and expanding market share may result in losing sight of the primary reason hospitals exist.

Undoubtedly, there will be increased price and nonprice competition among hospitals. Research has found higher costs in competitive areas compared to those without competition. Further, hospitals will both cooperate and compete with their medical staffs. Competition with members of the MSO began in earnest during the early 1980s when freestanding diagnostic and therapeutic treatment centers were established by physicians. These developments resulted from the effects of certificate-of-need programs, changes in reimbursement, increasing portability of technology, and ready access of physicians to capital financing. An example of hospital-physician cooperation is a joint venture such as a magnetic resonance imaging installation; an example of competition is a physician-sponsored ambulatory surgery center. The long-term effect of these activities on hospital-physician relationships is unclear; it is likely, however, that they will add to the challenges of hospital management.

Channeling is a new concept in medical malpractice insurance. In channeling, the hospital's umbrella policy is used to insure care provided by private physicians whenever it is delivered in the facility. This has the advantages of reducing premium costs for physicians, tying physicians more closely to the hospital, and simplifying issues of liability should an untoward event occur. If channeling becomes commonplace, an immediate effect is that the physician's medical malpractice claims record will be increasingly important in MSO credentialing decisions. A long-term effect is that the hospital will be more attractive to physicians and thus be able to compete more effectively.

A policy change likely to significantly increase hospital internal competition occurred in 1985 when the JCAHO ended its prohibition on MSO membership for nonphysician and nondentist practitioners. Previously, JCAHO standards permitted independent allied health professionals (IAHPs) such as nurse midwives and clinical psychologists to have clinical duties and responsibilities as identified by the hospital and consistent with state law. Eliminating the membership barrier removes an important psychological constraint on hospital action. Although the JCAHO's change is permissive, not mandatory, the law in the District of Columbia is paradigmatic of developments likely in other jurisdictions. It prohibits hospitals from denying nonphysician practitioners the right to apply for staff membership and clinical privileges. Health care facilities must respond to applications on an individual basis and "apply reasonable, nondiscriminatory standards of evaluation."[21] Physicians are likely to object to allowing nonphysician MSO membership for IAHPs. Denials, however, risk violating the law, as well as resulting in legal actions using antitrust theories. The net result is likely to be significant change in the composition of hospital MSOs in the decade ahead.

Conclusion

Acute care hospitals continue to operate in a milieu of rapid change. They successfully met the challenge of a regulated environment in the 1970s. Now they must respond to the rigors of competition, coupled with the constraints of prospective pricing. Few entities want competition in the Darwinian sense. Only those in a dynamic growth mode can afford to be enthusiastic about it. At the beginning of the 1980s there were predictions that by 1990 a score of hospital chains, not-for-profit and investor-owned, would dominate the hospital system. Will the small and medium-sized community hospital go the way of the independent service station during the oil crises of the 1970s? Will the choice be to participate or perish, affiliate or atrophy? There are obvious advantages to having hospitals merge, cooperate, and coordinate. However, as with all solutions there are disadvantages that are either unknown or understated.

The post-1985 era will be similar to the preceding two decades: turbulent with occasional wrenching changes precipitated by policymakers forcing acute care hospitals to respond to initiatives and intrusions. Although analogous to education and welfare, health services are unique. When grand and noble experiments devised by federal policymakers fail, new initiatives are attempted. These, too, are usually effective only at the margin, if at all. No other industry or sector of the economy has suffered the extent of policy tampering on both the supply and the demand side of the equation that health services have. Regrettably, the end is not in sight. This may be a result of the complexity of a system where changes in one part cause dysfunction and undesirable results in another. One point is clear, however: Hospital managers will continue to face an array of forces and interventions. A professional prerequisite is to respond within constraints. This makes managing the acute care hospital one of the most demanding and challenging tasks in society.

Notes

1. Committee on the Costs of Medical Care, *Medical Care for the American People*, Final Report adopted October 31, 1932 (Chicago: University of Chicago Press, 1932). Reprinted by U.S. Department of Health, Education, and Welfare, Public Health Service (Washington, DC: Government Printing Office, 1970).
2. Gilman Ostrander, *The Rights of Man in America, 1606-1861* (Columbia: University of Missouri Press, 1960), p. 88.
3. Dennis Lloyd, *The Idea of Law* (Baltimore: Penguin Books, 1970), p. 84.
4. Max Farrand, ed., *The Records of the Federal Convention of 1787*, vol. 2 (New Haven: Yale University Press, 1913), p. 202.
5. Max Farrand, *The Framing of the Constitution of the United States* (New Haven: Yale University Press, 1913), p. 202.
6. Farrand, ed., *Records of the Federal Convention*, vol. 2.
7. Farrand, *Framing of the Constitution*.
8. Albert Gallatin, speech in the U.S. House of Representatives, June 29, 1798, in Farrand, ed., *Records of the Federal Convention*, vol. 3, p. 379.
9. Farrand, ed., *Records of the Federal Convention*, vol. 5, pp. 352-365.
10. Chilperic Edwards, *The Hammurabi Code* (London: Watts and Co., 1921).
11. James A. Tobey, *Public Health Law* (New York: The Commonwealth Fund, 1947), pp. 9-10.
12. James a Tobey, "Public Health and the Police Power," *New York University Law Review* 4(1927): 126.
13. *Gibbons v. Ogden*, 22 U.S. 1 (1824). In this first commerce clause case to go to the Supreme Court, it was determined that congressional power to regulate commerce is unlimited except as prescribed by the Constitution.
14. Act of August 13, 1946, Ch. 958, 60 Stat. 1040-41.
15. National Association of Health Data Organizations, etc.
16. "Joint Ventures: Why do 7 Out of 10 Fail?" *Hospitals*, December 20, 1986, pp. 40-44.
17. "Hospitals Not Ready for Outpatient Surgery PPS," *Hospitals*, November 20, 1986, p. 81.
18. "Hospitals Becoming Driving Force in ACC Market," *Hospitals*, December 5, 1986, p. 67.
19. Sarah E. Stuart and Wilford E. Maldonado, "How PPS Is Changing Hospital-Physician Relations," *Trustee*, April 1986, pp. 14-15.
20. "Bowen's Catastrophic Plan Starts the Debate," *State Health Notes*. Intergovernmental Health Policy Project, The George Washington University, Washington, DC, No. 69, January 1987, pp. 3-4.
21. Michael E. Reed and Susan G. Feingold, "Hospital Privileges: State Law Comes to the Fore," *ACS Bulletin*, November 1986, p. 39.

Bibliography

Ackerman, F. Kenneth, Jr. "Competition and Regulation: The Consumer Choice Health Plan Alternative." *Medical Group Management* 27 (July-August): 58, 1980.

Allcorn, Seth. "A New Direction for Health Care Delivery in the United States." *Health Care Strategic Management* 4, No. 12 (December):25-28, 1986.

Altman, Drew. "The Politics of Health Care Regulation: The Case of the National Health Planning and Resources Development Act." *Journal of Health Politics, Policy and Law.* 2 (Winter): 560-580, 1978.

Arthur Anderson & Co. and the American College of Healthcare Executives. *The Future of Healthcare: Changes and Choices.* Chicago. Arthur Anderson, 1987, pp. 1-45.

Averill, Richard A. and Michael J. Kalison. "Present and Future: Predictions for the Healthcare Industry." *Healthcare Financial Management* 40, No. 3 (March): 50-54, 1986.

_____. "Experts Discuss the Future of the Healthcare Financial Manager in the Year 2000." *Healthcare Financial Management* 40, No. 9 (September):54-56+, 1986.

Baglia, B.R. and Brad Johnson. "Analysis of an Industry in Transition." *Health Care Strategic Management* 4, No. 12 (December):5-14, 1986.

Banta, David and Clyde J. Behney. "Medical Technology: Policies and Problems." *Health Care Management Review* 5 (Fall):45-52, 1980.

Batavia, Andrew I. "Preferred Provider Organizations: Antitrust Aspects and Implications for the Hospital Industry." *American Journal of Law and Medicine.* 10, No. 2, (Summer):169-188, 1984.

Battistella, Roger M. and Thomas G. Rundall, eds. *Health Care Policy in a Changing Environment.* Berkeley, CA: McCutchan Publishing, 1978.

Beauchamp, Tom L. and Seymour Perlin, eds. *Ethical Issues in Death and Dying.* Englewood Cliffs, NJ: Prentice-Hall, 1978.

Boland, Peter. "Questioning Assumptions About Preferred Provider Arrangements." *Inquiry* 22 (Summer):132-141, 1985.

Brady, Timothy S. and Ronn Kelsey. "What Hospital CEOs Can Do to Make Entrepreneurism Work." *Health Care Strategic Management* 4, No. 11 (November):10-13, 1986.

Brozovich, John P. and Stephen M. Shortell. "How to Create More Humane and Productive Health Care Environments." *Health Care Management Review* 9, No. 4 (Fall):43-53, 1984.

Charles, Robert. "Does the Non-Profit Firm Fit the Hospital Industry?" *Harvard Law Review* 93 (May):1416-1489, 1980.

Childress, James P. "Priorities in the Allocation of Health Care Resources." *Soundings* 62 (Fall):256-274, 1979.

Christianson, Jon B. and Walter McClure. "Competition in the Delivery of Medical Care." *The New England Journal of Medicine* 301 (October 11):812-818, 1979.

Clark, Lawrence J., Theodore L. Koontz, and Virginia L. Koontz. "The Impact of Hill-Burton: An Analysis of Hospital Bed and Physician Distribution in the United States, 1950-1970." *Medical Care* 18 (May):532-550, 1980.

Cohen, Wilbur J. "Looking Toward the Future." *Inquiry* 17 (Summer):115-119, 1980.

Coile, Russell C., Jr. "The Healthcare System in 2010: Trends for a Changing Industry." *Healthcare Executive* 1, No. 7 (November-December):14-16, 1986.

Davis, Carolyne K. "Healthcare Reforms: What Can We Expect?" *Nursing Economics* 4, No. 1 (January-December):10+, 1986.

Demkovich, Linda E. "A Strategy for Competition." *National Journal* 11 (December 8):2073, 1979.

Duval, Merlin K. "Nonprofit Multihospital Systems." *Health Matrix* 3, No. 1 (Spring):22-25, 1985.

Dye, Thomas R. *Understanding Public Policy.* 4th ed. Englewood Cliffs, NJ: Prentice-Hall, 1981.

Enthoven, Alain C. "The Competition Strategy: Status and Prospects." *The New England Journal of Medicine* 304 (January 8):109-112, 1981.

_____. "Managed Competition in Health Care and the Unfinished Agenda." *Health Care Financing Review* (annual supplement):105-119, 1986.

Feder, Judith and Jack Hadley. "The Economically Unattractive Patient: Who Cares?" *Bulletin of the New York Academy of Medicine* 61, No. 1 (January-February):68-74, 1985.

Fottler, Myron D., Howard L. Smith, and Helen J. Muller. "Retrenchment in Health Care Organizations: Theory and Practice." *Hospital & Health Services Administration.* 31, No. 5 (September-October):29-43, 1986.

Gifford, Richard D. and Nancy Davidson. "Gone Tomorrow? CEOs Speak Out on Institutional Survival." *Trustee* 38 (May):33-37, 1985.

Greene, Barry R. "Alexander's Dilemma: Conflict Between Professionalism and Entrepreneurialism in Health Services Administration." *The Journal of Health Services Administration* 4, No. 4 (Fall):581-589, 1986.

Hofmann, Paul B. "Business Ethics: Not an Oxymoron." *Healthcare Executive* 2, No. 5 (September-October):22-24, 1987.

Howell, Jon and Larry C. Wall. "Executive Leadership in an Organized Anarchy: The Case of HSOs." *Health Care Management Review* 8, No. 2 (Spring):17-26, 1983.

Hunt, Michie. "Managed Care in the 1990s." *Health Care Strategic Management* 3, No. 12 (December):20-24, 1985.

Iglehart, John K. "Medical Care of the Poor—A Growing Problem." *The New England Journal of Medicine* 313, No. 1 (July 4):59-63, 1985.

Jencks, Stephen F. and Allen Dobson. "Strategies for Reforming Medicare's Physicians' Payments." *The New England Journal of Medicine* 312, No. 23 (June 6):1492-1499, 1985.

Jeppson, David H. "The Competitive Health Care Marketplace: Bringing New Challenges to a Changing Field." *Health Care Strategic Planning* 4, No. 7 (July):10-13, 1986.

Johnson, Richard L. "Reorganizing the Organization: New Roles Lie Ahead." *Healthcare Executive* 1, No. 7 (Novemer-December):27-29, 1986.

_____. "Volatility and Opportunity: Industry Forecast." *Health Progress* 67, No. 9 (November):27-30, 1986.

Kaluzny, Arnold D. and Stephen M. Shortell. "Creating and Managing Our Ethical Future." *Healthcare Executive* 2, No. 5 (September-October):29-32, 1987.

Kramer, Marcia J. "Self-Inflicted Disease: Who Should Pay for Care?" *Journal of Health Politics, Policy and Law* 4 (Summer): 138-141, 1979.

Leveson, Irving. "Some Policy Implications of the Relationships Between Health Services and Health." *Inquiry* 16 (Spring):9-21, 1979.

Luft, Harold S. "Medical Care In A Changing Economic Environment." *The Pharos* 48, No. 1 (Winter):2-5, 1985.

MacRae, Duncan Jr. and James A. Wilde. *Policy Analysis for Public Decisions.* North Scituate, MA: Duxbury Press, 1979.

MacStravic, Robin E. "Planning Issues for the 80s." *Hospital Forum* 23 (June):3-7, 1980.

Mannisto, Marilyn. "Multis' 1984 Growth: Small in Numbers, Large in Impact." *Hospitals* (December 16):40-42, 1984.

McManis, Gerald L. "The Next Generation in Healthcare Management." *Healthcare Executive* 1, No. 7 (November-December):46-48, 1986.

Mulstein, Suzanne. "The Uninsured and the Financing of Uncompensated Care: Scope, Costs, and Policy Options." *Inquiry* 21 (Fall):214-229, 1984.

Nich, David L. and William V. Meyers. "Why the Traditional Hospital Won't Survive." *Health Care Strategic Management* 4, No. 9 (September):24-27, 1986.

Neilson, Dan. "Surviving the Healthcare Revolution, or Winners vs. Losers." *Osteopathic Hospital Leadership* 30, No. 4 (June):6-9+, 1986.

Pointer, Dennis D. "Transformers Wanted: The New Healthcare Executive." *Healthcare Executive* 1, No. 7 (November-December):22-23, 1986.

_____. "Responding to the Challenges of the New Healthcare Marketplace: Organizing for Creativity and Innovation." *Hospital & Health Services Administration* 30, No. 6 (November-December):10-25, 1985.

Rines, Joan T. "Prospective Payment: Unanswered Ethical Questions." *Journal of the American Medical Record Association* 56, No. 3 (March):20-24, 1985.

Robins, Leonard and Frank Thompson. "The National Government's Role in Health Planning: A Political Analysis." *Journal of Health and Human Resources Administration* 2 (May):491-504, 1980.

Rosenstein, Alan H. "Hospital Closure or Survival: Formula for Success." *Health Care Management Review* 11, No. 3 (Summer):29-35, 1986.

Shannon, Kathy. "Hopes of Earlier Diagnosis Spur Research, Despite Costs." *Hospitals* (December 16):68-69, 1984.

Showstack, Jonathon A., et al. "Fee-for-Service Physician Payment: Analysis of Current Methods and Their Development." *Inquiry* 16 (Fall):230-246, 1979.

Sloan, Frank and Bruce Steinwald. *Insurance, Regulation, and Hospital Costs.* Lexington, MA: Lexington Books, 1980.

_____. "Effects of Regulation on Hospital Costs and Input Use." *Journal of Law and Economics* 23 (April):81-109, 1980.

Somers, Anne R. "Regulating Personal Behavior: Health Promotion's Goal." *Hospital Progress* 61 (August):58-61, 1980.

Torrens, Paul. "What's Up Doc?" *Healthcare Executive* 1, No. 7 (November-December): 27-29, 1986.

Vladeck, Bruce C. "The Design of Failure: Health Policy and the Structure of Federalism." *Journal of Health Politics, Policy and Law* 4 (Fall):522-535, 1975.

_____. "Restructuring The Financing of Health Care: More Stringent Regulation of Utilization." *Bulletin of the New York Academy of Medicine* 60, No. 1 (January-February):89-97, 1984.

White, William D. "Regulating Competition in a Nonprofit Industry: The Problem of For-Profit Hospitals." *Inquiry* 16 (Spring):50-61, 1979.

_____. "Why is Regulation Introduced in the Health Sector? A Look at Occupational Licensure." *Journal of Health Politics, Policy and Law* 4 (Fall):536-552, 1979.

Zuckerman, Howard S. "Multi-Institutional Systems: Promise and Performance." *Inquiry* 16 (Winter):291-314, 1979.

Competition And Entrepreneurship

Selection 35, "The Destabilization of Health Care," by Eli Ginzberg, insightfully analyzes developments in the health care system of the past 15 years that resulted in a breakdown of established patterns. A specific dimension of that destabilization is "The Dilemma Between Competition and Community Service" in selection 36 by Bruce C. Vladeck. The author suggests that hospitals exist under an evolving social contract to ensure that health care services are provided to those who need them regardless of ability to pay.

Jeff C. Goldsmith discusses an important new issue for the hospital manager in selection 37, "Entrepreneurship: Its Place in Health Care." He argues that those who believe patient care will suffer because of entrepreneurship misunderstand the entrepreneur's motivation. A theme from Part I about physician-hospital partnerships is addressed in selection 38, "Hospital-Physician Joint Ventures: Who's Doing What?" by Michael A. Morrisey and Deal Chandler Brooks. The authors describe survey findings and suggest likely types of arrangements. A major new initiative for hospitals, "New Trends in Hospital-Based Services for the Elderly," is discussed in selection 39 by William A. Read and James L. O'Brien. Geriatric care and the services hospitals are likely to provide in the future are highlighted.

35

The Destabilization
of Health Care

Eli Ginzberg

Eli Ginzberg, Ph.D., is Professor Emeritus and Director of the Conservation
of Human Resources Project, Columbia University, New York City.

During the past 15 years, there have been many signs of the increasing
destabilization of the health care system in the United States. Between the
Flexner report in 1910 and the beginning of the 1970s, a period of six decades,
the system had been characterized by a remarkable stability that reflected
three factors: the dominance of the medical profession; local sponsorship of
community hospitals; and the practice of cross-subsidization, which enabled
physicians and hospitals to care for many of the poor by overcharging the affluent. The established system could adjust to new opportunities, and the underlying structure protected and fostered important societal values.

The flexibility of the established system was demonstrated by the transformation of community hospitals from institutions of care to institutions of
cure, the restructuring of the medical profession when general practitioners
were replaced by specialists, and the proliferation of academic health centers
heavily involved in biomedical research funded by liberal grants from the
federal government. Even with the advantage of hindsight, the processes by
which the established system accommodated these pervasive changes while
maintaining its underlying structure and organization are not understood.

In the past 20 years, however, since shortly after the laws establishing
Medicare and Medicaid were passed, the established institutions have been
increasingly buffeted and battered. Consider the following factors: a large and
growing proportion of the medical profession now consists of physician
employees of nonprofit hospitals or corporate enterprises, rather than private
practitioners;[1] for-profit and nonprofit hospital chains threaten the role of
many free-standing community hospitals; the broad risk pool that enabled
persons in poor health to acquire health insurance at a reasonable cost is
being increasingly segmented as more and more large employers move to self-
insurance;[2] and cross-subsidization is evaporating in the face of intensified

Reprinted by permission from *The New England Journal of Medicine,* 315(12) September 18,
1986, pages 757-760. Copyright 1986 by the Massachusetts Medical Society. All rights reserved.

price competition, with adverse consequences for the poor and the near poor.[3]

Efforts initiated by the federal government in the late 1960s and intensified since then by the government and other payers have attempted to control steeply rising health care expenditures. But in our frenetic pursuit of the elusive goal of cost containment, many important values in the established system have been lost or are at risk. Destabilization—the undermining of the existing structure—to accomplish cost control might be considered a reasonable trade-off. But to destabilize a functioning system of health care without achieving corresponding gains in controlling costs, as I believe to be the case,[4] is a dubious result.

In this article, I will present an analysis of the destabilization process, which was begun in the pre-Medicare era and was potentiated by forces unleashed by the Medicare-Medicaid reforms and by the policy changes implemented in recent years.

By the mid-1960s, when the federal government enacted Medicare and Medicaid, latent forces were at work that would, over time, contribute to the unsettling of the status quo. The two most important were the rapid increases in the numbers of physicians in the training pipeline and the consequences of broader and deeper hospital and health care insurance.

In the first decades after World War II, the states moved aggressively to establish new medical schools and to increase the number of graduates of existing schools. In the early 1960s, the federal government, after years of providing indirect support to medical schools by means of grants from the National Institutes of Health, moved directly and vigorously to enlarge the supply of physicians.[5]

One of the principal constraints that had slowed the rate of change in the existing system—the tightness of the physician supply—was thus undermined, although it would take a few years before the consequences of the increasing supply of physicians would be felt. Among the obstacles to the growth of prepayment plans during the early postwar decades were the desirable options of young physicians in the fee-for-service sector. But the doubling of the supply of new physicians in the 1970s would eventually introduce changes in modes of practice.[6]

The second force that threatened the extant system was the rapid increase in health and hospital insurance characterized by "first-dollar" coverage. In 1971, Martin Feldstein called attention to the danger that broad insurance would result in "overutilization," which would lead in turn to waste and cost inflation.[7] Some years later, Alain Enthoven explored this issue in depth and called attention to the federal tax subsidy for employers and employees that further reduced incentives to economize in buying health care insurance and in using health care services.[8]

Each of these developments—a larger supply of physicians and improved insurance coverage—was likely to alter the health care system, but neither factor alone nor both together were sufficient to destabilize it.

The Medicare Era

The Medicare-Medicaid reforms and their direct and unanticipated consequences introduced a number of new forces that precipitated the process of destabilization. With regard to hospitals, the following direct consequences were felt. First, third-party payments rose from 77 to 91 percent of total costs,[9] and this lessened the longstanding preoccupation of trustees and hospital administrators with financial matters. Second, the new strong cash flows, which promised to increase from year to year, enabled nonprofit hospitals to break away from the philanthropic sources that had in the past covered a large part of their capital outlays.[10] Large hospitals (and many smaller ones) were able to go to the tax-free bond market and, on the basis of their prospective reimbursements, borrow all the money they needed for expansion, improvements, and modernization.[11] The hospital sector was on easy street for the first time. One aspect of this situation that escaped notice, however, was the erosion of the interest, power, and influence of many boards of trustees. Hospital administrators, acting largely alone, could meet the needs of their professional staff for new and improved facilities and new technology and services. A major source of strength in the preexisting system, a concerned and committed community leadership, had been weakened.[12]

The new affluence did not remain restricted to the predominant nonprofit sector for long. Shortly after the passage of Medicare and Medicaid, a new player entered the field—the for-profit hospital chain. Since the health care sector was awash in dollars, the well-managed new for-profit companies had little difficulty in finding attractive niches, primarily in the South and West, where most states had a charge-reimbursement rather than a cost-reimbursement formula.[13,14] With the equity market looking favorably on their prospects, the growth companies were able to obtain additional capital that helped fuel their growth. Congress also lent a helping hand by permitting Medicare reimbursement to be based on inflated values that resulted from acquisitions and improvements. Congress also provided the for-profit hospital chains a generous return on their equity investments.[15]

In less than a decade, the for-profit hospital chains increased their ownership of acute care beds from 55,000 (in 1976) to 111,000 (in 1984); by 1984, they were also managing another 41,000 beds.[16] Some informed observers have prophesied that before the end of the century, the health care system will be dominated by 10 to 20 "megafirms."[17]

The Post-Medicare Era

During the 1970s and the first half of the 1980s, many forces old and new produced effects on the health care system that, in combination, led to its destabilization. During the 1970s, the emergence and substantial growth of for-profit hospital chains weakened the hegemony of the community hospital in many parts of the country, and the emergence of potential surpluses of both physicians and hospitals resulted in corresponding threats to the continued dominance of these two key power centers. The establishment of professional standards review organizations (PSROs) and certificate-of-need legislation in the early 1970s,[18] together with the failed attempts in the late 1970s of the Carter administration to place a ceiling on annual capital outlays for hospitals, were early warning signs of a more aggressive role of the federal government. When Medicare was first enacted, President Johnson had assured the American Medical Association that the federal government would not unsettle the established system by interfering with the traditional patient-physician relationship. The fact that President Nixon took the lead as early as 1971 to obtain congressional support for the expansion of health maintenance organizations shows how quickly Johnson's promise was broken.

The 1970s ended with the established system still very much in place, although the signs pointed to a weakening of its foundations. When President Reagan took office in 1981, the new administration announced that it would rely on the competitive market rather than on federal regulation to shape the nation's health care system.[19] Furthermore, it gave notice that it would seek early congressional support for a radical cutback in federal expenditures for health care. However, the administration secured congressional approval for only some on its cuts, and it never introduced a broad, strategic proposal for reform based on competition.

Nonetheless, competitive forces came to play a much larger part, principally because of the following factors: the rapid growth of entrepreneurial activities by both for-profit and nonprofit health care organizations, primarily in the area of ambulatory care facilities; the explosive growth of health maintenance organizations, preferred-provider organizations, and other forms of managed care; and the determined and largely successful efforts of the business sector to renegotiate its health benefit plans and, in the process, to provide incentives for its employees to enroll in alternatives to fee-for-service arrangements. Moreover, a growing proportion of large corporations moved to self-insurance.

It would be difficult to find another two-year period comparable to 1981-1983 with respect to the number of innovations in health care financing and delivery. But two more events must be noted because they contributed substantially to the processes of destabilization: the institution of prospective payment for the hospitalization of Medicare beneficiaries and the growing excess of two critical resources — physicians and hospital beds.

The cumulative interaction of these multiple trends and forces substantially destabilized the three foundation blocks of the established system — the nonprofit community hospital; the dominance of the physician in therapeutic decision making; and cross-subsidization, which had previously enabled many providers to care for substantial numbers of poor patients. Many community hospitals, faced with a rapidly declining patient census, joined one of the large chains, which soon claimed to have a membership encompassing one third of all nonprofit hospitals. Other hospitals organized a for-profit affiliate to help them keep afloat in a shrinking market for inpatient care, and still others merged or changed their missions.[20]

Many physicians entering practice found themselves confronting a market that was much more competitive than they had expected. In the face of steeply rising malpractice premiums and the dearth of opportunities for starting a practice, many recently certified physicians settled for salaried employment, often with a corporate enterprise that paid primary care physicians $35,000 to $40,000 a year.[21] Almost all physicians were affected by the rules of the newly organized peer review organizations and the guidelines for treatment that the hospitals in which they practiced promulgated in response to the system of payment based on diagnosis-related groups. Physicians also faced a difficult choice in 1983, when they had to decide whether to accept a Medicare fee freeze or risk a delay in the adjustment of their fee profile.

The combination of corporate self-insurance, the tightening of their payment practices by all insurers, and the growth of volume discounting by preferred-provider organizations reduced the revenues that earlier had enabled many providers to cross-subsidize the health care of the poor. Many hospitals that were no longer able to use cross-subsidization to cover the expenses of patients with limited or no insurance were more inclined to "dump" these patients in public hospitals—a practice that recent federal and state legislation has sought to control. The antidumping legislation relating to seriously ill patients that was recently passed by selected states and the federal government reflects the difficulties facing many hospitals confronted by patients without insurance coverage.

The Dialectics of Destabilization

The remaining question I will explore is whether the accelerating forces speeding destabilization that are cited above are likely to continue unchecked until most of the earlier system of health care fades into history, or whether such forces will be slowed down, arrested, or even reversed. It has been difficult to discern the constants within the confusions of the recent past, and it will be even more difficult to discern the thrust of the present, which will set the directions and limitations for the future.

As for the future of the nonprofit community hospitals, we need to note the following likely developments: the disappearance of many small hospitals and the resizing of the total hospital plant. I do not expect, however, that the continued growth of the for-profit hospital chains will have a serious effect. These chains have not enlarged their proportion of acute care beds since 1980, and they are not likely to do so in the future, since studies indicate that they do not operate more effectively or efficiently than nonprofit hospitals.[22] Moreover, there are signs that the trustees of many community hospitals are paying closer attention to their institutions' present and future roles. In addition, many broad-based business coalitions may be the harbingers of greater community commitment. It is surely premature at this time to contemplate the early demise of the community hospital.

The forces affecting the medical profession are more difficult to assess. Clearly, the earlier untrammeled freedom of the profession to determine how, where, and for how long patients would be treated is being circumscribed by new rules, regulations, and protocols. But it is too early to conclude that all "interferences" are necessarily bad for physicians or patients, even as they may save payers money.

On the other hand, several new factors—including the ever increasing numbers of physicians entering the profession, the decreased opportunities for residents to practice their specialties, the unchecked rise in malpractice insurance premiums, the standardization of medical practice in prepayment and managed care systems, the marketing tactics pursued by for-profit medical enterprises, and the financial stake of physicians through ownership or partnership in facilities and equipment to which they refer their patients—suggest that the environment and the ethics of medical care are changing and will continue to change. During this time of destabilization, there is a risk that important values may be lost. Whether they are lost will depend on the quality of the medical leadership and the response of the public.

Another serious concern is that the care of the poor can no longer be financed as broadly as in the past through cross-subsidization. It should be noted that after the cutbacks of 1981-1983, many states extended and improved their Medicaid coverage. A considerable number of states have also established all-payer pools out of which they reimburse hospitals that provide care to disproportionately large numbers of poor patients. The secretary of the Department of Health and Human Services is under a congressional directive to revise the payment schedule for Medicare to reflect the "disproportionate share" of charity care provided by selected hospitals.[3]

The foregoing review raises three questions that require at least tentative answers. Will the forces encouraging further destabilization overwhelm the points of resistance (identified above) that have begun to emerge? Why would it be bad if destabilization continued? What are the important values embedded in the inherited health care system that we should continue to protect?

In regard to the first question, it is difficult to estimate how large a segment of the middle class will join a managed care system, even if it is a little less expensive than fee for service. My own guess is that the managed care system will continue to grow, although not at a precipitous rate, and that it may level off in the range of 25 to 33 percent. If this guess proves to be correct, the forces for destabilization will begin to abate.

But suppose my estimate is much too low, and managed care comes to dominate the system. What would be so bad about trying to control costs, prevent unnecessary hospitalizations, and shorten hospital stays, insisting that physicians use reasonable (not excessive) amounts of resources, and making still other departures from the good old days, which surely constituted no utopia?

There would be little wrong with these departures if they represented the whole story. But it further destabilization resulted in a proliferation of corporate practices of medicine in which most physicians became employees, in a system in which protocol medicine was the norm, in an erosion of local voluntarism in hospital care, and in the elimination of cross-subsidization, creating additional obstacles to access for the poor, then a great deal would be lost.

My greatest concern is that we have been pursuing contradictory policies that are adding to our problems. The competitive market is an opponent, not an ally, of cost containment.[23] When capacity increases, advertising and marketing increase, the boundaries of the system are expanded, duplication of costly services is encouraged, and the public is pushed to consume more health care services than it needs. Companies that are self-insured and that press for experience-rated premiums make it more difficult to bring poor patients into the system and to keep them there. Neither competition nor cost containment will ensure the maintenance of medical research and medical education, on which further advances in therapeutics depend.[3] Continued destabilization must be slowed and then reversed if we are not to undermine what has proved to be a highly satisfactory and effective system of care for most Americans.

Acknowledgement

I am indebted to Miriam Ostow for assistance in the preparation of this paper.

Notes

1. Schwarz, M.R. Physician personnel and physician practice. In: Ginzberg E. ed. *From physician shortage to patient shortage; the uncertain future of medical practice.* Boulder, CO: Westview Press, 1986:35-74.

2. *Source book of health insurance data 1985-86.* Washington, DC: Health Insurance Association of America, 1985:6.

3. *Report of the Task Force on Academic Health Centers: Prescription for change.* New York: The Commonwealth Fund, 1985.

4. Ginzberg, E. Is cost containment for real? *JAMA* 1986; 256:254-5.

5. Millman, M.L. *Politics and the expanding physician supply.* Totowa, NJ: Allanheld, Osmun, 1980.

6. Tarlov, A.R. HMO enrollment growth and physicians: The third compartment. *Health Affairs* 1986; 5(1):23-35.

7. Feldstein, M.S. A new approach to national health insurance. *Public Interest* 1971; 23 (Spring):93-105.

8. Enthoven, A.C. Consumer-choice health plan. *N Engl J Med* 1978; 298:650-8, 709-20.

9. Gibson, R.M., Levit, K.R., Lazenby, H. and Waldo, D.R. National health expenditures, 1983. *Health Care Finance Rev* 1984; 6(2):1-29.

10. Bradford, C., Caldwell, G., and Goldsmith, J. The hospital capital crisis: Issues for trustees. *Harvard Bus Rev* 1982; 60(5):56-68.

11. Cohodes, D.R., Kinkead, B. *Hospital capital formation in the 1980s.* Baltimore: Johns Hopkins University Press, 1984.

12. Ginzberg, E. Conservation of Human Resources Project Staff. *From health dollars to health services: New York City 1965-1985.* Totowa, NJ: Rowman and Allanheld, 1986:54-62.

13. Institute of Medicine. *For-profit enterprise in health care.* Washington, DC: National Academy Press, 1986.

14. Gray, B.H. and McNerney, W.J. For-profit enterprise in health care: The Institute of Medicine study. *N Engl J Med* 1986; 314:1523-8.

15. United States General Accounting Office. *Hospital merger increased Medicare and Medicaid payment for capital costs.* Washington, DC: General Accounting Office, 1983. (Publication no. GAO/HRD-84-10.)

16. *Statistical profile of the investor-owned hospital industry.* Washington, DC: Federation of American Hospitals, 1979-80; 1981; 1982; 1983; 1984.

17. Iglehart, J.K. Kaiser, HMOs, and the public interest: A conversation with James A Vohs. *Health Affairs* 1986; 5(1):36-50.

18. U.S. Senate Committee on Finance. *The social security act as amended through January 4, 1975 and related laws.* Washington, DC: Government Printing Office, 1975.

19. Stockman, D.A. Premises for a medical marketplace: A neoconservative's vision of how to transform the health system. *Health Affairs* 1981; 1(1):5-18.

20. Goldsmith, J.C. The changing role of the hospital. In: Ginzberg, E., ed. *The U.S. health care system: A look to the 1990s.* Totowa, NJ: Rowman and Allanheld, 1985:48-69.

21. Trauner, J.B., Luft, H.S., and Hunt, S. A lifestyle decision: Facing the reality of physician oversupply in the San Francisco Bay area. In: Ginsberg, E., ed. *From physician shortage to patient shortage: The uncertain future of medical practice.* Boulder, CO: Westview Press, 1986: 119-34.

22. Renn, S.C., Schramm, C.J., Watt, D.M., and Derzon, R. The effects of ownership and system affiliation on the economic performance of hospitals. *Inquiry* 1985; 22:219-36.

23. Ginzberg, E. Review of: Strained mercy: The economics of Canadian health care. *N Engl J Med* 1986; 315:715-6.

36

The Dilemma Between Competition and Community Service

Bruce C. Vladeck

Bruce C. Vladeck, Ph.D., is President, United Hospital Fund of New York, New York City.

The growth of competitive behaviors—and, perhaps more importantly, competitive ideologies—in the nation's hospitals is widely perceived to create a conflict between competition and traditional patterns of community service. But in fact, there is no dilemma, at least not in the sense of having to choose between two relatively unpalatable alternatives. A rededication to community service is going to be the most effective competitive strategy hospitals can adopt. Community service is not a luxury hospitals can afford to abandon in the pursuit of a competitive strategy. It is, rather, the core of an effective competitive strategy.

To make this point, I want to address four different subjects: competition as a theoretical economic principle, competition from a historical perspective, the nature of the poor and the financing of care for this segment of the population, and the competition between hospitals and doctors. These topics may seem unconnected, and in some ways they are, but they can be drawn together to crystallize the central argument.

The Economics of Competition

First, I think we're really quite naive in the health care sector, or perhaps we're self-delusional in our concept of what competition is and how competitive markets are likely to work. In most real markets, with the exception of those for bulk commodities like grain or chemicals or oil, most competition is not about price. Most competition in a real economy is some variant of what for 40 years economists have called "monopolistic competition," in which competitors seek to distinguish themselves from one another on the basis of nonprice characteristics. It could be product differentiation; it could be location; it could be image; it could be marketing. But the capacity to differentiate the product by something other than price is seen by most real firms as the most effective strategy. Kodak is not the low-price producer or supplier of photographic film or equipment; Budweiser is not the low-price beer. But both of them have been concerned that their market shares would grow too great and that they would run into antitrust problems. Their successful long-term strategies have not been price competitive.

Second, much of what we are now describing as competition in the health care environment, be it PPOs or HMOs or related relationships, would probably in most other sectors of the economy be defined as illegal "tying" arrangements under the Robinson-Patman Act and antitrust law. Not that there's anything wrong with them from a legal point of view, or even from a health services point of view. It's just that it's a funny kind of competition.

What we're moving toward in many of the more so-called competitive sectors of the health system is a form of "bilateral monopoly," with a cartel of large purchasers on one side and some number of suppliers on the other. A lot of things can be said for that kind of relationship, but it certainly doesn't look like competition in the Economics 101 sense of pure markets under perfect market conditions. It's awfully hard to have a competitive market when one buyer has a 40 percent market share and insists on behaving like a very aggressive and largely indifferent monopolist.

The notion that the Medicare prospective payment system is procompetitive shows how confused we've become about what competition really is, and how willing we are to accept political rhetoric from an administration needing to justify a 180 degree turn in policy. The underlying reality in financing hospital care is that the single biggest guy on the block—the only one whose market share is growing—has decided that he's going to make his own rules and not really listen to anybody else. That's what's going to determine the shape of health care financing and service arrangements in coming years.

It's also hard to pursue classical competitive strategies when you start with an industry that's functioning at 65 percent capacity on the one hand, but is characterized by a lot of local monopolies on the other. Again, that leads to competitive strategies that look a lot different than price competition in the classical economics sense.

All this is not to say health care is not becoming more competitive—it clearly is—and not to say that institutions won't need to compete effectively to survive—certainly they will. But the narrow notion of competition as having something to do with price per se is highly misleading. A competitive market dominated by two very large, very noncompetitive payers implies certain things about what the effective strategies are likely to be. And while the biggest payer is not very susceptible to traditional economic inducements, it is very susceptible to short-term political forces, and that says something else about the strategies for hospitals in the years to come.

One last thing on this general point of competition and theory, in relation to care of the indigent: The problems of caring for both the "covered" and the "uncovered" indigent have been with us a long time. It's true that in the short run a lot of the forces that are creating this so-called competitive climate are going to shrink the margins that have been available in the past from other payers and make it more difficult to subsidize care for the nonpaying. But if one looks at where the margins customarily have been and at who's been providing care to nonpaying customers, it's hard to make the argument that that should have a direct effect either. It's something of a cop-out to attribute problems of meeting the needs of the medically indigent to a competitive environment. The problems take on a different character under current circumstances, but they're not new problems.

Some Historical Perspective

Hospitals, it's important to remember, were initially created to serve the poor. You don't have to go back many years to see that in most hospitals, most of the patients weren't paying. There was a very simple reason for that: Before roughly the time of the First World War, if you could afford to get medical care outside a hospital, you'd be crazy to go into one. There was very little the institution could do for you, and most of what it could do could be done in your own home just as well. Most of the older hospitals in this country were originally created as facilities for poor people who had nowhere else to go, whether they were very sick or not.

It's also only since the Second World War that we've come to expect that hospitals would be able to meet their costs from patient service revenues. Before the Second World War, more than half of hospital revenues came from charity and from direct public subsidies. The only exception to that pattern was in the 10 to 20 percent of the hospital market that involved physician-owned proprietary hospitals, which were supported largely by patient fees. But most nonprofit hospitals, like most public hospitals, until very recently did not count on patient revenue providing anything like all of their financial requirements.

They certainly didn't count on any surplus or debt capacity arising from patient service revenue to generate capital. Through the mid-1950s, the great bulk of all capital for hospital construction and modernization came either from charity or from public subsidies. The use of equity and debt, and the use of patient service revenue to finance hospital capital, is really only a phenomenon of the last 20 years or so.

What we've seen in this country is a substantial change in what might be called the social contract between government and other major forces in society, on the one hand, and hospitals, on the other. Before the Second World War, voluntary hospitals were granted a tax exemption and a variety of other subsidies as well as a number of other forms of favored legal treatment, including, for instance, until very recently, exemption from coverages of employers under labor laws or minimum wage laws.

Most voluntary hospitals in this country grew up with the mission of taking care of their own, whether their own constituted a religious community or an ethnic community or all of a smaller rural or suburban community. The expectation was that they would figure out how to take care of their own, and that they would provide services whenever they could within the limits of the revenue they could raise.

This social contract changed somewhat during the Second World War, as the population learned about the advances of modern medicine and the benefits available from it. The new social contract was embodied in the Hill-Burton program. Communities built hospitals with Hill-Burton grants and loans and, in exchange, made certain assurances to the federal government. One of the assurances was that they would continue service to the poor according to historic levels. It was only then that we really began to talk about hospitals as a community resource.

What happened next was an explosion of private insurance, an explosion in medical technology, the increasing recognition of hospitals as "houses of hope," in the language then used, and an increasing improvement in the kinds of health care services available to an increasingly insured middle class.

This process culminated in the enactment of Medicare and Medicaid, yet another new form of the social contract. What Medicare and Medicaid said to the hospital community was: "Take care of our clients exactly the same way as you take care of your private customers; let them have semiprivate rooms, don't discriminate on the basis of payment source, and we will pay the cost associated with that care."

What happened as a result hardly needs repeating, but it's fair to say that hospitals didn't entirely keep their end of the bargain. In retrospect, the post-Medicare and Medicaid growth in expense looks a lot greater than anyone can justify. The proliferation of capacity also looks a lot greater than anyone can justify. Competition among institutions was a primary source of both of these phenomena, and has a lot to do with the fix we're currently in. At least twice in the post-Medicare period, when public policy makers got particularly upset about increases in hospital costs, the hospital industry committed itself to voluntary efforts to reduce the rate of cost increase as a way of precluding other forms of public intervention. Neither was successful.

Hospitals' margins grew throughout that period as well, to the point where you really could question the extent to which the hospital community had played fair under the social contract established in 1965. The industry could not discipline itself because of competition within its ranks. Despite a 20-year dialogue between public and private sectors about the cost implications of the entitlements and the payment mechanisms created under Medicare and Medicaid, each time the industry recommitted itself to doing something without direct public intervention, cost growth accelerated still further. That led by the beginning of this decade to unacceptable budgetary problems. Everyone knows about the problems with the Medicare Trust Fund. And throughout the 1970s and into the early 1980s, Medicaid costs for state governments rose 30 percent faster than state revenues in general.

What really created PPS in its present form was the increasing irritation and anger with the hospital community on the part of policy makers. A lot of what has happened over the last couple of years—the Medicaid programs and

PPS and PROs and a variety of other things—is really a conscious effort on the part of policy makers to mount a punitive initiative toward hospitals. William Guy has talked about how hospitals missed their chance in 1972 and 1975 and 1978 to come to some better accommodation with Medi-Cal, which culminated in the selective contracting scramble in California. You hear much the same kind of rhetoric among a lot of the congressional staff: "It's time these guys got theirs" is basically the message they are giving us.

Part of that message is the newest social contract, reflected in the Tax Equity and Fiscal Responsibility Act of 1982, the 1983 revisions to the Social Security Act, and the various Medicaid programs. The big payers—the public payers and increasingly the private payers—are saying to hospitals collectively, "Here's how many dollars we're prepared to spend. We can call it a budget neutral amount; we can call it a total Medicaid budget amount; we can call it a capitation rate under a private plan. But this is the limit, the ceiling, the cap. This is all you have in the coming year, and do the best you can."

There's been substantial reaction from hospitals that this new attitude represents a withdrawal, a reneging, a going back on commitments made in the past, and to some extent it is. But it's important to recognize the extent to which the collapse of the preexisting understanding was really arrived at mutually by both sides to the deal.

It is particularly important that, rather than beating their breasts about it, hospitals recognize their obligation to respond as energetically and creatively as they can under this new set of rules—not to cop out by dumping community services, by dumping patients, by dumping populations, but to acknowledge that these are the rules of the game whether they like it or not for the foreseeable future, and to accept that their continuing obligation is to do the best they can under those rules.

Hospitals and the Poor

The most obvious observation about the problems of providing care to the medically indigent is that the poor are not distributed at random throughout the population. The poor are concentrated—perhaps increasingly concentrated—in a relatively small number of areas. What this means is that the problem of providing medical care to the poor is not equally everybody's problem. It's a particular problem—and a particularly serious problem—for some communities and for some providers. Much of the anxiety about the impact of competition on the health care system has arisen from the recognition that some institutions are in a substantially better position to ignore this population.

It seems unlikely, however, that society will accept permanently ignoring that population. As we've seen in at least four Northeastern states and in Florida, if the hospital community itself does not collectively undertaken some sort of redistributive response in terms of the haves subsidizing the have-nots, those redistributions will be imposed externally. If they are imposed externally, they will be a lot less comfortable for the hospitals involved than those that hospitals impose on themselves. Whether such nonregulatory, nonexternally imposed redistribution is possible in a competitive environment, I don't know. But it is the crux of what people are worried about in terms of the impact of competition on the poor.

It is useful, although terribly oversimple, to distinguish between those who have Medicaid and those who have no coverage at all for health care services—two groups that might be called the old poor and the new poor. Most of the old poor—children, the elderly, the disabled—are covered by Medicaid; they are, in our current notion, the deserving poor.

Much of the concern about the impact of Medi-Cal and other Medicaid payment cutbacks arises from the confusion we have created in hospital financial offices over the last few years in the distinction between average and marginal costs. In fact, hospitals are very high fixed-cost operations; marginal costs for most hospitals most of the time are only a small fraction of average costs. Many hospitals have learned from experience with Medi-Cal that, depending on other sources of revenue, a payer that has 10% or 15% of the market in an industry with a substantial excess of capacity over demand, and which meets marginal costs, is worth having. It is important to recognize the need—once you're up and going—to cover those marginal costs.

Another group of people, some 25 million of them, have no health care coverage at all. But that population, which includes many people who have lost health insurance benefits as a result of losing employment and a substantial number of unregistered aliens, is not always going to remain poor. The uninsured tend to go on and off insurance coverage. I wonder whether institutions that are unwilling to treat them when they're having problems are going to be looked at very favorably when they are back to being paying customers.

There's no question that in the current political environment, public and policy attitudes toward services to the poor are substantially less generous than they've been in the recent past. If you take a long enough historical perspective, however, this is not the inevitable course of history. This is the swing of a pendulum, and sooner or later it is going to swing back. The question is, how will hospitals be positioned when the pendulum starts to swing back? How will the institution be perceived by the public as the public becomes increasingly sympathetic to putting back in the necessary dollars to serve indigent populations?

Hospitals and Doctors

The real competition that hospitals face in the balance of this decade and the decades to come is not among one another, but from physicians. Between 1960 and 2000, the ratio of physicians to population will roughly double. This is happening in an environment where many parts of the country already have a relatively abundant supply of physicians.

What we are facing in the hospital industry, in health care in general, is a very serious shortage of patients. I don't know where that patient shortage is coming from. Maybe patients are responding to economic incentives as insurance benefits change, or maybe the population is getting healthier and using health services less. But it's going to be competition over those patients and who gets to do the expensive procedures that will be driving the system.

Again a bit of historical perspective is useful. It's only since the Second World War that doctors have become so dependent on hospitals. Young physicians perceive admitting privileges as an absolute necessity to the practice of medicine. One can associate this with the technologies that developed after the Second World War, but there were other social and political forces as well.

But the technologies are starting to shift, and the social and political forces are shifting as well. It's increasingly clear that ophthalmologists, plastic surgeons, and, increasingly, urologists and other types of surgeons are less and less dependent on hospitals for most of the work they do.

In the short run, as the physician supply continues to grow and as hospital utilization continues to fall, and as physicians and hospitals become more competitive with one another, the competition between physicians and hospitals will be oriented toward the most lucrative markets. But there aren't enough of those markets to go around. As the physician supply continues to grow, and as the major payers move away from fee for service to some form of either capitated or fee schedule payment, physicians, like hospitals, will get less and less picky about whether the patient is paying the average price and instead will become more and more concerned about whether they're paying anything at all.

Again, it's not so long ago that most physicians in private practice — and this is not just American Medical Association mythology — did treat some patients for free and did provide *de facto* sliding scales tied to patients' ability to pay. That all went out the window with the development of "uniform, customary, and reasonable" charges and Medicare and Medicaid. But the economic pressures for physicians to keep markets, even if it means discounting prices, remain, and will be reinforced both by physician supply phenomena and by the movement away from fee for service. While competition between hospitals and physicians now tends to be over the best-paying patients, it's only a matter of time before any patient will begin to be attractive.

At this point, I want to propound what I call "Vladeck's theorem": Full hospitals rarely close. I state this cognizant that a hospital is a political and social, as well as an economic, institution. Someone from New York can speak with a significant degree of expertise on the closing of hospitals. A lot of hospitals there that lost a lot of money in recent years have been quite busy and have remained open, and a lot of hospitals that have not lost much money have closed.

The key to survival is having a justification for survival, and that justification is not the bottom line. It's having patients who perceive you as a provider of a needed service. I think once we get by the first generation of anxiety about competitive forces, we will all come to recognize that a poorly paying patient or even a nonpaying patient may be better in a competitive environment than no patient at all. Certainly the revenue that the nonpaying patient generates is no less than that of the absent patient. But as we get more sophisticated in our cost accounting, we will realize that the cost to the institution of serving that nonpaying patient isn't a whole lot greater than that for the nonexistent patient either.

Summing Up

Where does this lead, particularly in the short to medium run? First, the pivot to the whole system has got to be Medicare, the one buyer that has 40 percent of the market on the hospital side and that's pushing a third of the physician market and a lot bigger share of the market for certain kinds of specialists and for general practitioners, family doctors, and general internists in particular communities.

The Medicare population is going to be the only source of increasing demand for services in the years ahead. There are only three cohorts in the population that are likely to grow substantially over the next decade. These are children, as a result of the little bubble on the population curve, who are going to be healthier than they've ever been and who have never used a lot of inpatient services to begin with. We baby boomers are beginning to age into an era in which we will use slightly more health care services, but that's running against the trend of the decline in utilization in the 35-64 population. There is going to be explosive growth in the over-75 population, people who use a lot of institutional services and are going to continue to do so. So that 40 percent market share we're looking at for Medicare as a floor is going to continue to grow. All the net growth in demand, certainly for inpatient services, and probably for outpatient services as well, is going to come from that sector.

This means two things. One is we've got to fix the prospective payment system. There's a lot to be said for PPS, but I have yet to hear any rational justification whatsoever for uniform national rates. I've never seen a federal policy that is so extraordinarily redistributive in terms of dollars from one part of the country to another be enacted into law and implemented—all without the kind of screaming that I expect we'll begin to hear next year.

The second thing we have to do is to relegitimate the hospital in the eyes of the public and of policy makers. It is critical to recognize the extent to which public perceptions of hospitals, which have historically been quite favorable, have changed in recent years, and the extent to which those changes in perceptions have colored public policy developments. I don't think we can do that solely by advertising. It's very difficult to convince the public of a proposition that fundamentally isn't true.

The way to legitimate the hospital in the eyes of the public is to go back, in a sense, to the era in which hospitals were valued and were looked up to and were protected by public policy because they were perceived as providing an essential community service that no one else would—because they existed for the purpose of providing community service, rather than because the vice-president for marketing and strategic planning told them that was a good thing to do. To the extent that hospitals are perceived as necessary community resources, they will be supported and maintained as necessary community resources. To the extent that they are not, the kind of risk hospitals are facing now will only get worse.

You can't compete effectively under any set of rules in any sort of game if you don't know who you are and what you are and why you're there. The hospital industry has become particularly susceptible to a substantial degree of faddism. As it passed the $100-billion-a-year level several years ago, a whole new army of consultants and vendors and newsletter peddlers sprung up, whose stock in trade is to scare the hell out of potential customers so they will buy what they are selling. A little fear is probably good for the soul, but it has created a climate in which it's all too easy to lose sight of why hospitals are in business in the first place.

We've all been saving for a rainy day. I would suggest that in some communities the rainy day might be here already. What surpluses are for in the first place are to meet a basic institutional mission, not to worry entirely about the next generation. We also need to rediscover the most effective competitive strategies — ways of generating revenue from other than patient care.

I think it's critical that we rediscover the role of philanthropy in support of hospitals. There are a lot of philanthropic dollars out there. Americans are very generous; they give a lot of money to health care. But they give increasingly smaller shares of it to hospitals. The reason they do, as I've found over the last year or so, is that people won't give you money unless you can effectively make a case why they should. The dollars are out there if you can convince people that you have a case for them. To do that you have to have a case.

We are talking about a phenomenon that is not purely a phenomenon of economics, that is at root a social and very political phenomenon. We live in a political economy, not a textbook economy, and the most effective strategies for survival in a political economy involve the attitudes of the public and of important decision makers and policy makers about the legitimacy of the institutions involved. That's really the basic message.

The worst mistake hospitals can make is to confuse a swing of the social policy pendulum with the path of history. If hospitals don't do everything they can, as hospitals always have, to serve their communities in the tough times, when times get a little less tough the community may not care as much about them as it did in the past.

Note

This paper is a slightly revised version of a speech on "The Dilemma Between Competition and Community Service" presented at the annual meeting of the California Hospital Association on Oct. 18, 1984. I am extremely grateful to CHA for having invited this unreconstructed Easterner to make such a presentation and for having permitted, even encouraged, its republication in this form. Special thanks are due to Michael Nolen, director of education and conference planning at CHA, and to Allen Toon, publications editor. An earlier version of this paper appeared in *CHA Insight*, Nov. 28, 1984.

37

Entrepreneurship: Its Place in Health Care

Jeff C. Goldsmith

Jeff C. Goldsmith, Ph.D., is President, Health Futures, Inc., Bannockburn, Illinois.

After nearly 20 years of effortless growth and relative stability, health care managers, trustees, and physicians have been catapulted into a new world of uncertainty and change. The forces which have given rise to this change are familiar to us by now: changing payment schemes for government and private insurers alike; growing "enfranchisement" of the patient in the economic consequences of health care use; increasing plenitude of physicians in most parts of the country and developing glut in others; and the emergence of many new, lower cost forms of health care delivery and technology. Acting in combination, these forces have significantly diminished hospital use rates in most parts of the country, as well as reduced demand for physician office visits.

The resultant sharp increase in competitive pressures both for physician and hospital services has forced both managers and physicians to alter their behavior. However, successful adaptation to a more competitive world—to a "buyer's market" for health services—will require something more fundamental. It will necessitate a change in values and motivations which many in health care will find difficult to accept, let alone achieve: the adoption and cultivation of entrepreneurial values.

A Flick of the Financial Officer's Pen

In a seller's market, where physician and hospital services have been in relatively scarce supply, providers of care were buffered from market pressures by queuing for services and by an almost narcotic payment scheme based on cost or cost-plus reimbursement. It was barely necessary to have a strategy, financial or competitive, in an environment where the consequences of poor decision-making could be passed on to the taxpayer or the private in-

Reprinted with permission from *Healthcare Forum Journal.* Vol. 27, March/April, 1984. Copyright The Healthcare Forum.

sured employer with a simple flick of the financial officer's pen. The principal problem was how rapidly to grow and what services and technology to add. The result of these conditions was the evolution of a health care marketplace poorly attuned to the needs of the consumer or payer, and a managerial style far closer to that of a bureaucracy than to a business.

As the market has begun to tighten, and the payment system has become considerably less forgiving, hospitals and physicians who persist in the seller's market mentality of "we have what the public needs—let them come" will find their economic and professional fates increasingly determined by others. The marketplace—mass purchasers and patients as well as investors—is hungry for new products and services that will save money while preserving quality of care, for services that meet patient rather than provider needs. To respond to these increasingly insistent demands, providers of care will be compelled to become entrepreneurs in the best sense of the term, champions of new ideas that solve human problems.

This transformation will not be easy, particularly for hospital managers. Health care management under cost reimbursement took on an almost custodial quality, of managing conflict while "keeping the ball rolling." In the process, hospitals became substantial economic enterprises. Even small hospital budgets reached into eight figures. Larger institutions attained aircraft-carrier-sized mass and corresponding inertia.

The contrast between the style of management these institutions demanded and entrepreneurship could not be sharper. The entrepreneur is not a bureaucrat, but a visionary and a marketer. Driven by a vision of an unmet need or an emerging technology, the entrepreneur is consumed by the struggle to convert that vision into an enterprise. To accomplish this conversion requires getting others to share the vision and to invest capital, time, or other resources in bringing it to fruition as a new product or service. To do this requires the assumption of economic risk, not only by the entrepreneur but by those who support him or her.

Intelligent Risk-Taking

Unlike traditional hospital management, which sought to minimize risk, entrepreneurship is founded on intelligent risk-taking. Here is meant not wagering one's retirement savings at the baccarat table, but weighing the economic risk assumed by supporting the entrepreneurial idea against the likely reward, *as well as* against the alternative uses of the capital or time foregone in the process. In order to do this, the strength of the entrepreneur's vision must be weighed against what is known about the market and competitive structure the product is seeking to penetrate. Since there is almost no undefended territory in the health care marketplace, those who sponsor or support the health care entrepreneur must discipline themselves to subject the idea to the kind of rigorous empirical analysis they would any proposed allocation of scarce capital.

Having committed the organization or sponsors to proceed, the real difficulties begin. Management of entrepreneurship inevitably begins with a small, very fragile enterprise that must be nurtured through its takeoff with constant adjustments in strategy and progressive changes in management. Starting up and managing a small business, something with annual revenues that may be in the six- to seven-figure range, requires a completely different kind of discipline and approach than managing the eight- to nine-figure ongoing enterprise. It requires the willingness to adjust and change, but the discipline to avoid tinkering. It requires rapid decision-making, which is rarely produced by committees, multiple layers of approval and high-level pondering. It requires periodic infusions of capital, and the patience to wait to achieve positive cash flow at the appropriate time during the takeoff period. This type of management is an anxious, day-by-day proposition that must be sheltered from the routinized, relatively stable decision and management framework of the larger enterprise.

Large corporations have struggled for decades to nurture entrepreneurs in their organizations. Much of the book *In Search of Excellence* is focussed on the successful efforts to shelter the creative spark in large business enterprises dependent on capturing the benefits of new technologies.

Visionaries in Health Care

Entrepreneurship is no stranger to health care. Indeed, it has given rise to some distinguished examplars. Dr. James Campbell of Rush-Presbyterian-St. Lukes Medical Center in Chicago was an entrepreneur and institution builder committed to a vision of voluntary systems of health care. Drs. Thomas Frist, Sr. and Jr., the founders of HCA, were likewise entrepreneurs of a new form of organization of hospital services, the investor-owned hospital system. Drs. Wallace Reed, of the Phoenix Surgicenter, and Bruce Flashner, of the Doctor's Emergency Officenter chain, were visionaries who pried two key hospital services, surgery and emergency care, loose from the hospital and brought them directly to patients. Some, such as Paul Ellwood, MD, were entrepreneurs not of products, but of ideas—in Ellwood's case, that of prepaid, "managed" health care. They sold their vision not to investors or patients but to the policymakers and policy shapers who most affected the framework needed to bring about the idea.

These individuals achieved their success in bringing the vision to the marketplace in many cases over the passive and active resistance of institutional and professional rivals, and initial public skepticism. They bucked the bureaucrats and professional cliques that inhibited change, infuriating many of them in the process. And the society benefited from their success.

Critics Misunderstand Motivations of the Entrepreneur

The rise of entrepreneurship in health care has spawned a vigorous reaction from the fading centers of influence in medicine. Dire warnings about the rise of corporate medicine, and the "medical-industrial complex" are emanating from the public health/public policy and academic worlds. These critics misunderstand the motivations of the entrepreneur.

Unquestionably, successful entrepreneurship brings economic reward. The promise of easy reward attracts individuals who are motivated in some measure by greed, not by social needs. Hospitals and physicians who embark on entrepreneurial ventures, however, are as likely to be motivated by a search for a defensible economic framework to continue to serve their communities as they are by the pursuit of wealth for its own sake. There are far easier ways to become wealthy than continuing to seek to serve people.

What the entrepreneur ultimately seeks is the vindication of an idea. And that vindication, not the resultant economic consequences, is the true reward of successful entrepreneurship. As government commitment to support of health care wanes, the ability to preserve quality and continue to advance the state of the art in medicine and medical practice may hinge upon how successfully health care institutions and professionals can cultivate and support the entrepreneurs among us.

38

Hospital-Physician Joint Ventures: Who's Doing What

Michael A. Morrisey and Deal Chandler Brooks

Michael A. Morrisey, Ph.D., is Senior Economist and Assistant Director, Hospital Research and Educational Trust, American Hospital Association, Chicago.

Deal Chandler Brooks, M.A., is Director, Programs for Hospital Governing Boards, American Hospital Association, Chicago.

Joint ventures, essentially market-driven business agreements between hospitals and physicians, are intended to reduce conflict and foster cooperation between hospitals and physicians through the sharing of economic risks and rewards. Other than anecdotal information and selected case studies, little is known about the extent and nature of hospital-physician joint ventures. But the results of a 1984 American Hospital Association survey on hospital-medical staff relationships are beginning to fill the void.*

The survey, which focuses on 10 commonly cited joint-venture opportunities, reveals that only 11.76 percent of responding hospitals had a functioning joint venture in January 1984 (see Table 38-1). Preferred provider organizations (PPOs), medical office buildings, and ambulatory care centers were the most common joint ventures, although none of these were operated by more than 4 percent of the surveyed hospitals.

Sparsity of Ventures

There are several reasons for the relative sparsity of joint ventures, defined in the survey as existing when a hospital or its holding company and

---

*The survey questionnaire was mailed to 5,808 nonfederal, short-term, general acute care hospitals in July and September 1984. Hospitals returned 3,601 usable surveys, for a response rate of 62 percent. Investor-owned, small, rural, and south central hospitals were somewhat underrepresented in the final data.

Table 38-1. Percentage Of Hospitals Engaged In Hospital-Physician Joint Ventures, 1984.

Joint Venture	Percentage
Preferred provider organization	4.00 %
HMO	2.23
Individual practice association	2.14
Ambulatory surgical center	.88
Primary or ambulatory care center	2.20
Freestanding minor emergency center	1.54
Home health agency	.51
Freestanding laboratory	.77
Freestanding imaging center	1.11
Medical office building	3.34
Any of the above joint ventures	11.76

Source: Hospital Research and Educational Trust, American Hospital Association.

one or more members of its medical staff have a shared financial responsibility for an organization, facility, or service.

First, joint ventures are relatively new and require trust and active interest of both the hospital and medical staff members as well as some evidences of success. The story of how Baylor University Medical Center, Dallas, developed its joint ventures is a good example of the rethinking process that occurs among a joint venture's players (see p. 68, *Hospitals*, December 1, 1984).

Second, the survey data reflect a snapshot taken in January 1984 (hospitals were asked to respond as of January 1, 1984, and only with respect to ventures located within the hospital's service area and dealing with members of their own medical staffs). This picture is undoubtedly an understatement of the current number of operational joint ventures. However, even if the number of ventures had doubled, the number of hospitals involved would only be about 1,200.

A third reason relates to the economics of particular joint ventures. For example, urgent care centers may not be the successful joint venture originally imagined, because success apparently depends upon patient volumes about 15 percent greater than in a typical physician office. Further, the economics of advertising suggest that the hospital should establish six to eight locations in the community (see "Urgent care centers," p. 31, *Multis*, February 1, 1985). And the cost of failure is high—not only in the capital and staff time expended, but also in the ill-will created between the hospital and its medical staff.

A fourth reason relates to the appropriateness of a joint venture. In many instances, other arrangements may better suit the circumstances. For example, it may not be as desirable to establish a freestanding imaging center as a joint venture if established radiology groups in the area can purchase the necessary equipment themselves and sell their services to several hospitals through exclusive contract arrangements. This alternative approach would be particularly appealing in localities where hospital participation might trigger a certificate-of-need requirement.

And with 76.7 percent of hospitals reporting that they have exclusive contracts with radiologists, it may be that the goal of a closer relationship with selected members of the medical staff has already been achieved, at least in the radiology department.

A final reason for the sparsity of ventures reported is that a number of less prevalent joint venture opportunities were not included, such as birthing centers, women's health centers, eyeglass dispensaries, answering services, and group purchasing arrangements. Of course, joint ventures with other hospitals or insurers were not included in the survey.

As the influence of competitive and other environmental forces increase, the response of hospitals and physicians in the joint venture arena is likely to be as varied as the characteristics of the partners involved. Thus, any survey is likely to be less than complete.

Locations and Players

The bulk of joint venture activity is occurring in four geographic areas: the Pacific, Mountain, New England, and East North Central regions (Fig. 38-1). However, the types of services offered through joint ventures vary significantly across the regions.

In the Pacific and Mountain regions, PPOs are the most common joint ventures, with 9.6 percent and 7.0 percent respectively of surveyed hospitals in these areas responding that they have such agreements with members of their medical staff.

In New England, individual practice associations (IPAs) and HMOs are the most common forms of hospital-physician joint ventures. In the East North Central region, the joint venture activity is split between PPOs and medical office buildings.

Regional differences are consistent with other data on trends in health care competition. Recent working papers note, for example, that 38 percent of operational PPOs are located in California, and Denver is often cited as one of the homes of the first PPOs.

PPO, HMO, and IPA joint ventures were least likely to be found in the Middle Atlantic states (New Jersey, New York, and Pennsylvania). It may be, as some have suggested, that state rate-setting has blunted the development of competitive options. However, this speculation has not been subjected to rigorous study. Most of the joint venture activity in the Middle Atlantic states

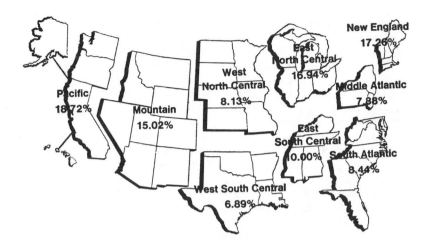

Figure 38-1. Percentage of Hospitals Engaged in Any Hospital-Physician Joint Venture, By Region, 1984. Source: The Hospital Research and Educational Trust. The American Hospital Association.

was found in primary or ambulatory care centers, where 3.7 percent of hospitals indicated that they had a joint venture in operation.

The analysis of hospital involvement used mutlivariate regression techniques that allowed control for several factors at once. In addition to region, differences were examined by size of the community and size of the hospital as well as hospital ownership and teaching status.

Cities with populations of 250,000 or more were most likely to have hospitals with established joint ventures. This supports the theory that relatively high volumes of activity are necessary to make many ventures profitable. More generally, if joint ventures are arising as a response to competition, it is likely that those hospitals located in communities with several hospitals, high physician-population ratios, and many cost-conscience public and private payers will be among the first to develop joint ventures.

The number of such hospitals, however, may be limited. A recent report indicates that 40.7 percent of U.S. hospitals have no more than one neighboring hospital in a 15-mile radius and 61.7 percent have no more than four such hospitals (see p. 89, *Contemporary Policy Issues*, Winter 1984-85). Depending upon physician density and changes in health insurance benefits, these relatively isolated hospitals may not ever actively pursue joint ventures.

After adjusting for community size and other factors, our results indicate that larger hospitals — those with 200 or more beds — are more likely to have developed joint ventures with their medical staff. This may reflect a particular need the larger hospital has — to find a mechanism for active cooperation with that subset of its medical staff that is essential for the hospital's survival.

While more private voluntary hospitals participate in joint ventures, after controlling for bed-size, region, community size, and teaching status, we found no appreciable differences between investor-owned and private voluntary hospital patterns of participation in joint ventures. This is somewhat surprising, because a joint venture with a not-for-profit hospital offers the hospital access to nondebt capital and the physician access to tax shelter opportunities. The fact that some nonproprietary institutions find for-profit ventures inconsistent with their missions may partially explain the lack of differences in our results.

Not surprisingly, state or local government-run hospitals and major teaching hospitals were less likely to have established joint ventures. One reason for this is the more complex decisionmaking processes in place at these institutions. In the teaching facilities it is often the case that the medial staff is composed of paid members of the academic faculty. Also, research and teaching physicians are often less interested in the entrepreneurial side of maintaining a medical practice.

The Future

It is difficult to judge the future even by the past. The past data suggest, however, that large, nongovernmental, nonteaching hospitals in large urban areas — particularly in the West, New England, and East North Central regions — will continue to develop joint ventures. It is the nature of competition that those who do not develop or imitate successful innovations fall by the wayside. The changing financing environment and the increasing supply of physicians suggest that profitable joint ventures will be imitated wherever competition demands them.

39

New Trends in Hospital-Based Services for the Elderly

William A. Read and James L. O'Brien

William A. Read, Ph.D., is Director, Section for Aging and Long-term Care, American Hospital Association, Chicago.

James L. O'Brien is Research Associate, Office on Aging and Long-term Care, Hospital Research and Educational Trust, American Hospital Association, Chicago.

The decision of an individual hospital to enter into long-term care is highly complex. The specific array of services delivered and coordinated through a long-term care program depends on numerous factors, such as the availability and accessibility of existing community services, the needs and resources of the elderly within the community, and the hospital's own financial resources. For those services on which we have data, the past five years have been characterized by dynamic growth in long-term care services — approximately 20 percent in home care, 8 percent in skilled nursing facilities, and 5 percent in hospice care. The flurry of program development, especially since 1983, will continue into the immediate future.

A survey of community hospitals by the American Hospital Association in 1985 and 1986 shows that the long-range plans of 66 percent of the 3,529 responding hospitals include the development or expansion of services for the elderly. Overall, the survey results show extensive hospital involvement in aging and long-term care services.

Hospital-Owned and Operated Services

Hospitals now own many innovative and unique programs — innovative in terms of the types of programs traditionally available to the chronically ill, and unique in comparison with the traditional array of hospital services. On average, community hospitals directly own and operate four different long-

Reprinted by permission from *Trustee*, Vol. 39, No. 9, September 1986. Copyright 1986, American Hospital Publishing, Inc.

term care services, and 85 percent of the hospitals surveyed provide at least one such service.

The long-term care service that hospitals most frequently operate is a patient and family educational program (54.4 percent of respondents). Although such an educational program is not a long-term care service per se, family caregivers are the most frequent source of long-term care. Effective education can ameliorate the stress associated with the extended care of a loved one, and it can minimize the need for institutional care.

The next five most common services for the aged are emergency response systems (35.8 percent of hospitals), home health (33.3 percent), information and referral services (33.2 percent), hospital-based skilled nursing facilities (SNFs) (19 percent), and durable medical equipment (17.3 percent).

Not surprisingly, the least available long-term care service is foster care (0.4 percent of hospitals). Foster care, in which a chronically ill patient is placed with a family on either a short- or long-term basis, has only recently been formulated as a service option, and it is not yet clear what its future will be.

Hospitals also infrequently provide alternate housing arrangements for the elderly. Only 2.3 percent of responding hospitals provided senior apartments and 0.8 percent offered either sheltered housing or continuing care retirement centers (CCRCs).

It should be noted that a small number of hospitals have entered into formal contractual arrangements with existing retirement centers. For instance, hospitals may contract to provide medical services for the residents of senior housing units. They may even establish an outpatient clinic at a center or operate on-site intermediate and skilled nursing beds.

The other services least frequently available at an institutional level are home visitors (3.3 percent of hospitals) and psychiatric long-term care (1.4 percent). Although the data collected in the survey provide no information on the reasons why this is so, one can speculate that the lack of payment, negative stereotypes associated with the services, and their uniqueness, have played some role in limiting their development.

Services Provided on a Contractual Basis

Typically, hospitals enter into formal contractual arrangements with other providers to ensure the accessibility of services. Formal contracts enable a hospital to supplement the services it provides through its own programs. Together, owned and contracted services may provide an indication of the typical services hospitals of the future will offer.

The most frequently contracted long-term care services are home health (21.5 percent of hospitals), and homemaker services (16.2 percent). Unlike hospital-owned services, the other most frequently contracted services are for alternate levels of institutional care, including freestanding skilled nursing facilities (15.1 percent), psychiatric long-term care (14.8 percent), hospice (12 percent), and intermediate care (12 percent).

Specialized Geriatric Programs

One operational strategy that has been suggested to effectively care for older adults is to provide services in separate, specially designed, distinct programs. For the purpose of the survey, specially designed services for the elderly were characterized as having staff trained in geriatrics, specific admission criteria limiting care to individuals over 65 years of age, and architectural adaptations that accommodate the functional and sensory decline of some older patients.

Although the proportion of hospitals that offer such services is small (see Figs. 39-1 and 39-2), one must remember that geriatric services were virtually unheard of until recently. Separate, distinct services for the elderly are being provided mostly in large, urban hospitals. Special services are also more likely to be provided in outpatient, health maintenance and assessment areas, and least likely to be provided as inpatient services. Although there are no firm data, there is probably less resistance to starting distinct programs in newer, less traditional areas.

Planning for the Future

Of particular interest are the steps hospitals have taken in planning services (see Fig. 39-3). Ideally, these steps are the first movement toward broadening community involvement in planning new services. Of the nearly 2,000 hospitals that are planning long-term care services, 72.5 percent have conducted a demographic analysis of the community; 47.8 percent have catalogued the services already available within the community; and 43.8 percent have conducted attitude surveys of potential consumers and/or their families to gather detailed information on patterns of use, satisfaction with existing services, and the need for new services.

Even more striking is the degree to which hospitals have begun discussing their plans with nonhospital groups (see Fig. 39-4). At least one quarter of the hospitals that are planning new services have talked with community agencies, the elderly, and other providers in the area. There is no evidence on the specific focus of such discussions, or on the meaningfulness of their input into the hospitals' final decisions about long-term care programs. However, anecdotal evidence gathered in conversations with many hospital planners indicates that such input has become increasingly vital to the success of long-term care programs, and is of great benefit to both the hospital and the other participants.

Inpatient
geriatric services

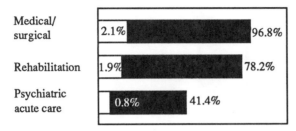

Medical/
surgical   2.1%   96.8%

Rehabilitation   1.9%   78.2%

Psychiatric   0.8%   41.4%
acute care

Ambulatory
geriatric services

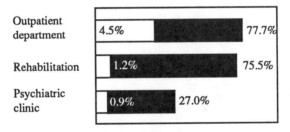

Outpatient
department   4.5%   77.7%

Rehabilitation   1.2%   75.5%

Psychiatric   0.9%   27.0%
clinic

☐ Separate services for the elderly
■ Service provided to patients of all ages

Figure 39-1.

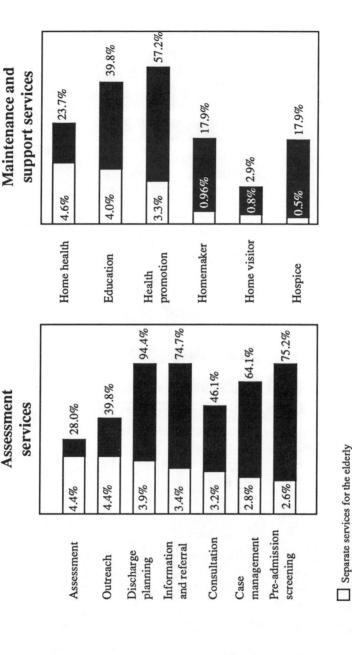

Figure 39-2.

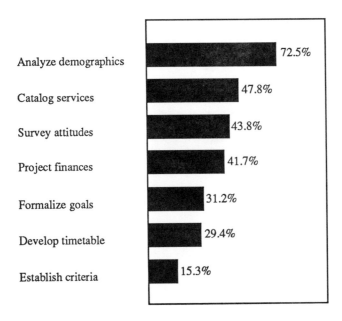

Figure 39-3. Hospitals' Planning for Future Services.

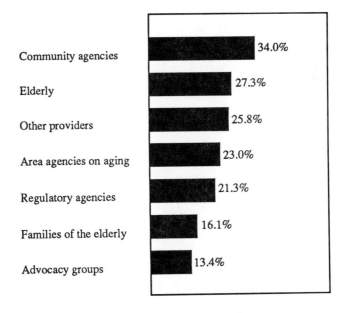

Figure 39-4. Hospitals' Planning Participants.

Policy Issues and Ethics

In selection 40, Kurt Darr, Beaufort B. Longest, Jr., and Jonathon S. Rakich analyze "The Ethical Imperative in Health Services Governance and Management." They identify administrative ethical issues likely to arise and discuss the role of managers as moral agents with an independent duty to protect patients and further patients' interests. Bruce C. Vladeck identifies the issues involved in answering the question "How Much Indigent Care Should Hospitals Provide?" in selection 41. The author argues that in the current environment, indigent care is more than a social responsibility; it is a competitive necessity.

In selection 42, "The Future of the Rural Hospital: Assessing the Alternatives," L. Fred Pounds and Jeffrey C. Bauer discuss new opportunities for rural hospitals. They argue that visionary governance is essential if these hospitals are to create health systems that mesh with their limitations as well as maximize their potential.

40

The Ethical Imperative in Health Services Governance and Management

Kurt Darr, Beaufort B. Longest, Jr., and Jonathon S. Rakich

Kurt Darr, J.D., Sc.D., FACHE, is Professor of Health Services Administration, and of Health Care Sciences, The George Washington University, Washington, DC.

Beaufort B. Longest, Jr., Ph.D., FACHE, is Professor and Director, Health Policy Institute, University of Pittsburgh, Pennsylvania.

Jonathon S. Rakich, Ph.D., is Professor of Management and Health Services Administration, The University of Akron, Ohio.

Introduction

What is ethical in this situation? Which interests should be considered? These questions increasingly affect those governing and managing health services organizations. This article suggests a construct in which to consider them.

Some may see a direct correspondence between law and ethics, that is to say, "Whatever is legal is also ethical, and vice versa." This need not be the case and isn't necessarily true for several reasons. The most important is that law provides only the minimum standard of performance, either positive or negative (but usually the latter), expected from members of society. Professions demand compliance with the law but add other duties and hold members to a higher standard. This means that even when the law does not require a certain activity of *any* citizen, including a specific group, a profession's code may. This makes an activity legal, but not necessarily ethical. A model showing the relationship of law to ethics has been developed by Verne Henderson.[1] Fig. 40-1 presents a matrix of the possible combinations of legal, illegal, ethical, and unethical.

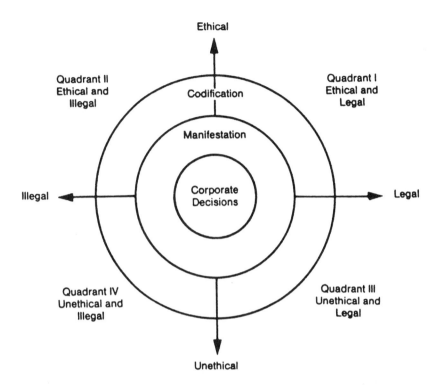

Figure 40-1. A Conceptual Framework. From Verne E. Henderson. "The Ethical Side of Enterprise," *Sloan Management Review*. Vol. 23, No. 3, Spring 1982, pp. 37-47.

This article discusses the administrative ethical aspects of issues, all of which have biomedical components as well. Issues analyzed and for which preventive measures or solutions are suggested are fiduciary duty, conflicts of interest, confidential information, resource allocation, and consent. Primarily biomedical ethical issues such as medical experimentation, death and dying, and abortion are not considered.

The technical and complex nature of medical care severely compromises the patient's ability to judge it and effectively interact with care givers. This highlights the need for everyone in the organization to protect and furthering the patients' interests, whether affected by biomedical or administrative ethics. Since all are moral agents whose decisions and actions have moral implications, this is the ethical imperative for those who govern and manage health services organizations.

Guidance for Leadership

Personal Ethic

Those in positions of leadership have already developed a personal morality—a *weltanschauung*—to guide their lives. This is their personal ethic, and those leading health services organizations consider this an important part of their professional lives. To effectively identify and understand, but most importantly to solve, ethical problems—whether biomedical or administrative—one must have a well-developed personal ethic. Leaders as well as followers in health services organizations apply this ethic in the context of their organization's philosophy—that statement of morality developed by the organization. A compatibility between the two is important to developing an affective corporate culture.

Principles

Implicit in any personal ethic adequate to effectively solve ethical problems will be the presence of four basic principles as they affect the patient: autonomy, beneficence, nonmaleficence, and justice.[2] It is patients the health services organization serves, and all actions must be measured against the goal of protecting them and furthering their interests.

Autonomy means that the wishes of self-legislating (competent) patients are followed, that they are involved in their own care to the extent they choose to be, and that when patients are not self-legislating because they are children or of diminished competence, the organization has special procedures for surrogate decision making or substituted judgments. Autonomous patients are treated with respect; it is unethical to lie to them. The principle of autonomy is especially important in terms of consent and use of confidential patient information.

Beneficence requires a positive duty to contribute to the patient's welfare. This principle has a long and noble tradition in the health professions and is equally applicable to the organization's governance and management. Tom Beauchamp and James Childress divide beneficence into two components: provision of benefit (including prevention and removal of harm) and balance benefits and harms. The latter can be used only to consider the costs and benefits of a treatment or action, not to override the other principles.[3]

The third principle to be included in a personal ethic is nonmaleficence, a duty that obliges us to refrain from inflicting harm. This harm can be mental as well as physical and is readily extended into an organizational setting to issues such as patient privacy. While beneficence is a positive duty, nonmaleficence is negative—refraining from doing something that harms. Beneficence and nonmaleficence affect governing body members and managers in issues such as fiduciary duty, use of confidential information, and conflicts of interest.

Justice is the final principle important to a personal ethic. A major problem is defining what is just or fair. Egalitarians say that it is just to provide like amounts of services to all with similar needs. Libertarians stress merit and achievement as measures of what is just. Aristotle asserted that "equals" should be treated equally, "unequals" unequally. An interpretation of Aristotle's view means that most medical care should go to those in greatest need, since in terms of health they are situated unequally. There is broad latitude in developing the specific content of the principle of justice, but there are limits, nonetheless. Considerations of justice have most apparent application in resource allocation.

These principles are found explicitly or implicitly in codes of ethics propounded by various professional groups. The American College of Healthcare Executives' Code of Ethics is among the most comprehensive, but even it is specific and precise *only* on conflicts of interest. Governing body members and managers should look to organizational philosophy and professional codes for assistance, but they can only be effective leaders if they have a well-developed personal ethic that includes attention to the principles of autonomy, beneficence, nonmaleficence, and justice.

Ethical Issues Affecting Governance and Management

Fiduciary Duty

Fiduciary is a concept that arose from Roman jurisprudence and means that certain obligations and duties are present in a relationship. A fiduciary is someone with superior knowledge or position, and neither may be used ethically for personal gain. This requires managers to act only in the organization's best interests, with the caveat that the independent duty of the moral agent toward the patient cannot be ignored.

Governing body members of both for-profit and not-for-profit corporations have a fiduciary duty. The legal standard for meeting this obligation is more demanding when governing body members are true trustees, i.e., they hold title to the assets and administer them to further the purposes of the trust.

Loyalty means that the individuals must put the interest of the corporation above all self-interest, a principle based on the biblical doctrine that no man can serve two masters. Specifically, no trustee is permitted to gain any secret profits for himself, to accept bribes, or to compete with the corporation.

The fiduciary duty of responsibility means that members of the governing board must exercise reasonable care, skill, and diligence proportionate to the circumstances in every activity of the board. In other words, the trustees can be held personally liable for negligence, which can be an affirmative act of commission, or omission.[4]

The legal standard sets the tone for ethical guidelines, but should be considered only a minimum. Managers are not fiduciaries in the same sense as are governing body members, but they have similar ethical responsibilities in the terms of loyalty and a duty to avoid conflicts of interest. The American College of Healthcare Executives' "Code" recognizes these duties.

Conflicts of Interest

Conflicts of interest are major sources of problems in health services organizations. They occur when someone has sets of obligations and duties that are inconsistent — they are in conflict — and meeting one set means abrogating another. Accepting extravagant gifts is an obvious example. Others are more subtle.

Has the manager acted ethically who uses a position of influence and power to gain personal aggrandizement of title, position, and salary at the expense of patient care or other organizational activities? Is the manager behaving ethically who is lax in implementing a more effective patient consent process? Is it ethical for a governing body member whose physical and mental capacities are diminished to remain on the board? Is the manager behaving ethically who insists that all reports to governance be prepared in a manner that inadequately shows negative results? Is it ethical for a governing body member or manager who suspects there are problems in the department of surgery to fail to prove or disprove this suspicion? While problems of these types *may* have legal implications, all raise ethical questions.

The difficulty with conflict of interest is that many types are very subtle and it takes continued questioning and self-analysis to identify them. They are likely to increase as competition intensifies. The College's "Code" and the American Hospital Association's statement on conflicts of interest suggest ways of reducing or eliminating the problem. They concentrate on disclosure of real or potential conflicts of interest, divestiture of outside interests that might cause a conflict to arise, seeking guidance from the governing body when questions arise, and not participating in or attempting to influence any matter in which conflicts might exist.

Confidential Information

Any unauthorized use of confidential information about the patient or organization is unethical. The most common misuse occurs when employees and medical staff gossip about patients. Thought this may seem innocent, it is not, and discussion of patients should be on a need-to-know basis only.

Careless internal use of patient information is the most common problem regarding confidential information, but misusing it in other ways receives more public attention. This latter abuse occurs when patient or organization confidential information is used to benefit an individual or other persons with whom that individual is associated or related. Examples include disclosing information about governing body decision making so associates can make advantageous sales or purchases; giving or selling patient medical information to the media or attorneys; and making marketing strategies available to competitors, whether for profit or revenge.

An example with potential for both conflicts of interest and misuse of confidential information is found when the health services manager serves on the governing body of another health services provider or planning agency. Allegiance to one's organization conflicts when another's certificate of need or marketing activity is considered. A more subtle problem arises when those in such a situation become privy to information important for business purposes or planning in their own organization. Regretfully, the importance of that type of confidential information in a competitive environment may necessitate that managers and governing body members avoid all involvement with any potentially competing organization.

The College's "Code" views misuse of confidential information broadly and prohibits all that are inappropriate. It is immaterial that the organization is unharmed.

Resource Allocation

The process of resource allocation has recently received more attention as an activity raising ethical issues. Whether macro or micro, it necessitates making decisions — literally who gets what, when and how. This means making judgments about importance, worth, usefulness, merit, need, societal value, and the like. Sometimes when the government is involved, decisions are also based on political motives and ideals.

Like governments, all health services organizations make macro allocation decisions. Micro allocation is usually a function of the physician's willingness to refer; the patient's access to services and technologies; and, sometimes, economic considerations. Often, micro decision making is guided (in a sense, prejudged) by policies and procedures of government as well as the organization.

Numerous theories have been developed about making macro allocation decisions. At one extreme are those who argue all technologies must be available to all persons; a corollary of this hyperegalitarian position is that if services or a technology are not available to all, none should receive them. This position is based on the concept that each human being has inherent dignity and thus a right to receive equal health services. Conversely, there are those for whom health services are not a right to be guaranteed by society; rather, they are an earned privilege. This hyperindividualistic position also holds that health services providers have no obligation to those who cannot pay, unless they choose of their own free will and humanitarian instinct to provide care. Between these extremes is a view that society is obligated to develop, encourage, and perhaps even provide health services in limited situations. Medicare and Medicaid are examples where such a position has been adopted.

Theories about allocating exotic life-saving treatments on a micro basis —
i.e., to individual patients—have been developed by James Childress and
Nicholas Rescher. These theories aid decision making about which patients
get what. Childress rejects subjective criteria such as future contributions and
past record of performance saying that such comparisons demean and run
counter to the inherent dignity of the human being. He argues that a system
which views as equals all persons needing a certain treatment recognizes
human worth, and once medical criteria are used to determine need, opportunities for a scarce treatment should be available first-come, first-served, or
alternatively, on a random selection basis, such as a lottery.[5]

Rescher's scheme is two-tiered: The first is basic screening and includes
factors such as constituency served (service area), progress of science (benefit
of advancing science), and prospect of success by type of treatment or
recipient, e.g., denying renal dialysis to the very young or old. The second tier
deals with individuals and uses biomedical factors (relative likelihood of success for that patient and life expectancy) and the social aspects such as family
role, potential future contributions, and past services rendered. If all factors
are equal, a random selection process is used for the final choice.[6] Social
aspects are the most difficult. They are heavily dependent on value judgments
and cause ethical dilemmas when true scarcity exists. For example, the
shortage of donor kidneys raises questions about the appropriateness of
foreign nationals on transplantation waiting lists.

Each micro allocation theory has advantages and disadvantages. Yet, it
provides guidelines that permit the issues to be addressed in an organized
and predictable fashion. This may not result in decisions which satisfy
everyone, but is has the advantage of systematizing the frameworks for
decision making. Public awareness of how choices are made is an important
attribute in a democracy.

Consent

The concept of consent began at law as a recognition of one's right to be
free from nonconsensual touching. The ethical relationship expands this right
and includes the principle of autonomy: self-determination. It also reflects the
special trust and confidence (a fiduciary relationship) between physician and
patient, as well as that between those who govern and manage the organization and the patient. Inherent in consent is a view of the equality and dignity
of human beings. Its emphasis on patients' rights or sovereignty is an idealized
view and contravenes long traditions of medical paternalism which put the
physician in the role of authoritarian figure who makes decisions in the
patient's best interests.[7] Such a history suggests the difficulties inherent in
perfecting the principle of autonomy.

The *legal* minimum requires full disclosure about the nature of the condition, all significant facts about it, and explanation of likely consequences that
might result from treatment or nontreatment. Ethical guidelines build on this
base. The principles described above suggest active patient participation.

Guidelines developed by the President's Commission for the Study of Ethical Problems in Medicine and Biomedical and Behavioral Research state that patient sovereignty with complete participation is preferred.[8] The Commission recognized such participation as a goal to be sought rather than a readily achievable relationship.

Organizations generally apply a legally-oriented consent process that focuses on self-protection. There is relatively little emphasis on the ethical relationship with the patient. This is legally prudent, but ignores the separate, positive ethical obligation to maximize involvement of patients out of respect for them and recognition of their autonomy.

Solving Administrative Ethical Issues

Organizational Philosophy

A crucial starting point for solving administrative ethical issues is that there be a specific statement of philosophy that defines the organization's reason for existence and the goals it seeks to achieve. Such a philosophy must be sufficiently precise and detailed so performance can be reviewed or, even more preferable, evaluated. Anecdotal information suggests that few health services organizations have an explicitly stated philosophy; fewer have philosophies with components specific enough to measure achievement of them. Nonetheless, an implicit philosophy is identifiable for all organizations.

Decisions and actions of governing body and management have a philosophical basis, even if vague or ill-defined. The lack of a stated philosophy providing a basic point of reference encourages inconsistency and a lack of continuity and may lead to contradictory policies and results. Furthermore, it diminishes the organization's ability to develop an effective corporate culture.

Responsible governing bodies will emphasize in their statements of philosophy and mission, as well as derivative policies, the importance of protecting patients and furthering their interests — an application of the principles of autonomy, beneficence, nonmaleficence, and justice. Accountability will be included as inherent in the independent relationship between organization and patient. This relationship results from the fiduciary duty owed the patient as well as the ethical responsibility to protect patients from harm.

This accountability is broad. Some argue it is sufficiently demanding that patients harmed through medical malpractice, but unaware of that harm, should be informed of it by representatives of the organization.[9] A radical view? Perhaps, but one consistent with the high degree of trust the public places in health services organizations and an appropriate measure of the duty that those who govern and manage them should execute in return.

The strategic planning process is also a function of the organization's philosophy, a primary manifestation of which is the mission statement. An organizational philosophy must be articulated before planning objectives can be established. The organization's mission statement reflects ideals — ends thought unattainable — but progress toward which is believed possible.[10] In this respect, perhaps the most difficult aspect is selection of an appropriate balance between social responsibility and economic performance.[11]

Governance and management are responsible for developing the organization's philosophy and deriving the mission and specific operational plans. In addition, management interprets and implements the plans. The dynamic is clear. The probability of an organization's moral survival is enhanced to the extent there is maximum congruity between its philosophy and expressions of the personal ethic of governance and management. This is not to say professional managers cannot work effectively in an organization where there are variances between personal and organizational ethics. But the duty of loyalty and allegiance to the organization requires governing body members and managers to uphold the organizational philosophy until it is at variance with their personal ethic.

None can disregard their role as moral agents whose actions have consequences for patients and others. If they act unethically even at the behest of organization or superior, it is no defense to argue they were only following orders.

Institutional Ethics Committees

As conceived, institutional ethics committees considered a terminally-ill patient's prognosis and assisted in answering the question about ending life support. This concern with biomedical ethical problems was reflected in their membership and purposes. Here, it is recommended they be used to assist in developing and implementing an organizational philosophy and to assist governance and management in identifying and solving administrative ethical problems.

Robert Veatch argues ethics committees can and should have various roles, many of them mutually exclusive.[12] Adopting this view, it is apparent that a committee most likely to be effective in administrative ethics will have fewer clinical personnel and more representatives from governance and management. Clinical personnel must be included because research suggesting organizations are most effective when they involve clinicians in management decision making is also likely to apply to solving problems of administrative ethics.

A national study conducted by the President's Commission about the structure, procedures, activities, and effectiveness of biomedical ethics committees in hospitals suggests some useful parallels as well as pitfalls to be avoided in establishing administrative ethics committees. The Commission reported biomedical ethics committees facilitated decision making when they clarified important issues, shaped consistent hospital policies with regard to life support, and provided opportunities for professionals to air disagreements.[13] The committees were not found particularly effective for educating professionals about issues relevant to life support decisions.

The study also found that only one percent of hospitals had committees; on average they reviewed only one case per year. Although specialized ethics committees, specifically infant care review committees, are rapidly growing in number, anecdotal information suggests there are fewer new biomedical ethics committees with general functions than had been predicted.

One President's Commission finding suggests there are problems with patient autonomy.

> The composition and function of committees identified . . . would not allay many of the concerns of patients' rights advocates about patient representation and control. Committees were clearly dominated by physicians and other health professionals. The majority of committees did not allow patients to attend or request meetings, although family members were more often permitted to do so.[14]

This is a matter affecting resource allocation and consent and should be of vital concern to governance and management.

There is evidence that biomedical ethics committees are most effective when they wait to be consulted rather than interposing themselves. A consultative role means committees make recommendations, not final decisions.[15]

Similar limitations may apply in administrative ethics—depending on the specific facts and issues under consideration. Generally, the committee should be proactive in developing and revising the organizational philosophy and in considering macro resource allocation questions. Similarly, it should take the initiative in reviewing and revising the consent process. However, it may choose a more passive role and wait to be consulted in specific instances of conflicts of interest and misuse of confidential information.

The President's Commission's finding as to the relative ineffectiveness of biomedical ethics committees in educational activities is puzzling and may be an aberration. The composition and experience of an administrative ethics committee will make it a reservoir of knowledge and expertise, and these resources should be made available to the staff. This will generally add sophistication and improve the quality of ethical decision making. Two recent books provide useful information about establishing institutional ethics committees.[16]

Ethicists

Many large teaching hospitals, typically those with university affiliations, include ethicists on their staffs. Ethicists are usually doctorally-qualified philosophers who are teaching faculty at a university or medical school. Primarily, they participate in solving biomedical ethical issues. There is no reason, however, why their involvement should be limited in that fashion. Ethicists could aid governance and management as well.

Health services organizations interested in obtaining the assistance of an ethicist should not limit their search to medical schools, but should consider all persons with specialized preparation in ethics and its application in the health field. The literature reports that physicians are more likely to ask assistance of an ethicist than an ethics committee. One reason suggested for this is that committees are not seen as cost effective. Similarly, and beyond considerations of efficiency, it may be more palatable for the typical manager to consult with an ethicist to assist in identifying and analyzing the moral obligations and rights and responsibilities bearing on a case than to seek guidance from a committee.

Summary

Organizational philosophies, ethics committees, and ethicists provide assistance to governance and management. But, as with all tools, those who use them must know when there is a problem and when assistance is needed. This requires governing body members and managers to be sophisticated about the presence of ethical problems. Such knowledge comes with education and experience. More importantly, those who would implement their personal ethic and meet their duties as moral agents must be willing to act. Lacking this, all else is futile.

Conclusion

All decision making and activities of health services organizations contain ethical dimensions, whether administrative or biomedical. In this regard, two problems confront managers and governing bodies. The first is to recognize the presence of administrative ethical issues. The second is to apply analytical and reasoning processes to address them, thereby enhancing the quality of decision making. Applied ethics is an emerging aspect of health services management. Its effective use enhances the purpose for which health services organizations exist.

Economic pressure from cost cutting by third-party payors and increased competitiveness affect all health services organizations, but especially hospitals. Governing bodies and managers may be tempted or feel compelled to take actions that negatively affect patients in terms of the principles of autonomy, beneficence, nonmaleficence, and justice. To do so puts them in derogation of their independent moral duty to protect the patient; and, in so doing, they fail to honor the ethical imperative. The potential conflict between economic interests and patient care considerations are not far below the surface in the patient relationship; for those who govern and manage health services organizations, the ethical implications are enormous.

Notes

1. Verne E. Henderson, "The Ethical Side of Enterprise," *Sloan Management Review* Vol. 23, No. 3 (1982): 41-42.
2. Tom L. Beauchamp and James F. Childress, *Principles of Biomedical Ethics*, 2d (New York: Oxford University Press, 1983).
3. *Ibid.*, p. 149.
4. Arthur F. Southwick, *The Law of Hospital and Health Care Administration* (Ann Arbor, MI: Health Administration Press, 1978), p. 47 and 50.
5. James F. Childress, "Who Shall Live When Not All Can Live?" *Soundings, An Interdisciplinary Journal* Vol. 53, No. 4 (Winter 1970).
6. Nicholas Rescher, "The Allocation of Exotic Medical Lifesaving Therapy," *Ethics* Vol. 79 (April 1969).
7. *Making Health Care Decisions,* Vol. 1, President's Commission for the Study of Ethical Problems in Medicine and Biomedical and Behavioral Research. Washington, DC: U.S. Government Printing Office, October 1982, pp. 2-6.
8. *Ibid.*
9. Kenneth Williams and Paul Donnelly, *Medical Care Quality and the Public Trust* (Chicago: Pluribus Press, 1982).
10. Russell L. Ackoff, *Creating the Corporate Future* (New York: John Wiley & Sons, 1981).
11. James B. Webber, "Planning," *Hospitals* Vol. 56, No. 7 (April 1, 1982): 69-70.
12. Robert M. Veatch, Ph.D., quoted in "Ethics Committees Proliferation in Hospitals Predicted," *Hospitals* (July 1, 1983): 48-49.
13. *Deciding to Forego Life-Sustaining Treatment,* President's Commission for the Study of Ethical Problems in Medicine and Biomedical and Behavioral Research, Washington, DC: U.S. Government Printing Office, March 1983, p. 447.
14. *Ibid*, p. 448.
15. Benjamin Freedman, "One Philosopher's Experience on an Ethics Committee," *Hastings Center Report* Vol. 11 (April 1981): 20-22.
16. William Read, *Ethical Dilemmas in a Changing Health Care Environment: Hospital Ethics Committees* (Chicago: The Hospital Research and Educational Trust, 1983).
17. Ronald E. Cranford and A. Edward Doudera, eds., *Institutional Ethics Committees and Health Care Decision Making* (Ann Arbor, MI: Health Administration Press, 1984).

41

How Much Indigent Care
Should Hospitals Provide?

Bruce C. Vladeck

Bruce C. Vladeck, Ph.D., is President, United Hospital Fund of New York, New York City.

While the public is not enthusiastic about paying higher taxes or increasing federal social programs, its tolerance for visible episodes in which vulnerable people are denied care is very, very limited. In other words, the extent to which indigent care is an issue for public debate is directly proportionate to the extent to which people are denied service – and, more specifically, the extent to which that denial takes place in the public eye.

Scenarios for the Future

There is no question that the current political environment has produced public policy and attitudes that are substantially less generous toward care for the poor than they have been in the recent past. In its efforts to master inflation and shrink the federal deficit, the Reagan Administration has cut back federal entitlement programs – in some cases asking states to assume a larger portion of the burden.

But consider two plausible scenarios for health care in the event of another recession. Given a current base of 30 to 35 million uninsured (Feder, Hadley and Mullner, 1984), it's not unrealistic to project a post-recession figure of 50 to 55 million. At that point, the people now determining economic policy will be discredited, and an angry Congress will be looking to control hospital costs with radical – but politically acceptable – remedies beyond Ted Kennedy's wildest dreams.

Some industry leaders believe that systems like the New Jersey all-payer program position hospitals as a public utility. But if this first scenario comes to pass, we'll all find out what it means to be a *true* public utility. A true public

Reprinted by permission from *Health Management Quarterly*, Summer 1985, pages 2-4. Copyright 1985 by American Hospital Supply Corporation Foundation. All rights reserved.

utility system could see hospitals declared "common carriers," with a government agency carving up market share, assigning patients to designated providers and enforcing rigid price controls.

The alternate scenario conjures up a swing toward universally affordable coverage, as defined by monopolistic price-setting on the part of the government. Universal coverage is analogous to the Canadian experience — except that Canadian providers began living with price controls long before the inflationary spirals of the 1970s struck the system. Given the inflated base from which price-setting would start here in the United States, American hospitals are likely to find such a system less than acceptable.

The Real Cost of Uninsured Care

Given the current political environment and the specter of things to come, can hospitals afford to provide a reasonable volume of services to poor people? At present, a relatively small proportion of all institutions is losing money while providing a great majority of the free care. The bulk of institutions are making money while providing relatively small volumes of free care (Feder, Hadley and Mullner, 1984).

Today, the average American hospital maintains an occupancy rate of the 60 to 70 percent range, and it's making more money as a proportion of total revenues than ever before. In fact, 1984 profits in the hospital industry totaled at least 25 percent more than the total amount of free care being given (AHA Trends, 1985). Yet some hospitals undertook to drastically reduce the volume of care they provided to nonpaying patients as a result of changes taking place in the health-care system.

Historically, hospitals expected a 2 percent margin: Such a margin was a triumph for a hospital CFO. Today, despite reduced demand, margins far exceed 2 percent. How much additional free care could hospitals deliver if they returned to the 2 percent standard?

The Facts Don't Justify Panic

Rapid changes in the health-care environment appear to have panicked the hospital industry. The shift from retrospective to prospective payment brought about the first wave of panic — even though it appears that the long-time prediction of advocates of prospective payment is about to come true: Hospitals have a more realistic chance of making money with prospective payment than they did under the old retrospective system.

Correspondingly, the facts about uncompensated care simply do not justify the panic response from hospitals. The medically indigent aren't putting hospitals out of business. Except for 100 or so public or inner-city, voluntary hospitals, the typical indigent care load runs in the area of 5 percent to 8 percent of total patient-care volume — that's 5 percent to 8 percent of *average* costs and a much smaller proportion of *incremental* costs.

Yet despite hospital managers' and CFOs' claims to heightened sophistication and more businesslike, competitive instincts, a startling number of them continue to confuse the average cost of delivery care to paying patients with the incremental costs of delivering care to nonpaying patients.

The average cost of delivering emergency-room services, for example, is the fixed cost of maintaining the service fully staffed, 24 hours per day divided by the number of paying patients you need to treat in order to meet those costs. After that base is met, the nonpaying customer who walks in the door isn't increasing the emergency room's fixed cost. He's only costing $11 or $9 or whatever the incremental cost is for materials used—because fixed costs are spread across the paying population. When the services you provide nonpaying patients are incremental relative to your paying service base, you must assess the cost of care to the poor by assessing the incremental cost—not the average cost.

The real issue behind all the number crunching is this: If a third of the business in your hospital's emergency room is non-paying customers, are you going to close your emergency room? The answer is no. From a marketing perspective, you can't afford to do so.

Who Will Fill the Beds in the Future?

Another thing that scares hospital people—and it should scare them—is that the demand for inpatient hospital services has dropped. We have an industry that was at over-capacity to begin with, and now there are fewer and fewer patients to go around.

If the major problem the hospital industry faces in the current environment is that, on the one hand, people no longer are prepared to pay the price set by hospitals, and on the other hand, the supply of services exceeds demand—the last thing you want to do is turn *any* demand away.

Utilization among the middle-class, insured population is dropping, and it will continue to drop. For the rest of this century, the Medicare population will provide the only growth in demand for hospital services. That demand, per enrollee, is going to fall, but because our population is aging, the sheer volume of enrollees will produce the industry's only net increase in demand.

Survival in the Inpatient Business

This means that to survive in the inpatient business, either you must create a very distinctive market niche that attracts private customers—of whom there are fewer and fewer to go around—or the core of your business is going to have to be Medicare business.

Now, sitting around your board room, it's easy to say your hospital is going to market itself exclusively to younger, high-income Medicare customers who want elective procedures. But, in today's environment, such a marketing strategy can create a backlash. The community that demands lower hospital costs could be the same community that censures a hospital that is perceived as denying care to indigent citizens.

Beyond questions of humaneness, turning people away is a very short-sighted act. It probably will come back to haunt you when the public begins to examine the legitimacy and positioning of your hospital within the community. On the other hand, what is it worth in the grand scheme of things to be viewed by the community as the sole provider of essential, under-compensated, charitable services? – Probably a lot more than the incremental costs of providing services to nonpaying patients.

Some hospitals have taken this long-term perspective, and they're discovering that providing health-care services to the poor can be their means of survival. In inner-city areas of New York and New Jersey, hospitals that are in trouble are beating the bushes for nonpaying customers. They've figured out that from both political and marketing perspectives, positioning themselves as the sole providers of services to the poor in their communities will have a major impact on their capacity to survive.

If, however, hospitals develop a reputation of taking paying customers, only, many local communities – which have supported hospitals in tangible and significant ways for a long time – are simply going to withdraw their support.

Can You Make a Case for Philanthropy?

Already, community support of hospitals has declined. It wasn't very long ago – immediately prior to World War II – that the typical community hospital in the United States simply assumed that 10 or 15 percent of its operating budget and all of its capital would be generated from local philanthropy. But in the late 1960s and early 1970s, hospitals were largely indifferent to philanthropy because Medicare and Blue Cross dollars met their needs.

Public perceptions reflect that indifference. Since the advent of Medicare, hospitals which used to be the primary object of local philanthropic support, have lost out in the competition for community-level philanthropic dollars. The public perceives that, with plenty of third-party money around to pay for health care, hospitals are rich and fat and happy, and most institutions haven't made a plausible case for philanthropic support.

Aggregate philanthropic dollars are, in fact, growing faster in the United States than is the population at large or the economy as a whole. In some areas – the arts, for example – philanthropy has replaced lost government dollars effectively.

As times get tougher, dollars get scarcer and competition intensifies, hospitals will look longingly at these potential sources of revenue. But few hospitals will be able to provide community philanthropists with plausible reasons to give.

Marketing Traditional Values

In a very profound sense, decisions about financing care for the poor indicate the kind of society we want to have. Hospitals' current preoccupation with competition sometimes obscures the fact that they exist to heal the sick, to provide comfort to the afflicted, and to delay or prevent untimely death. Given this mission, caring for the poor could be the Achilles heel of competition. Those hospitals that survive in the current competitive environment will be those hospitals that adopt the traditional values of hospital care as their market position.

42

The Future of the Rural Hospital: Assessing the Alternatives

L. Fred Pounds and Jeffrey C. Bauer

L. Fred Pounds is President, Avanti Health Systems, Houston.

Jeffrey C. Bauer, Ph.D., is an independent healthcare consultant, Brush, Colorado.

The most persistent problem of the last decade for rural hospitals (finding a doctor) pales in comparison with today's concern for survival. While its essential mission may endure, the rural hospital may require fundamental change if it is to fulfill that mission.

The typical hospital mission statement ("The hospital shall ensure the delivery of health care services to the local community") is as relevant today as ever. Rural residents continue to need health services. However, to provide safe and appropriate inpatient care in the future, hospitals will need a minimum critical mass: 30 beds with an average occupancy rate of 60 percent, an active medical staff of 10 physicians, and a market area of more than 18,000 residents. Our initial estimates are derived from our ongoing studies to determine the minimum size of an acute care hospital that meets joint criteria of financial self-sufficiency and clinical quality. If a hospital falls short in one or more of these areas, the pursuit of alternatives may be the only way to fulfill its mission.

Like their urban counterparts, rural hospitals are increasingly less dependent on inpatient services to provide health care to the local population. Because patient care is shifting toward the outpatient setting, efforts to reverse a declining census may actually hasten the hospital's closure by diverting the rural trustee's attention from the real issues and relevant opportunities.

Building for the Future

While the continued existence of the hospital as a building with beds is a matter of rural community pride, it is no longer a medical necessity, and trustees are only deceiving themselves if they think utilization will return to the comfortable levels of the past two decades. The rural hospital of the future should be more of a diversified business entity and less of an inpatient facility. Forward-looking trustees must therefore focus community pride on safe, appropriate, and locally accessible health services.

A few rural hospitals may be able to survive unchanged as traditional acute care institutions, but the majority will not. Before clinging to a "business as usual" attitude, trustees must assess their alternatives—closure or change. They can begin by comparing their hospitals with characteristics of those that are failing (Table 42-1) and those on the road to success (Table 42-2).

By measuring their hospital against these criteria, trustees can determine if their facility is heading toward failure or survival. If the hospital is doomed on its present course, then change is the only alternative. Even if the hospital exhibits the characteristics of success, change should still be considered to ensure that the hospital is achieving its full potential.

The future of rural hospitals is limited only by the imagination of trustees, who must respond to the limits and possibilities of local circumstances. The following key concepts are provided as a framework for assessing alternative directions.

Appropriate and Timely Data

Unless trustees and administrators wish to rely on luck, they will need better data to support decisionmaking and management. A management information system is essential to promote the flexibility hospitals need today. The system should support marketing, planning, and pricing decisions and must provide the sophisticated cost information managers need to operate in an increasingly competitive environment.

Modern approaches to clinical data storage and retrieval are essential components of promising new rural delivery systems. For example, the paperless medical record will be a necessity for rural facilities that become part of a comprehensive system, and important improvements in quality can be captured through development of online telecommunications capabilities to link rural providers to national data bases (e.g., TOXLINE, MEDLINE, computer-assisted diagnostic support services, etc.).

Managerial and Production Efficiency

Since rural hospitals can no longer rely on cost-based reimbursement to defray the expenses of resources that are less than fully utilized, efficiency—production without waste—is essential to survival. Alternatives to traditional approaches to personnel and capital include multitask, cross-trained

Table 42-1. Characteristics of Failing Rural Hospitals.

Insensitivity to the marketplace
Hospital leaders do not notice and or do not respond appropriately to change (competition from distant providers, new reimbursement mechanisms and policies, better informed consumers, adverse rumors, etc.). They tend to believe that marketing is nothing more than advertising: they fail to understand that marketing requires trustees to view their hospital "from the customer's point of view."

Inadequate medical staff development strategies
The medical staff issue has two dimensions, quantity and quality. Simply having enough doctors does not ensure hospital survival; rural residents have demonstrated their willingness to drive to the city if they do not have confidence in the local doctors.

Weak financial management
Insolvency is not always caused by lack of money; many failed hospitals might have remained open if they had adhered to sound financial principles such as budgeting, cash flow analysis, sophisticated billing policies and procedures, product line analysis, cost accounting, and risk management.

Weak management/board direction
Trustees and administrators of failing hospitals either do not have or fail to follow a relevant long-range plan. They lack meaningful policies and procedures for operations, and measurable objectives with appropriate feedback.

Inappropriate diversification
Many hospitals attempt to compensate for poor results by developing new products such as wellness centers, home health agencies, durable equipment rental services, and unrelated for-profit businesses. Such diversification cannot work unless it is based on sound planning and marketing.

Overstaffing
Some of the first hospitals to close were those with excessive staff patient ratios — usually more than four employees per adjusted occupied bed. (On the other hand, many successful rural hospitals operate with 3:1 ratios.) Administrators and trustees of failing hospitals may be aware of the problem, but are unable to identify and terminate excess employees.

Source: *Survival Diagnostic Process.* Price Waterhouse, 1986.

employees (e.g., a laboratory/radiology technician, a medical records librarian/data manager) and new "downsized" replacement facilities (e.g., an infirmary with 24-hour observation beds) for use where the population of the market area is no longer large enough to support a conventional acute care hospital.

Table 42-2. Characteristics of Successful Rural Hospitals.

Flexible corporate structure
A rapidly changing environment means rapidly changing opportunities. The most successful hospitals are those with an open-minded governing board; a flexible legal structure that facilitates rapid decisionmaking; and the ability to affiliate and enter into joint ventures with other organizations.

Active governance by qualified trustees
Successful rural hospitals are those with actively involved trustees who represent a variety of expertise. Active involvement means "doing your homework," not just attending meetings. Desirable qualifications include backgrounds in accounting and finance, risk management, banking, investments, legal matters, and general business.

Competent management
Administrators of today's top rural hospitals have more than unquestioned, aggressive commitment to their jobs; they also have proven abilities in day-to-day management, communications, marketing, planning, and finance. They are decisionmakers and achievers and are compensated accordingly, often with performance-based incentive payments.

Identifiable and relevant market strategy
Successful hospitals know their market area(s) and the desires of their constituencies (patients, doctors, communities). They have an ongoing, market-driven strategic planning process that evaluates alternatives and quickly results in focused programs.

Measured financial performance
Budgets are used for planning and control; variances are analyzed carefully. Billing and accounts receivable are managed according to predetermined standards. Cost accounting and personnel systems are carefully applied to ensure efficiency and effectiveness.

Qualified and involved medical staff
A rural hospital cannot succeed without the support of competent physicians who work unselfishly for the hospital, often by serving on the board of trustees; these doctors do not play one hospital against another.

Source: *Survival Diagnostic Process*. Price Waterhouse, 1986.

Effective Community Leadership

Rural communities need hospital trustees who understand the full significance of the recent changes in health care and can communicate this understanding to citizens who believe the community cannot have health care without a traditional (inpatient) hospital. In other words, today's rural trustee must be prepared to bring modern approaches to health care in much the same way local school board members brought modern educational opportunities to rural America 20 to 30 years ago.

As a practical and political matter, trustees must have vision and leadership to promote alternatives that benefit the community, although this may occasionally result in confrontation between future-looking trustees and tradition-bound administrators. For example, if trustees determine that the existing hospital is no longer the appropriate resource for meeting community needs, they must protect jobs and prevent rural blight (boarded up windows and unmown grass) by finding another use for the hospital building. Nursing homes, specialty care centers, and offices are examples of possible alternate use.

Enforced Standards of Quality

Trustees must honestly assess the quality of care provided by the medical and nursing staffs. Local residents select health care providers on the basis of quality. The high number of rural residents who go out of town for health care suggests that quality frequently prevails over community pride. As a precondition of buying their health care locally, rural residents want better care, not just convenient care.

Meaningful and mandatory peer review, both external and internal, is a necessary first step toward quality assurance. Trustees may need to explore locally relevant continuing education requirements and definitions of minimum, experience-based competencies as complementary approaches to quality.

Adequate Capitalization

Any change in a rural hospital's response to its mission will assuredly require money. With the growing competition for funding, trustees will increasingly need to explore joint ventures with investors, taxable bonds, commercial loans, and other instruments that are not within the financial heritage of not-for-profit hospitals. In other words, they need to think like for-profit entrepreneurs, a concept that is not forbidden under Section 501(c)3 of the Internal Revenue Code.

Comprehensive Delivery Systems

Most rural hospitals serve too few people to cover the growing expense of providing a full range of health services. However, through affiliation with other rural facilities and/or urban tertiary care hospitals, rural hospitals can create relationships to ensure local access to a full-service health care system. Indeed, the pursuit and negotiation of cooperative agreements with other institutional providers may be one of the most important new obligations of a rural hospital trustee.

Since a full-service system will almost certainly require an agreement with an urban provider, rural trustees must protect their own interests when reaching agreements with their big-city counterparts. Any agreement must work both ways; the rural hospital should receive something it needs (doctors, access to capital and technology, management support, etc.) in exchange for the valuable patients it will channel to the urban provider.

The Future

Robert H. Ebert discusses "The New Health Era" in Selection 43. He examines the unique factors shaping the current health care system and those that are likely to mold it for the future. In selection 44, "Re-Organizing the Organization: New Roles Lie Ahead," Richard Johnson prognosticates about the future of the health care system and how the successful organization will respond to the changes the future will bring.

The final article in the book, selection 45, is a long-range look at the health care system 50 years hence. In "2036: A Health Care Odyssey," Jeff C. Goldsmith projects current technology and the effect it is likely to have on the health services system.

43

The New Health Era

Robert H. Ebert

Robert H. Ebert, M.D., is Special Advisor to the President, Robert Wood Johnson Foundation, Princeton, New Jersey.

Introduction

Unlike any other service or commodity, medical care's demand is only partially sensitive to price, and government has assumed responsibility for certain diseases and population groups. For those who have full insurance coverage, price is of little consequence, but for those who are uninsured or underinsured, price can be crucial. The difference is well illustrated in the case of candidates for coronary bypass surgery. Very simply, those who can pay for the services receive them, and those who cannot, do not. In contrast, rich and poor alike are entitled to renal dialysis for end-stage renal disease as the result of an idiosyncratic legislative action taken by Congress. In addition, medical care differs from other services and commodities because the consumption of medical services seems to be almost infinitely expansible. The public can consume only a finite amount of food, or banking services, but it is possible and perhaps even useful to provide more medical care, particularly at the beginning and end of life.

If the final analysis, however, what happens to our health care system in terms of who receives care, and in what manner it is provided, will depend on how much we are willing to spend on medical care individually and collectively. Some closely related factors to consider include:

- The degree to which medical care alters mortality, morbidity, and the quality of life, or how it is *perceived* to make a difference.

- The speed with which medical science can introduce new cost-effective technologies for the diagnosis and treatment of disease. Medical science is capable of providing solutions to medical problems that will reduce cost, but is more likely to find answers that will increase costs, at least in the short term.

Reprinted by permission from *Health Matrix*, 4(4), Winter 1986-1987, pages 3-6. Copyright 1986 by Rynd Communications. All rights reserved.

- The public's commitment to equality of access to a single standard of medical care.

Some External Factors Will Determine What We Spend

According to a study (in progress) for the Commonwealth Foundation and the Robert Wood Johnson Foundation by the Institute for the Future, five factors are predicted to affect the nation's health care expenditures in the next decades. The study, incorporating interviews with over 20 renowned economists, political scientists, engineers, and physicians, revealed the following:

1. The first and most significant factor is demography. The key issues will focus on the balance of self-interest between the so-called "baby-boomers" and the elderly. The "baby-boomers," a bulge in the population from 1945 to 1965, will range in age from 25 to 45 in 1990. As a group they are relatively well-educated, 50 percent having attended one or more years of college, and 25 percent having attended at least four years of college. During the 1990s they will assume dominant roles in the professions and in business. Their attitudes and spending priorities will have an important influence on public policy. As better educated consumers, they will be more critical of the quality and cost of medical care than the older generation and are likely to place a higher priority on education and housing than on medical services.

During this same period, the number of elderly will increase, and by 1990 there will be more than 31 million people over the age of 65. As the largest consumers of medical care, the elderly will certainly favor expansion of services to include home care, insurance coverage for nursing home care, and continuing care communities to provide medical services. They will resist cutbacks in Medicare and will continue to be a powerful lobby at both the state and federal level.

2. The state of the national economy over the next 10 to 15 years will also be an important factor. The rate of expansion will have an important impact on what business and government are willing to spend on health care. None of the economists interviewed by the staff of the Institute for the Future thought there would be dramatic changes in the rate of real growth of the gross national product (GNP), and the majority thought growth would be slow—in the 2-2 1/2 percent range. There could, of course, be surprises, particularly in the international arena, but no one predicted either boom or bust.

3. Interest and inflation rates will also have a bearing upon health care expenditures. Interest rates, in the long term, will reflect the degree to which we are able to deal with the federal deficit. All of the economists interviewed were cautious about predicting rates of inflation because of the variables involved, but they were cautiously optimistic and believed we would not leave double-digit inflation in the future.

4. Government policy toward spending and taxation, and what we do about spending cuts and tax increases will be an important cornerstone for future services. Tomorrow's government policy will be determined by how aggressively the executive and legislative branches of government are able to deal with the current federal deficit. The containment of health care costs will be an important part of this agenda.

5. Public attitudes about the importance of health care, and quality of care, and how aggressively we treat the terminally ill will be an important factor in determining future expenditures.

Environmental Factors Affecting Health Care

Even experts are unable to predict with any precision what will happen to the economy, inflation, interest rates, public attitudes, or government policy toward spending and taxation. To a significant degree, however, we react, individually and collectively, to what we *think* is going to happen. The majority of individuals and institutions involved in providing health care believe that efforts to contain cost will dominate public policy toward medicine in the future. Whether this is accomplished by competition, regulation, or more likely by a combination of both, is less important than the perception that the cost of medical care is out of control and that measures to contain it must be found.

Certainly this is the perception of those who pay for health care directly—namely, government and business—even though it is less of a concern to the consumers who ultimately pay the bill. The analgesia of the indirect payment mechanism for the majority of consumers temporarily shields them from the pain of paying out-of-pocket the total cost of either medical insurance or medical care. Government has a powerful stake in controlling the rapid inflation of medical care cost since it pays over 40 percent of the bill. Business has also become acutely aware of the fact that providing health insurance for employees has not only become a major cost of doing business, but is one of those costs that is the least controllable.

Health care providers are keenly aware of these attitudes, and it is speculated that the anxieties and frantic actions of these hospitals, HMOs, and physicians are more the symptoms of what might happen than what has actually happened. DRGs have had a greater impact on hospital occupancy than would have been expected, especially since only payment by the Health Care Financing Administration (HCFA) is involved. Falling hospital occupancy has had a ripple effect in other unanticipated ways. Hospitals are unsure whether to compete with neighboring institutions or to merge with them. The only way competition could be maintained is to encourage the admission of more patients by the physicians already on staff or to recruit other physicians. Just a few years ago, it was difficult for HMOs to obtain admitting privileges in community hospitals for their staff physicians. Now many community hospitals are actively looking for HMOs with which to contract for the provision of inpatient services.

Doctors are equally uneasy and uncertain of the future. Although the majority of physicians have always considered themselves individualists, wedded to the principles of a free marketplace, collectively they have never liked competition and have usually attempted to avoid it. Until recently, the medical staff of a hospital could veto the admitting privileges for physicians working with an HMO even though the administration of the hospital and the board of the hospital favored such an agreement. Few medical staffs would attempt to do so today, knowing that they would almost certainly fail. Instead, they are cooperating with those who manage individual practice associations (IPAs) and are willing to accept the payment mechanism and other controls offered by this brand of HMO.

The anxieties felt by physicians about the future are understandable. They continually face the skyrocketing costs of malpractice insurance, the oversupply of physician, and the changing pattern of medical practice. The traditional alliances of organized medicine are incapable of maintaining the status quo and seem unable to exert any influence on the direction of change. It is this uncertainty about the outcome of revolution, set in motion by cost containment, that is most unsettling of all. Most people can adapt to change if they can anticipate the outcome, but anxiety flourishes when the outcome is uncertain, and physicians know that they cannot predict the future. It is not surprising, therefore, that most physicians feel uneasy about their own future.

In addition, insurers are not confident of the impact of cost containment. There seems to be a confusion of role between some large HMOs and for-profit hospital chains that appear to be in the insurance business and those in-surers that are sponsoring various kinds of practice arrangements, including HMOs. It is becoming more and more difficult today to tell who is an insurer and who is a provider.

Perhaps medical schools and so-called academic health centers have the greatest cause for anxiety. In addition to the various aspects of cost control that may affect the practice of medicine, they have four other things to worry about: whether teaching costs will be reimbursed; whether HCFA and private insurers reduce payments for residency training; whether they will be able to maintain their competitive edge as tertiary care institutions over the competi-tion of community hospitals; and whether the federal government will further reduce its support of research, particularly clinical research. For decades, medical schools and teaching hospitals found it useful to obscure the cost of medical education by promoting the belief that the costs of education, re-search, and patient care were inseparable. Payers, although never really ac-cepting this belief, did nothing to alter this belief until they were faced with the need to halt the inflation of medical care costs. The result is that both payers and teaching hospitals are unable to answer the question: what does medical education really cost?

Clearly, the major cost of this eduction involves the training of residents and fellows, not the education of medical students in the classroom. It is precisely for this reason that there is so much concern about reimbursement for graduate medical education. Will it be limited to three years for medicine and pediatrics and five years for surgery, and will insurers, led by the HCFA, refuse to pay for training in the subspecialties? Will there be a reduction in the number of residency slots paid for, and will these be limited to approximately the size of the graduating classes of American medical schools? These are worries in their own right, but they are also related to maintaining a competitive edge in tertiary care. Teaching hospitals are faced with a dilemma. On the one hand they are better able to provide intensive care when there is a full staff of residents and fellows; on the other hand, they are training the competition.

The New Era

When making predictions about what will happen in health care over the next 10 to 15 years, one must survey the situations from all perspectives; those of the patient, the physician, and the social scientist. Each of these individuals views medicine from a different point of view. Here are a few of the author's own thoughts:

Cost Containment

Despite efforts to contain costs it is unlikely that the cost of medical care as a percentage of GNP will remain at 10 percent. The rate of increase may be slow, but by the year 2000 the cost of medical care as a percent of GNP will probably be in the 11-12 percent range. This is not to suggest that we will return to an open-ended system of reimbursement, but that the pressures to increase the amount and intensity of care provided will exceed our efforts to control costs. This conclusion is reached for the following reasons:

- We will continue to have a mixed public-private system of payment for medical care, yielding the efforts to control costs uncoordinated, as they will be exercised by a variety of payers.

- Although the "baby-boomers" may wish to see more money spent on education and housing than on medical care, they will find it difficult to resist the demands of the elderly for more and better quality care. Since the elderly will include the parents of the "baby-boomers," the latter will be favorably inclined toward the extension of services to the impaired elderly who require either custodial or nursing care. Few in middle age will wish to provide those services in their own homes for their parents. For many families, it will be impossible to do so, since both husband and wife will be working full-time.

- Reduction in hospital utilization has produced some savings, but it will soon become apparent that complex procedures performed on an ambulatory basis are also expensive, particularly if they are combined with home care. We may even discover that in certain situations it is more efficient and cheaper to diagnose and treat the patient in the hospital than in the clinic or at home.

- Americans are fascinated by technology and are likely to equate quality of care with the availability of the latest technology, be it magnetic resonance imaging or laser treatment of atherosclerotic plaques in the coronary arteries. We may ultimately be taxed on some part of our health care benefits, including Medicare, but this will not be a sufficient deterrent to slow the introduction of the latest advances of medical science.

- Although physicians' fees may rise more slowly than in the past, partly as a result of competition and partly because of regulation, the total amount spent on physician services will rise significantly because we will have more doctors to provide more services.

Quality Assurance

Two forces will combine to foster assurance that the quality of care provided is high: the first is a better educated public, and the second will be the insistence by big payers — namely, government and business — that money provided for health care benefits is well spent. Large variations in practice patterns within and among regions are being examined in a systematic way. It is likely that more regional standards of care will be supplanted by a national basis.

The Uninsured

The problem of the uninsured and underinsured has been accentuated by our efforts to control cost and will not be easily solved in the next 10-15 years. It is probably feasible to do something about insuring employees of small businesses, and collective approaches to bad debts in the hospital have been shown to work. There may even be some sort of national legislation to protect against the financial consequences of catastrophic illness. But, it is doubtful that we will solve the problem of the medically indigent in any other way than with a two-tiered system of medical care. That is what we have now, and it is quite likely that public hospitals will continue to provide care for the majority of the poor. I doubt that anything short of national health insurance or a national health service is likely to assure a single standard of care. Unfortunately, those who suffer the most are mothers and children and, to a lesser extent, the elderly. The only good news is that between the ages of 20 and 50, less care may be better.

Prevention

To a large extent, prevention is an individual matter and is more dependent on individual habits — good or bad — than on physician intervention. While vaccination and secondary prevention accomplished by treating such diseases as hypertension and diabetes are important, individual health is more likely to be affected by such things as smoking, alcohol consumption, diet, and exercise. The better educated the public, the more likely it is to take prevention seriously. Unfortunately, this means that the poor, who are usually less well-educated than the affluent, are doubly vulnerable. They are more likely to have habits detrimental to health and less likely to receive medical care when they need it.

Systems of Care

In the future we are far more likely to have several systems of medical care. This means that we will continue to have both fee-for-service and prepayment; for-profit and not-for-profit providers; public and private care; integrated systems and solo practitioners. This is mainly because the public likes to have a choice, and what suits one person is an anathema to another. Younger, better educated professionals seem attracted to prepaid group practices, whereas older individuals are more likely to identify with a particular doctor or hospital than with a system. It has become fashionable to say that everyone should have a primary care physician or a case manager, yet many patients with chronic disease prefer the care of specialists.

In addition, no system has a permanent financial advantage over another. HMOs were able to reduce the rate of hospitalization and, therefore, reduce cost. But, there are other ways to reduce hospitalization rates, and HMOs are not necessarily more efficient providers of ambulatory care than their competition. Finally, the nature of medical care is such that it will always be provided on a one-to-one basis, and in our culture most care will be given by physicians. This means that very large organizations have little advantage over smaller ones, except for access to capital. One suspects that there will be an increase in the number of integrated systems of care, but these are likely to be a mixture of tightly organized systems and systems that are loose federations.

For-Profits

Do for-profits govern the practice of medicine and the provision of hospital care? Neither the for-profits nor the not-for-profits have an absolute advantage over the other. Although the first has better access to capital, the latter has tax-exempt status. Both systems are capable of developing integrated care at the local or regional level. Neither has a monopoly in the best managers. Both are capable of responding to the demands of cost containment, and both can work in a fee-for-service or prepaid mode.

Salaried Physicians and Managed Care

Whatever the variety of systems that evolve, there will likely be an increase in the number of salaried physicians, both full- and part-time. Presently, more salaried positions are available, partly as the result of the increase in HMOs and other managed care. The security of a salary would be tempting in a time of uncertainty.

One consequence of the increase in the number of salaried physicians and the growth of managed care systems will be tension between physicians and managers. During most of this century, physicians have controlled the system, and managers merely facilitated the work of physicians. Now many physicians resent "working for" the managers. Tension is lessened to some degree by an increase in the percentage of women entering the medical profession, since many are also homemakers and prefer to work on a salary in a managed system. It is also possible that the kind of person attracted to medicine is changing, and that the strong individualist is being gradually replaced by the organizational man or woman.

The Academic Health Center

One apparent trend is the drifting apart of universities and their academic health centers. It is becoming increasingly evident that the preoccupation of these centers with income generation and competition for the major market share of tertiary care has very little to do with university functions. Those universities that own teaching hospitals have also discovered that they have a huge potential liability for significant financial losses. What is unclear is where the medical school will emerge in our future system. Will it split with the first two years absorbed by the university and the clinical years by the academic health center? Will the entire medical school align itself with the AHC and further separate itself from the university? Or will the medical school align itself with the university and distance itself from the caregiving function by contracting with hospitals, HMOs, and others to provide the clinical environment for teaching? Only time will tell, but the present situation is unstable, and a major change is likely.

Conclusion

The new era in health care is likely to be a mixture of the old and the new. A revolution has been set in motion, and in the long term the changes will be profound. These changes will probably occur before the year 2000, a short time in which to effect great change, given the inertia of both institutions and generations. By the year 2020, many predict that there will be some kind of universal insurance guaranteeing a minimum level of care for everyone. Quality would be maintained by providing health care within integrated systems. Most physicians would be salaried, and the distribution of physicians among the specialties would be controlled by the number of training slots. It is doubtful that our care system will be nationalized, but it will almost certainly be regulated. The competition that persists will be between systems, not between individuals. For these reasons, caution must be taken in our decision-making regarding health care.

44

Re-Organizing the Organization: New Roles Lie Ahead

Richard Johnson

Richard Johnson, M.B.A., is President of the Tribrook Group, Inc., Oakbrook, Illinois.

Fundamental changes in board structure lie ahead. Up to now, boards have represented community interests. Increasingly, boards will redefine the boundaries of community obligation as funding (revenues) becomes more restrictive. Large hospital boards will become small boards under a parent/subsidiary organizational model. They will be composed of knowledgeable, experienced health professionals and a limited number of outsiders with specialized talents.

Most likely, the CEO will be the leader of the governing board. An outside chairman will likely be in place, but that person will be compatible with the CEO. The traditional master-servant relationship will be replaced with a collegial relationship of experts.

Governance structures will raise many new issues: How does board structure and composition impact the pursuit of new markets? How involved will boards become in risk taking versus conservation of assets?

Representative boards have been production driven, but expert boards will be consumer driven. In the future, boards will focus on market share and market penetration. The new focus: customer convenience, primary care, and stabilizing the marketplace through HMO ownership.

Success Ratios

DRGs will be failing by 1989. Currently, DRGs are a blend of a 55 percent national rate and a 45 percent hospital-specific rate. In 1987, they'll move to a 75 percent national and a 25 percent hospital-specific rate; by 1988 the rate will be a 100 percent national one. Currently, 43 percent of patient days are paid for by Medicare, a figure that will grow close to 50 percent by the end of the decade. The result is that the rate of payment for Medicare patients will impact half of the total hospital revenue by 1988. With the curtailment in adjustments to the base rate to hospitals because of high federal deficits, hospitals will have to jeopardize quality of care or restrict the number of Medicare patients they accept.

Capitation will fail to grow at the rate predicted by industry pundits. By 1995, we should see approximately 25 percent of the population covered by capitated plans, including the Medicare population. And when the Medicare population gets involved, we'll be talking about some 60 million people under capitation. In another eight to ten years, that figure will level off with a net increase of 2 million to 5 million additional people enrolled each year. But it will probably be well into the 21st century before we see the majority of our population capitated, which will result in a sustained competitive environment in which economics will dominate and quality of care will become, and remain, secondary.

The era of runaway formation and management of HMOs by inexperienced professionals will give way to a period of massive shake-outs and consolidations in the next five to ten years. Well-heeled HMOs will survive. Two to three HMOs may go national; but local, independent HMOs — owned by hospitals and physicians offering capitation, preferred provider coverage and indemnity (triple options) — will be the winners. In selecting an HMO, the public is asking three questions, and they will continue to ask them in the years ahead: What's it going to cost per month? What is the range of benefits? What hospitals do you use?

The number of hospital beds will continue to decline. Over the next decade, approximately 1,000 hospitals will disappear and, with them, 17 percent of the healthcare labor force. While there may be fewer employees in toto, those that leave will become involved in ambulatory care.

Supermeds will fail to take over the healthcare system. Medicine has been and will continue to be a local phenomenon. Large financing schemes will be popular, but their roots will be local. Well-managed local healthcare corporations can still look forward to dominant positions in the marketplace. The result: large and significant local healthcare corporations with their own capitated schemes, hospitals, nursing homes, and home health agencies, in association with physician group practices.

Docs Out of the Box

The majority of physicians may not be on salaries as anticipated. Today, about 24 percent of physicians are on payroll, but that includes hospital-based physicians and those still in residency training. But the number of salaried physicians may grow to 50 percent in 10 years.

In 20 years, physicians just coming out of residency programs will likely take a salaried position in a location of their choice. After a few years, they'll move out and develop a three-part income: fee for service, salary for part-time work in a hospital or HMO, and capitated payments. In general, physicians will have multiple sources of revenue.

Another significant trend involves women. Thirteen percent of practicing physicians are women, but this will grow to 25 percent. Many of them in their child bearing years will probably seek regular hours, opting for a salaried group practice or a hospital-based position.

But as the trend toward ambulatory care continues to escalate, so will the battle between hospitals and physicians over economic turf. While physicians want to keep hospitals economically neutral, hospitals will have to undertake services and programs that are in direct competition with physicians on their medical staffs.

Despite predictions, a nursing shortage will not materialize. In the face of a surplus, hospital executives will employ nurses as permanent part-time staff, already a popular trend in business. In addition, there will be more cross-training of healthcare personnel. Nurses, for example, will be trained to do simple X-rays and lab tests in ambulatory settings in order to provide cost-effective services.

Who Will Win?

Not-for-profit alliances may have already experienced their days in the sun. In 10 to 15 years, organizations like the VHA and Sun Health will have faded from public visibility unless they consolidate the balance sheets of their member organizations. Without substantial equity positions in capitated plans, they will have limited opportunities for long-term success.

The financing of teaching hospitals will remain unresolved. Very likely, they will be avoided by HMOs because of their high costs and will have to be financed through tax dollars from public sources. In return, they will be responsible for indigents, a return to the old public hospital type. Ultimately, block grants out of federal coffers may be needed to fund both teaching and research.

As Medicare continues to restrict its payments to community hospitals, they will restrict services to the elderly. Cost shifting will disappear and limitations will be placed on the number of Medicare patients these hospitals will accept.

Financially strapped cities and counties will probably have to shoulder much of the burden of indigent care. This will be a difficult burden because of the reductions in revenue sharing that are underway and will continue in the years ahead. This won't be offset by tax hikes at the local level because of the public resistance that will be encountered.

Of these cross currents, several scenarios are possible. But one seems most likely. The indigent may enter capitated plans paid for by public funds, with the federal government mandating benefit levels so that the needy obtain at least minimum standards of care.

Today a balance exists between doing good (the social ethic) and operating like a business (the economic ethic). Social ethics are in balance with business ethics. But as economics tighten and HMOs proliferate, a more hard-nosed bottom-line orientation may come to dominate, if not overtake, the ethos of care and compassion. By the time the 21st century is entered, the pendulum may have started to swing back and restore the balance.

45

2036: A Health Care Odyssey

Jeff Goldsmith

Jeff Goldsmith, Ph.D., is President, Health Futures, Inc., Bannockburn, Illinois.

Thinking creatively about what health care delivery will be like 50 years from now is difficult at a time when the next 6 to 18 months are fraught with so much uncertainty. It is, however, much safer than short-term prognostication, if only because the inevitable (and embarrassing) confrontation with the facts is postponed beyond immediate memory.

This much is certain: Many of the elements of a mid-21st century delivery system are in germinal stages today. The two most uncertain elements in predicting what the system of the future will be like are how far the current vectors for change will extend into the years ahead, and how they will interact in our complex society to reshape health care delivery.

The Direction of Change

The major vectors for change in U.S. health care delivery are:

- Scientific progress in biomedical research

- Technological innovations in diagnosis, treatment, and clinical information systems

- Changing clinical practice (as influenced by the two forces listed above)

- Institutional and managerial strategies that bring innovation to the patient.

The most powerful long-term vector for change may be the maturation of scientific inquiry in cell biology and genetics; progress in these areas could

Reprinted by permission from *Hospitals,* Vol. 60, No. 9, May 5, 1986. Copyright 1986, American Hospital Publishing, Inc.

generate the most far-reaching effects in reshaping the delivery system. But these also are the areas of greatest uncertainty—although perhaps there is more uncertainty about the timing of the payoffs of biomedical research investments than about the ultimate outcomes.

For example, scientific progress borne of research investments during the past 30 years gave rise to a burgeoning biotechnology industry. Although it likely will take several decades to mature, this industry may well produce not only screens for genetically determined or genetically influenced conditions—such as diabetes, cancer, and mental illness—but also methods of genetic therapy that will alter genetic structures to reduce *or even eliminate* vulnerability to these illnesses. Biotechnology also will bring new biological entities, bred in the laboratory, to fight illness—including conditions caused by viral agents that eluded past therapy.

A Brave New World Unfolds

Many of the technologies described 50 years ago by author Aldous Huxley in his classic *Brave New World*—technologies such as in vitro fertilization and genetic engineering—either are already here or within realization. Also within realization, however, are the moral and ethical dilemmas inherent in using these technologies to alter the human future. These dilemmas include, for example, the decision to abort a fetus because it shows a genetic predisposition to a costly or a fatal illness, or the invasion of workers' privacy by insurers and employers anxious to limit their future health care liabilities.

Progress in arresting illness at its root cause would enable society to avoid further massive social investments in what scientist and author Lewis Thomas, M.D., calls "halfway technologies"—artificial hearts, organ transplants, and the like. If society realistically can expect to conquer genetically programmed diseases and viral illnesses by the middle of the next century, then the remaining causes of death may be either purely social in character (homicides, suicides, accidents, and self-abuse from unhealthy habits like cigarette smoking) or related to the inevitable wearing out of the body.

Liberation from "phantom killer" illness could profoundly alter social attitudes toward health care spending. It may become, for example, socially acceptable for patients to bear most of the costs of illnesses that they had major roles in causing.

Americans also may come to believe that social resources should not be lavished on medical problems that inevitably lead to degeneration or death. Society may decide not to finance the "bionic body," leaving access to artificial means of mobility or life extension to those few individuals with the resources to afford them. Reallocating social dollars from these classes of medical problems to unmet needs—such as alleviating the social causes of illness and providing better access to medical care for less fortunate Americans—may be an important dividend of shifting societal values.

Today's Advances, Tomorrow's World

Developments in medical technology will create a more immediate impact on the shape of the U.S. health care system. But the most profound long-term effects may not come from the highly visible, big-ticket technologies (such as artificial organs) that receive the most media attention. Instead, advances in anesthesia and in less-invasive surgical technologies (both of which will dramatically broaden the scope of ambulatory surgery), plus improved diagnostic imaging and enhanced clinical information systems, may collectively produce a more significant impact in reshaping the delivery system.

Thanks to improved anesthesia and to advances such as laser surgery, fiberoptics, and high-tech catheters, entire surgical disciplines will be transformed into specialized forms of "bioplumbing." For example, ophthalmology has virtually disappeared from the inpatient hospital setting, followed by urology, plastic surgery, and gynecology. Advances in catheter technology not only have enhanced the safety of critical care monitoring but also are transforming cardiology from a primarily diagnostic discipline to an invasive, curative discipline. By the early part of the next century, *only the frailest or sickest patients will require inpatient hospitalization for surgery.*

At the same time, technologies that took off during the 1970s—technologies such as continuous-action peritoneal dialysis and enteral and parenteral nutrition—will be joined by new generations of technologies, enabling more patients with serious illnesses to be sent home safely. Remarkable progress with implantable devices already has produced implantable insulin pumps and implantable defibrillators; combining miniaturization with advances in microprocessor technology will enable sophisticated chemotherapy to be administered safely at sites remote from the hospital.

Meanwhile, other advances will produce remote fetal monitoring systems that can transmit signals over the telephone or via telemetry to indicate threats to the fetus. Parallel advances in monitoring technology will produce sophisticated multifunction monitoring systems, such as the ambulatory computer—a "super-Holter" monitor that can monitor, evaluate, store, and send signals that indicate patient distress or risk to remote locations.

These technologies will enable physicians to extend their therapeutic and protective powers beyond the walls of their offices and hospitals. Systems providing continuous medication and patient monitoring will reduce the need to hospitalize patients, perhaps dramatically. The patients of the 21st century will be connected to their physicians or hospitals by webs of telemetry similar to those used in cellular communications; perhaps these communication webs will be coordinated or monitored by computer systems that could trigger responses in advance of crises.

Thus, changing medical technology will make it possible for the home or the residential community to reemerge as the primary site of clinical care—just as it was at the beginning of the 20th century. As a result, medical care in 2036 may become less obtrusive and more woven into the fabric of everyday life.

Making the Most of the Man-Made Mind

At the same time, the maturation of artificial intelligence applications in medicine may enhance, perhaps dramatically, productivity of physicians and nurses, and it may improve patient safety as well. Although research into the medical applications of artificial intelligence (the use of large clinical data bases and interactive software for support of diagnostic decisions) has been under way for more than 20 years, 1984 marked the first time that a commercially available product incorporating artificial intelligence became available for hospital use.

In the years ahead, "intelligent" clinical information systems will become the hospital's operating core, interacting with physicians and nurses in diagnostic decisionmaking and patient management. These systems will monitor patient conditions on a real-time basis, tracking physiological signs and incorporating test results, comparing patient responses against profiles gleaned from vast clinical data bases, and assisting the patient care team in evaluating and planning care. The most rigorous application of computer-assisted care will be in the intensive care unit, where monitoring technologies are most sophisticated and where integration of patient information and decisionmaking is most critically needed.

Physicians will use artificial intelligence systems to complement and to extend their diagnostic capabilities. By the early 1990s, a patient's first encounter with a new physician or health plan may take the form of responding to a diagnostic inquiry program linked by telephone or home computer to the physician's office. This will frame the first face-to-face meeting between patient and physician with a detailed, structured clinical background.

Referrals of patients to specialists or admitting patients to hospitals will be accompanied by machine-to-machine transmittal of clinical information that's necessary for therapy. Clinical information systems will combine text and images in new storage and retrieval modes, such as the writable laser disc, that will replace paper medical records. Information transmittals will contain both high-resolution visual images of specimens or affected body parts as well as oral or written commentary from the consultant.

Welcome to the Hospital of 2036

As treatment advances divert large numbers of patients from the inpatient hospital setting, and as life-support and maintenance technologies enable patients to carry on their lives away from hospitals and nursing homes, the hospitalized population will shrink to perhaps half its current size by the early part of the next century, despite an aging population. The hospitalized population will be incredibly frail and costly to treat, exhibiting acuity levels comparable to or higher than patients in today's hospital intensive care units.

The physical hospital will be much smaller and infinitely more complex technically. A 400-bed facility will be considered large, and the young people of the future will marvel at the 1,000- to 1,500-bed facilities that began empty-ing out during the 1980s.

By 2036, today's hospital will be converted (by technology and by chang-ing delivery patterns) into the high-tech, critical care hub of a dispersed net-work of smaller clinical facilities, physician offices, and remote care sites. These networks will be knit together by "intelligent" clinical information sys-tems and by both air and ground critical care transportation systems. The economic boundaries of the system will be defined by the coverage of financ-ing packages tied to the provision of care within the system. Each metropolitan area will boast multiple competing systems, whose networks may stretch out as far as 200 miles from the core facility.

The Baby Boomers: Boom or Bust?

After a crisis of fiscal adjustment during the late 1980s, government spending for health services will grow at a less rapid rate than either personal or corporate health care spending. By the early 21st century, government financing may be a distant third as a source of U.S. health funds, behind (in order) individual patients and corporate employers.

Why? Because as concerns mounted in the late 1980s about the adequacy of the system for financing the nation's growing need for long-term and chronic care services, privately financed annuity mechanisms—supported by tax preferences similar to those for individual retirement accounts (IRAs)—were put in place to finance these services. Paired with IRA mechanisms for income support, the availability of health-related IRAs justified government retrenchment from supporting middle-class retirement and health services needs, thus permitting a reallocation of funding for those who lack either government or corporate insurance coverage.

However, both the provisions for advance funding of chronic care costs and the available financial support for acute care will prove grossly inade-quate later on, despite unprecedented scientific and technological progress made during the previous 50 years. During the decade 2030 and beyond, the U.S. health care system will be locked in its most serious economic crisis in 100 years, as the 78 million postwar baby boomers begin to die.

Despite the reduced volume of inpatient services, the cost of caring for a growing number of hospitalized patients will progressively outstrip public and private resources, creating serious fiscal problems for patients and care providers alike. Having failed to replace themselves demographically, the baby-boom elderly will not be able, as did their elders, to use their political power to tax the young to subsidize their care.

Despite active life-styles and healthy diets, the baby-boom generation may experience a lengthy and unsatisfying twilight of enforced leisure, reduced mobility, and emotional involution. Ironically, the active life-styles pursued by baby boomers during mid-life may extend their lives, but at the price of worn-out musculoskeletal systems that only a few will have the finan-cial resources to alleviate.

Ultimately, society will become rigidly age segregated, with the elderly living in retirement colonies outside the mainstream of their communities; many communities may have no young people at all. The biggest problems faced by American society will be restoring the vitality it experienced in the late 20th century and mobilizing its resources to plan for a brighter tomorrow.

Index